# No Place Like Home

Columbia Studies of Social Gerontology and Aging
Abraham Monk, General Editor

---

*Nicholas L. Danigelis and Alfred P. Fengler*

# No Place Like Home
## Intergenerational Homesharing Through Social Exchange

Columbia University Press
New York

363.58
D18n

Columbia University Press
New York   Oxford
Copyright © 1991 Columbia University Press
All rights reserved

Library of Congress Cataloging-in-Publication Data

Danigelis, Nicholas L.
   No place like home : intergenerational homesharing through social
exchange / Nicholas L. Danigelis and Alfred P. Fengler.
       p.   cm.—(Columbia studies of social gerontology and aging)
   Includes bibliographical references and index.
   ISBN 0-231-07404-2
   1. Aged—Home care—Vermont—Case studies.   2. Shared housing—
Vermont—Case studies.   3. Volunteer workers in social service—
Vermont—Case studies.   4. Project HOME (Chittenden County, Vt.)
I. Fengler, Alfred P.   II. Title.   III. Series.
HV1468.V4D36   1991
363.5'8—dc20                                                        91-11460
                                                                          CIP

For providing us homes in which we could be nurtured to seek a better understanding of the human condition, we dedicate this book with love and affection to our mothers, Anna Danigelis and Alice Fengler, and to the memories of our fathers, Louis Danigelis and William Fengler.

# Contents

# Acknowledgments

A number of individuals and organizations have facilitated our efforts to study Project HOME over the last seven years We wish to thank first those who have been a formal part of the Project HOME program, including all the paid and unpaid staff and all the clients who so graciously provided us with the information on which this book is based We are especially indebted to Suzie Button, Helen Head, Dot Black, Sally Conrad, Janet Graber, Suzen Larsen, and Polly Rowe.

Second, we thank those who have been our research assistants: Joy Hammond, Katherine Malle, Ruth Miller, Steph Robert, Janet Sluzenski, Jennifer Strickler, Susan Wildman, and Laurie Steffenhagen Witham. Their most visible contributions are described in chapter 4, but the countless hours they spent doing the mundane tasks upon which any large-scale project like ours is based are here also acknowledged with gratitude.

Third, we are deeply indebted to the AARP Andrus Foundation and the University of Vermont Graduate School for financial support at the critical times when our research required more of our time and resources than we otherwise could have given.

Fourth, we want to thank Dale Jaffe, Steve Cutler, and the two anonymous Columbia University Press reviewers who provided many useful suggestions for improving the manuscript.

Finally, to our families and colleagues, we thank you for putting up with us these many years during which Project HOME has fluctuated between being a research project and an obsession.

# No Place Like Home

# 1
# Homesharing and the Continuum of Care

## THE ATTACHMENT TO HOME

When Dorothy said to Aunty Em after her odyssey in the land of Oz "there's no place like home," she was echoing a sentiment that is widespread among young and old alike. The home is likely to have particular meaning for older persons, 70 percent of whom own their own place. For one thing, it has material significance. Most older homeowners have paid off their mortgages, and so their home represents a major, if not entirely liquid, economic asset. Perhaps even more important for older persons, their home also has emotional significance. It is a familiar and loved surrounding. Symbolically, home represents a life history of attachments, reminiscences and past relationships.

Arguments emphasizing the power of psychological attachment to home come from a variety of sources. As O'Bryant (1983) puts it, the reasons for this attraction to home have less to do with the physical condition of the home, the proportion of a person's income that is needed for its maintenance, or the health condition of the occupant. Instead, housing satisfaction varies directly with the occupant's age and time spent living in the home. Why are age and length of time in residence so important? The answer is emotional significance. O'Bryant and Wolf (1983) believe that, even if improved alternative housing is available, homeowners will choose to remain in their own homes because of the increased psychological importance attached to home that grows stronger the longer individuals live in the same place.

Holcomb and Parkoff articulate the particular psychological attractions when they describe home as a place "which is familiar, to which one is attached, a place of love and roots, of security and one in which pretensions can be relaxed and one can be 'closer to oneself.' Home is a place to live, to relax in, a possession and/or a repository of possessions, a place for privacy and both companionship and alone-ness" (1980:5).

They further argue that, compared with younger people, the elderly are more likely to see home as a "locus of personal history which fosters identity" and as a "show place for the possessions and memorabilia of a lifetime" (Holcomb and Parkoff 1980:6). This attachment to home is particularly true for women, who comprise most single elderly homeowners, since they have spent a larger proportion of their lifetime at home. "Their roles as wife, mother and neighbor were played there; their creativity and tastes are reflected in the material products of a lifetime of 'nesting behavior' "(Holcomb and Parkoff 1980:6–7).

Whatever its objective deficiencies, one becomes intimately familiar with one's own home and so can adapt and adjust to its shortcomings. Because it is a known and valued quantity, the occupant is understandably reluctant to leave "familiar and loved surroundings or to consider coping with the challenge of searching for a new home and the stress consequent to a radical change in the social and physical environment" (Lawton 1977:21).

Finally, evidence of the attachment to home cuts across national boundaries. For example, in the United Kingdom the term "staying put" has been coined in recent years to describe a social policy designed to facilitate elders remaining at home (Wheeler 1982). The policy reflects not only a concern for caring for elders as inexpensively as possible but also an implicit emphasis on the value of independence. This policy of "staying put" is not unlike the policies of other countries. An eight nation study has found that "the aged prefer remaining in the homes within the community in which they have lived for most of their lives; that they live longer and happier in their own homes; and that their continuing to live at home with community assistance is less expensive than institutionalization" (Doron 1979:62). For many elders, therefore, continuing to live in one's own home makes both psychological and economic sense.

# COMPETENCE AND ENVIRONMENTAL PRESS

## Environmental Demands on Elders

Elders are more likely than the nonelderly to experience losses of significant others, increased housing expenses, and deterioration in physical and mental health. All of these indicators of loss suggest that elders will also experience increased difficulty remaining in their own home. Although there is enormous individual variation, collectively the elderly are increasingly likely to experience illness and impairment as they age, and this difference between old and young seems to have become more pronounced during the last few decades.

According to the most recent government reports, for example, bed-disability days[1] are over twice as prevalent among those 65 years old and over. At the same time, the bed-disability days among elders has been increasing, while comparable figures for those under 65 have been relatively constant. Specifically, in 1970, bed-disability days per person were 5.3 per person per year for those under sixty-five but 13.8 per person per year for those sixty-five and over; by 1983, the younger group's rate was relatively unchanged at 5.4, while the older group's rate had risen to 16.7 (U.S. Bureau of the Census 1986:101, table 160).

The above figures are averages, of course, and a large proportion of the elderly population loses very little activity due to disability. Nevertheless, the increase in the average number of bed-disability days among elders is noteworthy, because it suggests that increasing numbers of elders are being incapacitated in one way or another. Given the increases of individuals living well into their eighties and beyond, it is not surprising to see this trend toward higher levels of disability. Studies in other western societies have found comparable trends in disease and impairment (Shanas and Maddox 1985).

With regard to mental impairment, a review of the research by Shanas and Maddox (1985) has led them to conclude that incidence of mental illness tends to increase with age. Estimates of the frequency of senile dementia range from 5 per 100 for all persons sixty-five years of age and older to 20 per 100 for those eighty and older. The rate of hospitalization for mental disorders increases with age, as older persons account for about one fourth of the new admissions to state mental hospitals (Shanas and Maddox 1985). The inability of many older persons to function in the community is shown by the high proportion of depressive disorders among older people in nursing homes, which ranges from 50 to over 60 percent (Shanas and Maddox 1985).

Another limitation in the ability of older persons to remain in their own home is the increased expense associated with home maintenance. Older people tend to live in housing that is older than the housing occupied by younger people (Struyk and Soldo 1980). Although there is some variation depending on which measures of adequacy are used, the elderly also tend to live in inferior housing to a greater extent than the nonelderly (Lawton 1980). Since elderly occupied homes are older and of poorer quality than those of nonelderly homeowners, it is perhaps surprising that major home improvements are reported less often. Even small repairs tend to occur less often (Struyk and Soldo 1980). When major repairs are made, older people tend to pay more than younger people, perhaps reflecting the higher costs of repairing older housing.

Golant (1984) has found that the four most frequently mentioned problems in caring for a home include heavy chores, home financial difficulties, doing routine cleaning, and difficulty finding professional workers. Although these four problems are frequently mentioned, only one is associated with reduced likelihood of satisfaction with dwelling: "burdensome financial expense of home care." It is not the fatiguing or time consuming aspects of home care but rather the impact of housing expense that makes old people feel less satisfied with their dwellings.

Another occurrence more likely to afflict the elderly and which con- tributes to a less sanguine and comfortable home environment is the death of a spouse. Not only does one experience bereavement from the loss of a companion and confidante, but one also will likely miss a partner who shares in the physical care of the home.

Given the tendency of men to marry women who, on average, are two years younger than themselves and given the eight or so years longer life expectancy of women over men, the older woman is likely to experience a period of grieving plus a significant number of years living by herself. Few choose or are able to live with children, and the incidence of widows living alone has increased significantly in the last several decades.

Although the family continues to be an important support system, a shortage of unmarried aunts and the competing responsibilities of family and job for middle aged women are likely to limit their availability as companions and caregivers (Treas 1977). Few elders wish to live with their children as reflected in the steady decline over the last thirty-five years in the numbers of elders who live in households with other kin (Mindel 1979). The popular phrase "intimacy at a distance" represents the preferred nature of the relationship between older parents and their children. Family members, particularly daughters, do provide considerable care when it is needed, but separate living residences are the preferred arrangement.

Given the strong desire of many elders to remain in their own homes, the question is whether the home environment can support and accommodate the older person experiencing these economic, physical, and social losses. The older the person becomes, the greater is the likelihood of experiencing one or more of these problems.

## Staying Home as an Adjustment to Environmental Demands

One way elders respond to social loss and physical and mental deterioration is to cling with more fervor to those parts of the environment that appear more permanent. Too many changes occurring simultaneously result in severe stress, as much of the literature on the effects of residential relocation from community to institution suggest. Regnier (1981:180) in summarizing Pastalan's age-loss continuum, notes that elders try to increase their control and certainty over the environment "by seeking to maximize physical and psychological attachment to those items that are stable and familiar." The home, while becoming less manageable in one sense, simultaneously also represents a haven of security and continuity at a time when deterioration is taking place within the physical body.

Unfortunately, those internal changes affecting health may make one's current living environment increasingly unsuitable for the older person. The average home was built and designed for a family whose members are healthy, active, and reasonably well off financially. Late in life, after children have departed and often after the male provider for the family has died, the aged are left with considerable unused space that must be maintained and heated. Although mortgage payments are typically completed, the home may not be readily converted to cash. Property taxes can make severe economic demands on already limited finances. As noted earlier, the housing of elders also tends to be older and to require more maintenance. The home itself, therefore, begins to have costs as well as benefits, as it ages along with its occupant(s).

## The Home and Environmental Press

The occupant's aging also often produces problems. Tasks centering about homecare and upkeep that were once manageable by a healthy body or shared with a spouse become increasingly demanding as the person ages and experiences declines in physical capacity. Lawton's (1980) concept of environmental press is relevant here. When the individual's physical or mental competence declines, the environment can appear threatening and begin to "press" on the person's awareness. "As press level increases above a certain level, the limits set by the person's competence are surpassed, and the behavioral and affective outcomes are no longer positive; the stress threshold has been exceeded" (Lawton 1980:13). The higher one's competence, the wider the range of press from the environment one is able to cope with in a positive manner.

With declining capacity and competence due to illness or disability, domestic chores such as cleaning and cooking, which may have been routine activities earlier in life, now become daily obstacles to overcome. Cupboards become difficult to reach, light bulbs hard to unscrew, and windows resistant to easy closure. Arthritic hands and knees have difficulty opening doors and climbing stairs. The home, formerly a refuge and base for security, has become threatening and a liability. Fear of crime, particularly robbery, may have a confining effect on the life styles of older persons and thus restrict their movement in the community. The press of the environment now exceeds the individual's competencies and forces the consideration of alternatives. Lawton and Simon (1968) refer to this situation as an example of the "environmental docility hypothesis": The less competent the individual, the greater will be the impact of environmental factors on that individual. Ideally one wants to match environments and their "demand character" or "press" with the personal resources and competencies of the individual. Using this principle, a small improvement in environmental quality would bring "press" and "competencies-resources" into balance again.

In this continuous negotiation between competencies and environment, there are several options available to older homeowners as they try to reduce the press of the environment. They may want to sell their home and move either to a rented apartment or condominium in the private sector or into publicly subsidized housing. The availability of high quality affordable housing may be limited, however, and many elders may not be able to wait until spaces become available in either community or congregate housing. Particularly in communities with colleges and universities and other institutions hiking the demands for rental units, apartments may be difficult to find and afford. Most elderly apartment renters tend to live "in older buildings in older parts of cities where rents are relatively low but amenities are few, safety poor and tenure often insecure" (Carp 1976:251). Discussion now turns to two other kinds of options available to elders: intermediate housing and homesharing.

## INTERMEDIATE HOUSING

Recent efforts to find housing alternatives to the economic and social burden of living alone and the often greater problems encountered in unnecessary institutionalization have produced various kinds of intermediate housing. These range from large planned public housing units to small group homes, approximating successive points on a theoretical continuum from institutional care on the one hand to private family residence on the other.

The primary goal of public housing is to provide a high quality living environment at low cost for older people with low incomes. According to Lawton (1980), public housing is primarily a housing stock program rather than a service-delivery program. Nevertheless, there is often a congregate dimension, frequently taking the form of a central kitchen and meal services, in these housing projects. A major advantage of congregate housing is the sociability fostered by assembling many tenants in the dining hall for taking meals together (Lawton 1980:81).

### Types of Congregate Housing

In Great Britain, sheltered housing or grouped housing specifically designed for the elderly and served by a resident warden has become extremely successful. The units are usually located on only one or two levels and fewer in number than the larger multilevel congregate housing schemes in the United States. The problems of such sheltered housing derive from its success. People are living in schemes much longer than was ever anticipated and, as a result, are reluctant to move to other more supportive levels of care (Hobman 1981).

Another kind of intermediate living arrangement is called small group or community housing. Group homes for the elderly are defined "as a small number of unrelated older adults living together as a supportive family group" (Peace 1981b:16). Such housing is usually divided into separate units but includes some shared living space such as a living room. A variety of services such as janitorial and building maintenance may be included in the rental fee. This arrangement efficiently utilizes living space since many older homeowners are living in housing that exceeds their spatial needs (Welfield and Struyk 1979). It also provides a less institutional-type setting than congregate housing and does not require its tenants to make major adaptations to new life styles. Finally, it is an arrangement that closely approximates "normal living" (International Federation on Ageing 1979:24). Where it is successful, it "fosters a sense of personal connectedness, intimacy and interdependency" (Peace 1981a:14). The Philadelphia Geriatric Center reports that movement into smaller dwelling units "were changes for the positive perhaps related to the fact that smaller units were easier to take care of" (International Federation on Ageing 1979:24).

Share-A-Home of Florida is committed to a family-like atmosphere that strives to maximize independence without institutional constraints. Therefore, for example, there is little staff scheduling of resident's time. Streib et al. (1984) note that this kind of living arrangement can offer nurturing, support, affection, and concern much like a traditional family environment. However, such a family-like environment is less supportive during a crisis, because neither the residents nor the staff can act as long-term caretakers for the seriously impaired as many families do.

Yet another kind of congregate housing is found in Great Britain: Abbeyfield Homes. These are usually "family houses in established residential neighborhoods each accommodating six to eight residents and a housekeeper" (Peace 1981b:16). Each resident has his or her own bedsitting room, a wash basin and cooking ring while all other facilities are shared communally. The resident housekeeper does all the household shopping, cooks meals and generally looks after the communal parts of the home. The sheltered housing Abbeyfield dwellings are now facing the problem of what to do with long-term residents who have deteriorated too much to function independently in such homes.

As a means of reducing the press of environment, small group housing approaches would appear to have much to recommend them when resources can be found to organize them. At the individual level, Peace (1981b) summarizes important factors predicting success in these housing schemes. Most important is compatibility between residents. Careful matching of residents increases the likelihood of compatibility by focusing on matching shared interests in order to increase social support and thus compatibility. Three other predictors found to increase the likelihood of successful adjustments to small group housing arrangements are dependence on roommates for assistance, lack of mental confusion, and safety of neighborhood. Overall, therefore, like other social arrangements in family, business, and leisure, small group housing initiatives are as good as the degree to which their participants get along with one another.

## Relocation

Do elders *want* to move into small groups housing arrangements? The evidence is preliminary, but some generalizations are suggested. For example, although there are often long waiting lists for these kinds of intermediate housing, it is also true that most elderly prefer to remain in their own homes for as long as possible. Home has many attractions for the elderly homeowner. The sense of history and family tradition as expressed through memories and possessions; the feeling of familiarity and resulting security from a long tenancy in this residence; privacy, and above all the sense of mastery and control over environment all combine to make home an attractive place to live out one's life.

Group living is still an unfamiliar experience for the majority of elders. Most who come to Share-A-Home, for example, do so because their failing health makes living alone impossible or because someone who was caring for them is unable to continue this care. They do not come because they share the family ideology of the organization; in fact, more than half believe either that they have no alternative or that the only alternative is institutional care of some sort (Streib et al. 1984).

In another study of elderly homeowners in England, it has been found that many have at one time or other thought about moving from their present home (Fengler et al. 1984). Few, however, think they will do so in the immediate future, and others never plan on moving. Some have had their names on waiting lists and even visited alternative living environments, but generally the elders interviewed express negative feelings toward most of these alternatives. Overall, their feeling is probably best summed up as follows: Perhaps a move will be necessary in the future, but one should delay this event as long as possible and maybe never have to leave home.

Although the majority of elderly homeowners in the Fengler et al. study know something about residential homes and sheltered housing, few see these alternative living arrangements as allowing them to maintain those aspects of "home" they value most. They may recognize the value of a more supportive environment for those who really need it but hope that it will not be necessary for themselves. Alternative "homes" are basically viewed as representing a loss of something they now possess and value. As O'Bryant and Wolf (1983:231) conclude from their re-search, for most homeowners "alternative housing will not attract older persons if it does not also incorporate the psychological values they have come to enjoy as a result of owning their own home."

Most comments made in the British study regarding relocation empha-size "meaning of home" orientations such as the value of privacy, inde-pendence, and personal belongings. Most of these qualities are perceived to be absent in alternative living environments. Loss of space to store valued possessions and too much enforced communal interaction are two fears elders have of moving. Privacy is a highly valued component of home and would be reduced by a move. It is particularly interesting that several homeowners oppose a move, because they fear they will have to associate too much with other older people.

Concerns about moving center around the likelihood of retaining valued furniture, having to share with people one doesn't get along with, or having too little to do. Regimentation and routinization are also frequently associated with relocation. They perceive less freedom, inde-pendence and choice in a group setting. Finally, for some, moving would involve distance from valued friends. No one views relocation as a chance to develop new friends, but several see it as resulting in the loss or attenuation of old friendships.

Obviously these views by elders may reflect a great deal of ignorance and misinformation about nonhome living environments. To what ex-tent the homeowners' perceptions accurately portray alternative living environments and whether the experience of living in such environments will actually be as disruptive as they anticipate are questions which this study could not answer. Nevertheless, such attitudes and fears cannot be dismissed by service providers and housing planners whose jobs are to assist elders in making intelligent decisions about their housing options —especially since alternatives now exist allowing elders to remain at home. The most important one is homesharing.

## HOMESHARING

In its most basic form, house-sharing involves two unrelated individuals shar-ing a single-family dwelling that is owned by one of them. Sharing may range from a simple boarding house arrangement in which a non-homeowner occu-pies bedroom space only to a communal arrangement in which financial, social and household chores are shared more or less equally among the participants. (McConnell and Usher 1980:1–2)

The idea behind homesharing is that an owner of a home with under-utilized space or rooms offers to share the home with an unrelated person who also wishes to share. The arrangement is handled through an intermediary agency that seeks to match compatible owners with sharers. This last quality of agency intervention distinguishes such households from naturally occurring shared elderly households. During 1977 in the United States alone there were some 89,000 shared households made up of two or more elderly persons (Mukherjee 1982).

## The Principle of Exchange

Homesharing operates on the principle of exchange theory, which says that individuals act to maximize rewards, minimize costs, and maintain interaction as long as the interaction is more rewarding than costly (Blau 1964; Dowd 1975, 1980a, 1980b; Homans 1961). Each of the participants has something to offer the other in a homesharing situation. The exchange can range from the simple boarder-owner arrangement in which rental payments are traded for a bedroom to the situation in which the provision of round-the-clock personal care services to the homeowner is traded for room, board, and a stipend.

Of course, in homesharing, not only are rewards exchanged but so too are costs. As a result, each participant must balance rewards and costs in any shared living situation. For example, an elderly homeowner may compromise some privacy in order to avoid a greater loss of privacy by a move to a more communal living arrangement such as a group home. In another case, a homeowner may be willing to sacrifice some independence in order to regain some other valued property of "home." Home may represent a sense of family, or people, and the interests their presence brings to the home. Or home may mean security and safety, a haven where one is rarely fearful of external predators.

The loss of spouse and former family members cannot be completely replaced by a live-in sharer, but perhaps some of the sense of "home is people" and "home is safety" can be restored. The cost of some lost privacy and independence is more than compensated for by the rewards of companionship and the felt security from criminal activity.

Homesharing has in common with other forms of intermediate housing the principle of joint living between nonrelatives through the offices of an agency that assists in matching the clients.[2] Beyond this, however, the homesharing living arrangement differs from other forms of intermediate housing both in kind and in emphasis. Because of the small size and location in the psychologically meaningful private "home" of one of the occupants and the absence of a housekeeper or warden, one may find a greater sense of interdependence and "life sharing" in homesharing than in other forms of group living. This enhances the importance of the matching process, since there will not be the variety of potential support-ers available to satisfy homesharers' needs as one finds in small group housing arrangements.

Homesharing agencies tend to "assist" rather than support. That is, their basic responsibility is to raise the public consciousness toward homesharing, process applicants, and arrange matches. Some follow-up services such as counseling, advice, and referral may be provided; but the agency's responsibility to arrange directly for support services to sustain the homesharing arrangement is usually minimal compared to most agency-assisted community housing arrangements, such as those developed in conjunction with the Philadelphia Geriatric Center or the Abbeyfield Society of Britain.

Nevertheless, if an agency matches a large number of frail homeowners with personal care providers who supply many needed services, it may find itself increasingly drawn into the consultant and caseworker roles. The agency staff may be asked to manage cases of homeowners who need several compatible live-in personal care companions or to coordinate the informal care and respite help offered by kin and the more formal care provided by service deliverers.

## Space in Homesharing

Although such "lifesharing" arrangements underscore the significance of careful matching and follow-up monitoring, it is also true that many large homes can accommodate another person easily, often with few shared spaces and facilities, so that the arrangement approximates that of paying lodger and homeowner. In such cases, homeowner and lodger may rarely interact with each other, because all daily living of each party is being done on separate floors of the home. For example, Help the Aged in England purchases private homes from elderly homeowners and remodels them so that several elders loosely matched by the agency can live in one of those units. The "homeowner" remains at home but chooses how much "lifesharing" to engage in with the other occupants.

In other cases, an older homeowner and younger lodger may physically share many spaces but spend most of their daily life apart from each other. Their lives would revolve around separate friends and activities, and they would share the same home spaces only for brief intervals.

There are thus two dimensions of "space" relating to the amount of privacy available to the homeowner and the live-in homesharer. Architectural space refers to the actual space available to the occupants in cubic feet. It also can refer to the sizes, numbers and locations of rooms in the homes. Lifestyle space, on the other hand, refers to the daily living patterns characterizing homeowner and sharer, which can determine the potential for social interaction, as well as the likelihood of in-home privacy.

A relatively healthy elderly homeowner living on the first floor of a good-sized home may rarely see a homesharer who works all day, uses a back entrance to the home, and has separate bath and bedroom facilities on the second floor. Nevertheless, for this homeowner, it may be necessary only that someone be available during the night time hours in case of emergency. Perhaps the live-in homesharer also agrees to do some infrequent heavy chores around the home, such as shoveling snow off the sidewalks or replacing screens with storm windows each winter, in exchange for lowered rental payments. In this arrangement, lives are quite separate and interaction may be infrequent. The sharers' separate daily lifestyles and the in-home spatial arrangements of the rooms lessen the need for and likelihood of frequent social interaction. They live their lives relatively independently of one another.

On the other hand, a homesharer might agree to cook one meal a day and run a few simple errands, like twice weekly grocery shopping. This would already necessitate more interaction and interdependence between homesharer and homeowner. Over time, the older homeowner might experience some deterioration in health and require more personal care from the homesharer, including the preparation of all meals as well as help with daily housecleaning and shopping. Because they share so much space and spend so much time in each other's company, the compatibility of the couple is likely to take on greater significance. As the competencies of the homeowner decline, the press of the environment can be reduced by the increasing assumption of daily tasks and personal care by the homesharer. The homeowner's live-in sharer may be either the original sharer who is willing and able to assume new caregiving responsibilities or a new caregiver who views the responsibilities as a full-time job. More than one caregiver may be employed at one time, operating in shifts, as the financial arrangement now changes from one in which the homeowner receives rent in exchange for letting out space to one in which the homeowner gives room and board and a stipend in exchange for personal care services.

## The Continuum of Care at Home

Thus the home itself may be viewed as representing a continuum of care living arrangement that requires different levels of service and personnel over time to sustain the older person in her or his own home. For example, beginning with a minimally integrative arrangement in which a college student simply pays rent for a second floor room, it is theoretically possible for a person to remain at home until death as a succession of homesharers, family members, and professional service providers are coordinated over a period of years by kin and the homesharing agency. Not only is such a continuum of care theoretically possible, but, as will be demonstrated later, it actually does occur in some homesharing arrangements.

The concept of "aging in place" represents an important issue for many group housing and sheltered schemes and for homesharing arrangements. In the former, the need to increase services to an increasingly frail population is an attempt to assist elders to avoid relocation out of the small group situation. Elders may enter a group home in relatively good health. Over time, however, the original population ages and needs new services. Either these people must relocate or new services must be provided to sustain the older person in place. In the United States, there are congregate housing programs in which living arrangements are subdivided into two or more types within the same complex to reflect the differing amounts of services provided to clients. In England, the need for new services has resulted in the construction of "special care" Abbeyfield Homes and "very sheltered" sheltered housing becoming available.

This same principle can apply to homesharing, as people age while still preferring to remain in place. Homesharing service agencies can either allow the elders to make their own arrangements or assume more responsibility for finding compatible homesharers who can provide the necessary level of care. If more agency responsibility is needed, they can increase services to homeowners by arranging for personal care homesharers, stimulating kin involvement, and utilizing professional service providers in proportion to the needs of the frail homeowners and the press of the environment. Usually, the homesharing arrangement is such a fluid and dynamic situation that much coordination of care between several caregivers and respite caregivers as well as family members and professional personnel is necessary, and more agency involvement is desirable.

At least in the early stages of a program, however, homesharing is one of the simplest and least bureaucratically assisted and sustained living arrangements among intermediate housing schemes. Other than arranging the match itself and, if needed, providing some early counseling, the agency basically allows the newly matched couple to decide the nature and form of their lifestyle and their responsibilities and relationship to each other. This is all done in an environment already familiar to one member of the pair. Moreover, as shall be seen, many if not the majority of matches are intergenerational, an arrangement rarely seen in other intermediate or small group living arrangements.

## Domiciliary Care: Another Form of Homesharing

As previously noted, what makes homesharing different from other shared living arrangements is that one of the sharers remains in his or her own home. In most cases, the shared living arrangement is limited to just pairs of people, while most other kinds of group living schemes involve three or more people sharing an agency-owned or -sponsored household.

There is, however, one other kind of shared living arrangement that involves the private home of one of the sharers and is usually limited to two to four people (Sherwood et al. 1980). In the United States, it is referred to as domiciliary care, while, in the United Kingdom, it is referred to as assisted lodgings or family placement. Family placements are arrangements in which the clients (usually but not exclusively elderly) live in private households as paying guests usually in exchange for room, board, and personal care services. In England, there are approximately two dozen such family placement schemes, the majority of which focus on short term placements of only a few weeks either to aid in rehabilitation of the client or to provide holiday relief for the client's caretaker family. Family placement schemes in the United States seem to focus more on long-term placements with foster families.

One way family placement arrangements differ from homesharing schemes is that the nature of exchange in the former is more formal and contractual, because money (usually a fixed amount) is exchanged for caregiving. By contrast, most homesharing schemes involve a fairly flexible type of bartering arrangement in which a financial exchange may be only one kind of transaction.

Another difference is that homesharing schemes are usually adminis-tered by voluntary or nonprofit agencies, while family placement or domiciliary care schemes are administered within statutory agencies such as the area agencies in the United States and the social service depart-ments in England and Wales (Peace 1984).

Furthermore, many homeowners in homesharing schemes in the United States are in poor health and are willing to exchange room and board for the caregiving services of the healthier homeseeker. In family placement schemes, the situation is usually reversed and the healthier homeowner provides all the resources of caregiving in exchange for financial remu-neration. The relationship is clearly less "equal" and less open to barter-ing, because all the major resources, not the least of which is homeown-ership, rest with the homeowner. The homeowner may even have had some professional training in caregiving—a service rarely included in homesharing schemes.

Nevertheless, both schemes do address the issue of underutilized space and deinstitutionalization, and both are committed to some kind of matching procedure for sharers. Few matching schemes of any kind use systematic matching procedures. In family placement schemes, there is considerable variation ranging from matching character traits, hobbies, likes and dislikes (Thornton and Moore 1980) to attempting to intuit the likelihood that clients would be appropriate for one another (Butler 1979).

The consequence of both family placement and shared-housing schemes is often the development of close expressive bonds between the sharers. This is true of even the more contractual relationships arranged through family placement schemes (Leat 1983). Thus, Mor et al. (1982) note that over 80 percent of their clients are involved in the family life of the home. Leat (1983:23) finds that "the feeling of being valued as an interesting or enjoyable person rather than a relative to whom one is grateful or has duties" is important for the one giving care.

For many such caregivers, although the pay is important, taking care of an elderly person allows them to continue in an occupation from which it is difficult to retire. Many of them are either married women whose children have left home or individuals who have previous experi-ence caring for an elderly person.

Finally, the element of choice or control by the elderly client appears at two levels for both homesharing and family placement schemes. At one level is the option of family placement or homesharing instead of an alternative from a range of other care and accommodation options. The other opportunity for choice comes at the time of placement when a particular individual is offered a choice of potential matches. In both schemes, clients often exercise some choice and control, but it is not unusual for family members to make inquiries or for social workers or other social providers to inform clients of various available options. Often, simply the necessity of an immediate placement or the availability of a certain kind of client in short supply, such as a person willing to move into a home, limits the range of choice exercised by the client. Clearly the homeowner in family placement schemes and the non-homeowner in homesharing schemes seem to be fewer in number and thus have more choices available to them.

# HOMESHARING PROGRAMS IN THE UNITED STATES

## The Extent of Homesharing

Although homesharing is not a common living arrangement for today's elderly population, the concept of sharing with nonrelatives is not an unfamiliar one for some elders. According to Mukherjee (1982), census reports indicate that, in America in the 1930s, 10 percent of all families had lodgers. Furthermore, based on the 1977 Annual Housing Survey, she has found that about 1.6 percent of all persons sixty-five years and older were sharing housing with unrelated people, some of whom were nonelderly. Schreter (1986) points out that by the 1980 census the numbers of such elders was over 300,000. Given the proliferation of homesharing programs in the United States during the 1980s, it is quite likely that this latter figure is now higher (see, e.g., Schreter and Turner 1986; Robins and Howe 1989).

Attempts to organize or formalize homesharing resulted in about a dozen homesharing agencies across the United States by the early 1980s (Peace 1984).[3] Since that time, there has been a rapid growth in such agencies from 106 formal match programs in 1983 to 169 in 1986, a 60 percent increase in three years (Robins and Howe 1989). The average age of such programs is four years. The great majority are located on the West and East Coasts, although more recent years have found an increase in homesharing agencies in the Midwest and Sunbelt.

*Community and Agency Characteristics.* Until recently, no systematic research had been undertaken to distinguish the kinds of communities in which homesharing programs have developed. In the first study of its kind,[4] Robins and Howe (1989) systematically examine thirty-eight randomly selected homesharing programs to determine what community characteristics are associated with the presence of homesharing programs. Their sample is stratified by region and drawn from the 1983 and 1986 editions of the National Directories of Shared Housing Programs for older people compiled by the Shared Housing Resource Center in Philadelphia.

Surprisingly, they discover that "superheated housing markets," or communities with low vacancy rates and high rents, are not predictors of homesharing programs. This is also the case for communities with many other social service agencies available. Rather, the best predictors of the existence of a homesharing program are city size and proportion of population over sixty-five years of age: The bigger the city and the greater the proportion of elderly in it, the more likely the city has a homesharing program.

Concerning sponsorship, they report that most programs are sponsored either by agencies supporting the elderly or by housing agencies. As of 1986, about 40 percent of homesharing programs are sponsored by programs such as area agencies on aging, retired senior volunteer programs, the Gray Panthers, or senior centers. Another 20 percent are sponsored by housing agencies. General social service agencies sponsor another 30 percent (Robins and Howe 1989).

Funding for homesharing programs often has been small scale and short term. The Robins and Howe report finds that the most common sources of funding are Community Development Block Grants and support through the Older Americans Act. Other sources mentioned include private foundations, United Ways, and state and local government grants. The median budget of a shared housing program is $50,000 with a range from no funding to $2,000,000.

The personnel profile in homesharing programs also is varied. Programs may be staffed by full-time or part-time directors and may or may not use volunteer staff. Robins and Howe (1989) have found that only 12 percent have three or more staff members. About one third of the programs have one or less than one full-time employee and are often made up of several part-time employees. In the most comprehensive survey of homesharing agencies to date, the Shared Housing Resource

Center (1988a) has found that the majority of the 167 programs for which they have data use at least one volunteer. The median number of volunteers is three.

Although follow-up supportive services for homesharing programs vary more than they do for family placement programs, those homesharing agencies using them attest to their value. Robins and Howe (1989) report that services range from simply providing a brochure or list of names of people willing to share, to reality counseling, checking references of applicants, and follow-up counseling.

Within a limited time in their collective existence, therefore, it appears that homesharing programs are a variegated group. Nevertheless, a common theme appears to be their existence in large communities with a significant number of elders and their use of both paid staff and volunteers in some capacity. These findings will be reconsidered in the next section when the rationale for studying one homesharing program in detail is offered.

*Client Characteristics.* General information on homesharing clients is nearly as scarce as data on the agencies. In their review of three agencies involved in homesharing, McConnell and Usher (1980) describe the typical homeowner as a widowed female living alone who is in good health and slightly higher in socioeconomic status than her tenants. Tenants are again mostly women, more mobile than homeowners and frequently divorced or separated. Through interviews with staff members of agencies, McConnell and Usher have found that the primary motives for homesharing are limited finances and a need for companionship. The larger Shared Housing Resource Center (1988a) survey has found that 87 percent of clients are Caucasian and that 50 percent of the agencies place no minorities at all. Women clients outnumber men 71 percent to 29 percent, and the majority of clients have incomes of less than $10,000.

Regarding client age, most programs are involved in at least some intergenerational matching. The Robins and Howe (1989) survey shows that 9 percent of the homesharing programs serve elders only, 50 percent of the programs are intergenerational, and the rest provide services for anyone. One program, Operation Match (Levinson 1982) in Boston, actually matches more nonelderly than elderly. In general, the older clients tend to be homeowners, while the younger ones are homeseekers.

While it is too early to assert client profiles without qualification, it does appear that homesharing is especially attractive to relatively healthy older female homeowners who, while having more money than individuals seeking a homeowner with whom to share, nevertheless have fairly modest incomes. Somewhat less is known about homeseekers, but clearly they generally appear to be younger and more mobile—geographically and socially—than the older homeowner clients.

## The Significance of Homesharing

The Larger Community. Little is known for certain about the effects of homesharing on the communities in which they exist, but clear financial benefits to the larger society have been noted. Stimulating more such living arrangements has been recognized as an important goal by the New York State Senate Committee on Aging in 1982. Senator Hugh T. Farley, the chairman, notes that "if funding were provided for shared housing the government could save approximately $2,400 a year per resident. This is based on the unit cost of new construction compared to a unit of shared homes."

Beyond the cost of constructing new housing, one can also point out how shared housing can ease a tight housing market in which individuals and families who cannot afford to buy homes find that they are also being priced out of the rental market, a problem noted above with respect to communities containing university or college students. Unfortunately, the data from Robins and Howe (1989) show that homesharing programs do not necessarily arise in tight housing markets; therefore, some individuals in especially dire housing circumstances are likely to be in communities containing no homesharing programs to help them out.

Clients. A clear measure of significance of homesharing programs to clients would appear to be whether clients actually find a homesharer or not. According to Robins and Howe (1989), the average number of matches per year per agency is 54 or approximately 38 percent of the pool of applicants. The average does mask a wide variation of between 3 and 450 matches per year. About two-thirds of the programs make fewer than the average of fifty-four matches per year.

Data concerning whether clients are matched or not are only part of the measure of a homesharing program's importance for clients, however. Agencies serve their unmatched clients in a variety of ways. For example, Levinson (1982) reports that, in Operation Match of Montgomery County, Maryland over a four-year period, 3,500 persons made inquiries and about 1,000 persons or 28 percent of the potential pool were matched. Yet all people applying or seeking information about the program had their choices expanded through the consideration of homesharing. That is, even if a client eventually chose not to pursue homesharing after making an inquiry (as many did), the act of contacting the agency tended to give the client a greater sense of affirmative control over the living environment at a time when choices might have seemed to be both threatening and decreasing.

A second benefit, which will be addressed later in this book, is the educational service homesharing agencies provide to clients who contact the agency. In addition to gaining the sense of control just described, the client also may gain important information about other related services toward which the agency can point the client.

Another presumed measure of significance of homesharing for clients is duration of match. There is more to a successful match than length of time, however. The director of one of the most "successful" programs, Project Match in San Jose, California, with over 2,000 matches in six years, concludes that success in matching clients cannot be evaluated solely by examining the duration of matches either. Some matches are designed for a short term for a variety of reasons: Desperate clients unable to find affordable housing and in need of work may need only temporary housing until they can get a job and begin to pay for traditional forms of housing. Or a college student may spend only a semester in a home residence and provide help with tasks around the yard and security at night in exchange for reduced rent.

Similar arguments about numbers of clients matched and duration of matches are made for family placement arrangements in England. Thornton and Moore (1980), in a review of twenty-three such schemes, point out that many are set up with small numbers of placements in mind, suggesting that the total number of clients served should *not* be used as the indicator of a program's effectiveness. Many family placement arrangements are only two or three weeks in length, but this affords the family an opportunity to go on holiday or the client a chance to recuperate sufficiently from accident or illness to return to their own home.

Psychological significance to clients of homesharing has been asserted on the basis of some fragmentary information like the McConnell and Usher (1980) study. The authors report that, for homeowners, sharing provides not only much desired companionship and help around the house but also "new ideas and intellectual stimulation" in cases in which the homeseeker is a younger person (McConnell and Usher 1980:20). There often are obstacles, however, and they are not limited to intergenerational sharing matches in which the "generation gap" can be a real problem. For example, a pilot program attempted in Miami, Florida failed because of incompatibility between sharers. According to Streib (1978), there were widely discrepant expectations between hosts who wanted help with chores and tenants who wanted help with activities of daily living, and so neither party could be satisfied by the homesharing arrangement.

Finally, it can be argued that homesharing is an extremely cost-effective program for its clients. The Shared Housing Resource Center Survey (1988a) shows the average cost of a match to be about $52 per month per person. If such a person would have to have been institutionalized, he or she might have paid $1,400 per month for a nursing home bed.

The preliminary indications are that homesharing has the potential for helping the local community it serves by attacking, in however modest a way, housing and rental shortages. More important, it appears, homesharing also has a great potential for educating and expanding the choices of its clients and for relieving the emotional and material press of environment on elders and on others (a good overview is Mantell and Gildea 1989).

## Gaps in Knowledge About Homesharing

The recent works by Robins and Howe (1989) and the Shared Housing Resource Center (1988a) have extended the earlier work of McConnell and Usher (1980) in productive ways to give a good descriptive overview of homesharing programs in the United States. Similarly, Jaffe's (1989b) typology of homesharers based on in-depth interviews of a sample from the Madison, Wisconsin program provides important information on actual homesharers that goes far beyond the early McConnell and Usher (1980) work and even the pathbreaking case study on homesharing by Pritchard (1983) (see also Pynoos and June 1989; Thuras 1989; and Underwood and Wulf 1989). Equally important, have been recent efforts by Pritchard and Perkocha (1989), Hwalek and Longley (1989), and Spence (1989) to assess the impact of homesharing in regional contexts.

At the same time, however, many gaps in knowledge remain. In particular, it is not clear how effective homesharing programs are in meeting the needs of healthy and frail elders alike. Corollary questions include: How can homesharing programs evolve in such a way as to maximize their effectiveness in serving clients—especially in light of decreased emphasis on public spending for human service programs? Who are homesharing programs' clients and who *ought* they to be? What, in terms both of organizational initiative and client characteristics, facilitates an applicant's chances of getting matched? Once matched, what are the dynamics characterizing the lives of the sharers, and what implications do these results have for the elderly and the frail for whom homesharing appears to be an important option on the continuum of care?

# PROJECT HOME

Because agency-sponsored homesharing arrangements to help elders remain at home are a recent phenomenon, it is not surprising that little systematic data are available to evaluate the impact of homesharing on both program clients and the larger community. This book aims to fill in some of the gaps in knowledge that currently exist regarding homesharing.

Central are two general sets of assumptions about homesharing that will be developed and documented: First, *homesharing is both an important housing alternative along the continuum of care for elders and a context in which a continuum of care can be provided elders within their own home.* Second, *homesharing represents an important application of exchange theory both for those who homeshare and for those agencies who are attempting to provide homesharing services.*

These general arguments will be addressed in the following specific ways: We will describe the genesis and first five years' operation of Project HOME (Housing to Match Elders), a homesharing program in Chittenden County, Vermont; explain the dynamics that allowed Project HOME to survive and succeed; describe the pool of potential homesharers who have applied to HOME; explain why some applicants are matched and others are not; examine in detail the dynamics of the homesharing relationship in several different kinds of homesharing arrangements; evaluate the effectiveness of Project HOME as an alternative for some elders to institutional care; and, finally, discuss in general the relevance of homesharing as an appealing, realistic, and cost-saving alternative to institutional care by comparing Project HOME to other homesharing programs and highlighting aspects of HOME that make it a model approach to housing, health, and income problems besetting this country's elders.

## Empirical Bases of the Book

This book derives from an intensive case study of one homesharing program in one county in the United States. The data to be analyzed represent a wide range of sources, including applicant questionnaires (N = 618), follow-up questionnaires of selected applicants (N = 153), in-depth interviews with selected matched applicants (N = 74), in-depth interviews with project directors and their staff, time-use diaries from one project director, and all available logs from the project office. The time frame includes the six-month period *prior* to the actual start of the program (fall 1981 through winter 1981–82) and the first five years of the program's existence (April 1982 through March 1987). Applicant data cover the first four years of program operation, while follow-up data from selected applicants, program director and staff interview data, and agency logs cover the first five-year period.

## Why a Case Study?

There are three reasons for devoting most of the space in this book to Project HOME. First, it is a program that has been systematically monitored since its inception by the authors. In addition to all the data gathering and data analysis summarized above, the authors have supplied Project HOME with questions for client application forms, trained project interviewers, and shared preliminary findings with the director and her staff. The ethical implications of such a close relationship will be addressed later in chapter 4, but the point to be stressed here is that this book is based on much inside knowledge about the program as well as information gleaned from the usual sources like interviews with staff, client application forms, and follow-up interviews of program clients.

A second reason for emphasizing the case study approach stems from the site of the program, Burlington, Vermont, and its surrounding area within Chittenden County. The greater Burlington area, recently designated as a Standard Metropolitan Statistical Area (SMSA), contains a little over 100,000 people, including a proportionate minority of elders, in both relatively urban and relatively rural settings. If one examines recent Current Population Reports, it is clear that nearly three-quarters of the country's population resides in rural areas, towns, or cities of 100,000 or less. Thus, the information about homesharing gleaned from a detailed study of Project HOME is potentially generalizable to many current or planned homesharing programs in locales similar in size to that covered by Project HOME. As a corollary, Project HOME's existence in a technical SMSA, its budget, its history of using both part-time and full-time staff, and its volunteer component make it a typical homesharing program in many ways.

Finally, and perhaps most important, the first five years of Project HOME has seen a series of changes in program orientation that represent a wide diversity of applicants and program foci. Starting with an exclusively elders-only focus, Project HOME began to promote intergenerational matches after the first year. By the third year, personal care companion matches for frail elders paying their homesharers had become as important as the traditional homesharing matches in which the homeowner received a rent or combination of rent and services. As a result, Project HOME's clientele represent most kinds of people who would want to homeshare: "young" elders in their sixties and seventies; "old" elders in their eighties and above; healthy elders; frail elders; disabled adults of all ages; college students; young adults out of school; middle-aged individuals who are widowed, divorced or separated; couples; and families with children. Whether homesharing agency service providers would want to serve as diverse a clientele as Project HOME's or focus on only a subset of the clients served by HOME, there will be many important insights from a detailed examination of the HOME experience.

Thus, at the end of this book, we hope to make some useful generalizations about the process of homesharing for the thousands who have already come forward, seeking help from the over one hundred agencies aiming to serve them, and for the thousands who have not but who could benefit from homesharing. While homesharing is not for everyone, it is our profound belief that elders need to have the option of homesharing offered to them as one alternative among several along the continuum of care. This book is written with the hope that its contents will help elders and the homesharing programs that would serve them to understand better the homesharing alternative.

# 2

# Project HOME

Beginning services in the spring of 1982, Project HOME has grown from a small program almost totally run by volunteers with no budget to a major community service organization with three full-time and one part-time paid staff members, about the same number of volunteer staff members, and a budget of over $100,000. Even now, as an established service organization complete with advisory board and as a recipient of United Way funds, Project HOME remains a curious hybrid: It operates within bureaucratic limitations of budgeting, procedures for operation, and some division of labor, while it continues to depend on a dedicated core of volunteers for its key service delivery functions.

The increase in the number of clients served, of course, parallels the dramatic increase in the organization's size. In its first year of operation 85 people applied to Project HOME, which was able to make only four matches. By the fifth year of operation there was a threefold increase in applicants to 251 and almost a twentyfold increase in matches to 75 for the year. In addition, there are currently over 500 counseling inquiries a year that involve people's requests for information about homesharing or related service requests, suggesting that Project HOME has become an important clearinghouse for information pertaining, but not limited, to elders' (and others') living situations. Thus Project HOME staff provide information and referral for other more appropriate agencies or services.

This case study of Project HOME is based on the premise that several themes characterizing the organization's evolution over its first five years have important implications for the development and maintenance of other service delivery programs aimed at elders and other vulnerable groups and for the assessment of the quality of their service. Chapter 4 will develop themes concerning organizational structure, leadership, and social exchange, but first it is important to have an understanding of the key actors, events, and processes in the program. In this chapter, description will first focus on the main characters and events during Project HOME's first five years, and then on the main elements in the matchmaking process. Then chapter 3 will examine one group of key actors, the volunteers whose wide-ranging contributions have made Project HOME a relatively unique organization.

## THE ORIGIN AND HISTORY OF PROJECT HOME

*Origins: Serving Two Groups of Elders*

The idea for Project HOME was developed in 1981 by members of the county Retired Senior Volunteer Program who saw dual needs that a single homesharing service could meet. One problem was the serious housing shortage in the county's major city. According to the Retired Senior Volunteer Program (RSVP) director at the time:

> The original purpose of HOME arose from the fact that we saw a 1% housing vacancy rate in Burlington and we were concerned with the long waiting list with congregate housing facilities. We wondered if there was a simple way older people might be put in touch with other older people who either had room in their own home to share or were desirous of a place to stay. We thought there might be many older people who might like this kind of service which bypassed newspapers or other conventional kinds of advertising like bulletins.

The second need, not critical given the numbers of projects in which RSVP volunteers were involved, but critical with respect to the direction the program would take in its development, reflected the mission of RSVP to provide meaningful activities for its volunteers. Indeed, the RSVP director and her staff had already identified several RSVP volunteers who were seeking more challenging and innovative assignments, such as the ones envisioned in connection with Project HOME. Thus the original idea behind Project HOME was to service two groups of people: elderly in need of shared housing and older RSVP volunteers who would help to match these elders with each other. The former group would receive an important service, while the latter, in providing that service, would be receiving a meaningful experience through RSVP.

How meaningful the experience would be for the volunteers was described by the RSVP director when she pointed out that the envisioned project would eventually be run almost entirely through the efforts of RSVP volunteers who would advertise, recruit, match, and generally administer the entire homesharing initiative: "Older volunteers could understand best the needs of homeowners and sharers to a greater degree than younger persons and thus would become advocates for the clients." To provide administrative continuity, a part-time RSVP staff person was temporarily assigned to this project to get it off the ground. Eventually, however, the anticipation was that volunteers would be running the service by themselves, so the part-time HOME director was to be involved in the beginning stages of the program only.

Shortly after RSVP decided to begin Project HOME, in the fall of 1981, the RSVP director contacted one of the authors (Fengler) whom she knew in a professional capacity and asked if he would be interested in helping to construct a homesharing application form in exchange for use of the information on the forms in research endeavors relating to homesharing. Fengler agreed, bringing in Danigelis, with whom he had been working on other collaborative matters, to work on construction of a homesharing application form.

During the early winter of 1982, the authors, after consulting with the RSVP director and the RSVP staff person assigned to coordinate Project HOME, developed a draft application form and shared it with the director and her coordinator. After much negotiating, a final draft was agreed to and copies of the form were made. Once copies were in hand, the authors held a training session for the RSVP volunteers who would be using the application form to interview prospective homesharers. Around April 1, 1982, Project HOME, through word of mouth and public service announcements, "opened its doors" and began to accept applications from elders in need of homesharers.

## The First Year: Learning How to Match Clients

For a few brief months Project HOME resembled a cottage industry in that it functioned as a part of the whole RSVP program, using a part-time staff member from RSVP, depending on RSVP volunteers, and operating out of RSVP office space. Its organizational profile, therefore, was not unlike a family deciding to sell the *objets d'art* that their children were producing during recreation time at home. Not surprisingly, like many cottage industries, Project HOME required much more attention than the early staffing resources could accommodate. The director of RSVP, in fact, noted that within the first six months of HOME

> we realized it was not going to be so simple. People needed a lot of assistance in becoming interested in the idea of homesharing in the first place because it was a new concept in the community. Secondly, people needed assistance in actually being matched. They needed an intermediary to help clarify the issues and negotiate whatever sharing arrangements there were. We realized there would have to be a lot more input from one person to coordinate the activities.

In order to develop a matching instrument, train the volunteers to interview potential applicants, recruit, advertise, and, of course, arrange the actual match, the homesharing initiative in RSVP would need "one person to coordinate the activities." Thus, in October of 1982, about six months after the program had begun accepting applicants, RSVP hired a part-time staff person with help from an $8,000 community service grant from IBM that provided for this part-time director to work some twenty to thirty hours a week for one year.

The new HOME director was employed through RSVP and was thus responsible to the RSVP director. At the same time, the HOME director was, in theory, quite separated from the daily operation of RSVP and unlikely to be compromised by the daily distractions of the larger organization. In practice, the HOME director's desk was in the same office as RSVP personnel and next door to the RSVP director's office. Since volunteers were involved in HOME as interviewers, the goals of RSVP and HOME were compatible and the needs of two groups—homeowners and volunteers—were being served through the same project.

A key problem facing the new director was that no matches had been made at the time she was hired. A great deal of the problem lay in the tremendous imbalance in the pool of applicants: Twenty-three of the first twenty-nine applicants to the program were home providers; there were hardly any elderly applicants willing to move, and the few there were could not be matched. For the university researchers, nevertheless, there was enough preliminary indication that the study of Project HOME and its service mission was important enough and could be based on a sufficiently strong database for an application to an outside agency to fund an evaluation of the program. Thus, in the fall of 1982 they applied to the Andrus Foundation for financial support to evaluate Project HOME.

During this first year of its existence, over a dozen RSVP volunteers worked for Project HOME, interviewing applicants. By the end of the first year, some eighty-three applications had been received, but only four matches were made. Nevertheless, Project HOME had begun and was making itself known in the community among service providers and clients alike.

## The Second Year: New Directions

The first part-time director of Project HOME served for only half of the one-year grant awarded by IBM, leaving the program near the end of Project HOME's first year in a move which was dictated by family considerations and not directly related to the very slow pace at which progress was being made. Nevertheless, the first year of Project HOME was a difficult period for the program: The part-time director and her volunteer staff were trying to sell the concept of homesharing to elders in the area, but they had little experience in matching applicants with one another and they had not yet developed a systematic matching procedure.

At the beginning of the second year a new part-time director was hired, and for several weeks both the old and new directors worked together. At this time, the RSVP director continued to stress the importance of the HOME directorship as a part-time position. She reasoned that if the director were full-time, the HOME director "would be doing things a volunteer could do. The only way to focus the use of volunteers to the fullest extent is to have a part-time director."

The new director had experiences and interests directly relevant to homesharing: She had worked with older people as a chaplain and had training as a journalist. Her grandmother and mother's various experiences in a variety of living conditions helped spark her interest in living environments for older people. At the time she became director, she was also homesharing herself. Finally, the job was asking her to do things she liked and felt she was good at such as interviewing, serving people, and being responsible for program development.

Also during the spring of 1983, the university researchers were informed that funding from the Andrus Foundation was forthcoming. As a result, they initiated a roundtable discussion in which the old and new HOME directors, the director of RSVP, and the original RSVP coordinator for Project HOME discussed the progress and direction of Project HOME.

This roundtable became the first in a series of conversations and semistructured interviews with the new HOME director that, along with later interviews with relevant volunteer staff, provided the investigators with important information about the functioning of Project HOME. At the same time, the conversations with the director became a means by which she and they "brainstormed" (her word) about various problems and possible new initiatives regarding the program.

Three important things happened during this critical second year: an expansion of the target population, a complete overhauling and expansion of the application form, and an expanded role for the director.

First, from the beginning, the new director believed that while Project HOME was a service for the benefit of elders, the program could not continue to depend on only elder homesharer clients; the very low numbers of matches attested to the fact that getting older people to leave their own homes was terribly difficult, if not impossible. As a result, she opened up applications to well and disabled nonelders who were in need of shared housing and who would be willing to share with elders.

Second, after service in the field for nearly one year, the original application form had showed itself to be inadequate for purposes of matching applicants, especially the new, younger group, and for evaluating the program's efforts to match individuals. Together the new director and the university researchers developed a much more comprehensive application instrument comprised of a separate application form and interview schedule for home providers and a separate form and schedule for home seekers.

In addition to providing important information for matching and evaluational purposes, it had the latent function of screening out people who were not particularly interested in the program, since the two-step process for applicants involved both filling out an application form and submitting to a personal interview with one of the program's RSVP volunteers. In addition the new director believed that the new questions concerning current lifestyle and homesharing expectations "made a great deal of difference because people are alerted to compromises they are going to be asked to make. It also alerted our interviewers to look for a dream and see if it is really possible." By filling out the application, prospective homesharers informed themselves about what kinds of choices and compromises homesharing might entail.

Finally, because the IBM grant was scheduled to run out during the middle of the program's second year, the RSVP and HOME directors discussed options for uncovering new sources of funding. Since the RSVP director believed that HOME needed to support itself in this respect, she maintained that the HOME director needed to take the initiative and proceed to make grant applications where appropriate, with the understanding that RSVP would help in any way it could.

Despite having no experience in grant writing, the HOME director set to her task, and, within only a few months of the lapse of the IBM grant, Project HOME received support from the state of Vermont's Independence Fund, a source of funding aimed at programs that seek to delay or prevent unnecessary and expensive institutionalization of Vermont residents. Between the time the IBM grant lapsed and the Independence Fund grant started RSVP provided monetary support to carry HOME's administrative costs, and, afterward, RSVP made up the difference between the Independence Fund grant and what HOME needed to operate.

While all these important changes were occurring during the second year, the number of volunteers fluctuated somewhat, but around a half-dozen were doing interviews on a regular basis and another half-dozen were supplementing these more active volunteers with interviews at less frequent intervals. By the end of the second year, Project HOME had received an additional eighty-six applications and had made eighteen more matches. Among the matches, three involved clients who had already homeshared through Project HOME earlier.

## The Third Year: Declaring Independence

The third year was characterized by a tremendous growth in the number of Project HOME clients in the wake of continuing financial pressures. In response to these stimuli, there evolved a restructuring of roles within HOME's small staff and, finally, independence of the program from RSVP.

During the third year, as the director and her volunteers stepped up advertising and successes with clients became known, the program received a large influx of applicants. At the same time, the problem of money continued to be an ongoing concern, especially during the summer of 1985 as the one-year Independence Fund grant was nearing an end. Simultaneously, therefore, the HOME director was being asked to spend more time serving an increasing number of clients while spending more time writing grant applications to insure that the program continued. The dilemma was solved by the HOME director spending more time on grant proposal writing, while a small core of experienced volunteers assumed greater responsibilities for matching applicants with one an-other.

At the same time that funding was getting to be an issue, the RSVP director was becoming increasingly concerned that Project HOME was outgrowing RSVP's original expectations:

> With a minimal amount of community education we had an overwhelming response—so much so we are beginning to wonder if RSVP can give the kind of support service to Project HOME that it actually needs. We need to explore other agencies in the community who serve housing needs. Because what we are really getting involved in is direct service and that is not the purpose of RSVP. We are facilitators and catalysts, a role we have played well.

Thus, during this very busy third year, both financial and organiza-tional strains were coming to the forefront in the minds of both the Project HOME and RSVP directors.

After a series of discussions concerning the alternatives, the two direc-tors agreed that Project HOME should become an independent program that, while continuing to cooperate with RSVP, would nevertheless be a separate entity. In the meantime, the HOME director would continue to seek funding to pay for (basically) her salary.[1]

During this third year, the number of Project HOME volunteers was reduced to no more than a half-dozen or so, but what was lost in number was made up for in quality of work. As the HOME director spent more time on grant writing and related administrative matters, the volunteers, in large part on their own initiative and with the blessing of the director, became involved in matching and following up matched clients as well as taking phone inquiries from and interviewing prospective clients and developing advertising strategies.

During the third year, Project HOME received new funding from the Vermont Independence Fund and, before the year was over, had become a separate entity from RSVP. During this third year also, 162 new applications were taken, and 43 new matches were made including new as well as previously matched clients. Seventeen of the matches involved previously matched clients.

## The Fourth Year: Discovering Client Needs

The fourth year was characterized by the program's formal recognition of an expansion of its mission and concomitant peaking of the number of its applicants, while the newly independent organization continued to struggle for financial support.

Regarding clients, Project HOME had, from the beginning, been attracting frail elders whose homesharing needs were much greater than the typical homeowner. Such frail elders required more than a lodger who either would provide chore-like services or pay for a space in which to live; they needed personal care from a homesharer who either had previous experience (e.g., through nursing) or a willingness to commit much time and patience to caring for another individual.

In either case, the frail elder was not going to get such help from the traditional sharer who preferred paying or doing minimal work or both in exchange for a place to stay. The only solution was for the homeowner to *pay* someone to provide the necessary personal care. Fortunately, enough frail elders were able to provide a stipend in addition to living space for their caregiving homesharers, and many younger and middle-aged sharers were found who were willing to provide caregiving services in exchange for a stipend and a place to live. In fact, during the fourth year, the number of personal care companion applicants exceeded the number of traditional homesharing applicants. Later chapters will compare descriptive profiles of personal care companion applicants and traditional sharers (chapter 5), analyze what facilitates matches for each group (chapter 6), and examine some personal care homesharing arrangements in detail (chapter 7).

Money, a concern from almost the beginning of the program, became especially acute after Project HOME became independent from RSVP. Still, with funding from the Vermont Independence Fund being renewed and other, smaller sources, like the city, being successfully tapped, Project HOME continued to scrape by with enough support to pay the director and provide administrative support.

Because the Independence Fund was intended to provide seed money for *new* programs and Project HOME was rapidly becoming "old," the director and her staff believed that a relatively permanent source of funding was needed if the program was going to be able to focus its energies on service provision rather than dissipate them in efforts to keep the program itself financially solvent. Despite the day-to-day work of the core volunteers described in the previous section, the director could ill afford to become a full-time grant writer because the program had become strongly identified with her name and because she had so much knowledge about all of the homesharing applicants that it was becoming increasingly difficult to share with her volunteer staff.

Thus it was a serious setback when Project HOME's first application to the United Way was turned down during this fourth year of operation. Compounding the uncertain financial future of the program was the decision by the director to resign from her position in order to attend Divinity School. While her decision to leave was firm, she kept her departure date open in hopes that the organization could get on firm footing financially before she left.

With all the uncertainty stemming from financial concerns and the forthcoming departure of the director, Project HOME continued to maintain a high profile in the community and, as described above, expand the kinds of clientele it was willing to serve. With a core staff of the director and between four and six volunteers, Project HOME processed 285 applications and made 87 matches, over half of which (46) involved previously matched clients.

## The Fifth Year: Becoming a Flexible Bureaucracy

Attacking the problem of uncertain financing in the face of ever-expanding service requests from the community and service provision for clients, the director, her volunteer staff, and the manager of the housing unit in which Project HOME was still housed decided to formalize the structure of the program by creating an advisory board of interested community members who could provide a variety of resources for the organization that it was having difficulty providing for itself.

One resource, of course, was the existence of the board itself, which would encourage outside funding agencies to view Project HOME as an established organization somewhat accountable to a group other than itself or its clients.

A second advantage came from the people who made up the board and the kind of specific help they were envisioned as providing. The director and her staff carefully chose board members who would provide a variety of services that it was becoming increasingly hard for Project HOME to do for itself. Thus, the board charter specified four committees: Planning and Evaluation, Volunteer Development, Public Relations, and Fund Raising. The authors were asked to serve on the board and cochair the Planning and Evaluation Committee; two HOME volunteers were asked to serve on the board and on the Volunteer Development Committee; others were asked to serve on the board because of their expertise in public relations or fund raising and were assigned to the appropriate committees.

Two major events after the creation of the advisory board occurred during this critical fifth year: First, during the spring and early summer of the fifth year, the director and board solicited applications and interviewed candidates for the position of new director. The current director, with an advisory board and funding in place, finally had announced her intention to leave by the end of the summer. During the interviewing process, the board decided that the new director needed to have a serious commitment to service for elders and others needing homesharers but that also he or she needed to be able to run Project HOME efficiently and *manage* it. The time for large-scale entrepreneurial growth had passed, and Project HOME needed to protect what it had achieved.

After some deliberation, the board chose a woman with a background in legal aid work who was interested in pursuing an advanced degree in public administration. In the words of one board member, the board had been looking for and, in fact, hired a "caring manager." The old entrepreneurial director and the new managerial director overlapped a month to facilitate the changing of the guard. By the end of August the old director had left and Project HOME symbolically had entered a new era.

The second major event was precipitated by work on a revised application to United Way, developed by the new director with the help of the board and the old director. In the fall of the fifth year, Project HOME's application to United Way was accepted, and the program was now a United Way agency. Project HOME continues to receive much (but not all) of its financial support from United Way.

During the fifth year of the program, Project HOME continued to run on volunteer power. A core of no more than five or six volunteers, along with the director, performed the usual clerical duties but also did intake and application interviews, discussed with coworkers and the director who to match with whom, and followed up on clients, and two volunteers, of course, served on the advisory board. Some 251 clients applied to Project HOME during its fifth year, and 75 matches were made—of which over half (45) involved previously matched clients.

*Postscript.* Finally, a major change has been the expansion of Project HOME's office space: In an ironic twist, Project HOME has moved into the more spacious offices vacated by the Retired Services Volunteer Program, which moved to a new location.

# THE MATCHMAKING PROCESS

*Advertising and Recruiting*

When HOME first began operating its presence was quickly noted by service providers, but the program was not yet known very well in the larger community—especially among potential mover applicants.[2] Therefore, most early clients were referrals with serious health problems and immediate needs. The view of Project HOME as an alternative to institutional care, at least in the early stages of the project, was inappropriate. Such individuals could not be matched given their level of disability, the immediacy of their need for a match, and the constraints imposed by an early small pool of applicants overrepresented by homeowners. In this respect, Project HOME was clearly a prisoner of its very low profile in the larger community, which is not surprising in light of the fact that this was the infancy of the program.

During the second year of its operation, Project HOME started to become better known throughout the city and its surrounding areas because of more aggressive public relations efforts. Through magazine and newspaper articles, television and radio announcements, church and meal site visits, and pamphlet canvassing in supermarkets the program had begun to reach an increasing number of elders and others in need of homesharing arrangements. The mass media, in particular, helped produce an increase in applicants for whom homesharing was an appropriate living arrangement option. According to the second director,

> Those who approached HOME directly and spontaneously have a greater investment and motivation and a greater likelihood of being matched. We found that those who need constant observation are not good candidates for home sharing. The best candidates are in good health but in search of financial sharing, transportation, task and rent sharing.

The new director felt that smaller, more frequent articles about homesharing in local newspapers would not only attract present homeowners and seekers in need of a match but would also serve to educate the whole community to the general idea and advantages of homesharing. Thus, the community would perceive homesharing as one more alternative along the general continuum of care, and this heightened awareness would result in future clients when the circumstances arose. Advertising on the college campuses was also attractive because by August 1983 the director realized the program "had a great deal of success with intergenerational type matches." She did caution, however, that "students in need of financial assistance must also be willing to give by sharing their lives. An older person doesn't just want someone to share space with them."

During this time, "the number one 'puller in' is an article in the paper," according to the director of HOME. Unfortunately, she continued, the problem is that HOME was not "controversial enough" to make the sort of feature story that would publicize the program's services, because people who were matched do not want to advertise their situation. "The reason they came to us and did not put an advertisement in the paper (for a housemate) is the same reason they won't allow us to capitalize on their present situation for publicity purposes. The idea of homesharing is a very 'private thing,' and they don't want to talk about it," she pointed out.

Before it became an independent agency, Project HOME was also restricted by its affiliation with RSVP concerning the kind of advertising it was able to do. The conservative philosophy of RSVP "is to keep everyone happy and they are never ever going to go out on a limb," stated the director of HOME.

During the third and fourth years, the director and her staff began an aggressive campaign of publicity on behalf of Project HOME, only partly because of the program's declaring its independence from RSVP. Another reason stemmed from the need by the program to recruit caregivers to share with frail homeowners. Project HOME had become a charter member of the area long-term care consortium and had referrals from the emergency shelter, the Visiting Nurses Association, the Area Agency on Aging, the Hospital Social Service, and the Job Service. Placing advertisements in newspapers and giving slide and talk presentations to a variety of community groups and organizations involved them in more diverse networks of individuals who had the kinds of various skills and the need to be caregivers.

Another significant publicity effort was the creation of a twenty-minute videotape explaining Project HOME and portraying diverse kinds of homesharing situations, from the traditional bartering arrangement between sharers to the caregiving arrangement that had become so prominent after the second year of the program. Interestingly, the HOME clients who were highlighted in the tape, far from feeling that their privacy had been violated, reacted quite positively to the experience and were formally recognized and thanked for their cooperation by the HOME staff at a special party honoring the video "stars."

## Matching Clients

*The Application Schedule(s).* To date there have been a variety of application forms used by HOME to gather important information for the director and staff so that they can find appropriate sharers for applicants and for the researchers to be able to summarize the characteristics of applicants and explain which ones facilitated an applicant's chances of getting matched (see appendix 1 for an example).

Reasons for the diversity of forms include, in chronological order: the change from the first to the second director and an agreement between the new director and the researchers to incorporate a larger evaluational component, a desire by interviewers to delete questions they deemed too personal and unimportant, and the disengagement of the researchers from the program. The first cause, described earlier in this chapter, resulted in an increase in the number and variety of questions. The latter two causes, not surprisingly, resulted in a condensing of the application information form.

As new concerns over the intrusiveness and relevance of current questions became highlighted and, at the same time, a need for additional questions concerning previously uncovered areas became evident,[3] the application questionnaire became revised again. It is fair to say that there have been about as many application questionnaire changes as years that Project HOME has been in existence. (Chapter 4 will discuss the benefits and obvious costs of so many changes in the application questionnaire.)

*The Application Process.* During the first year of the program, after a potential client called the office, a volunteer interviewer in the client's geographic area was contacted. The interviewer in turn called the client to arrange for a mutually convenient interview, usually within a week of the initial call. Most interviewers worked as pairs, primarily because there were so many volunteers and so few applicants and the director wanted all volunteers to participate. Secondarily, the presence of a partner gave the volunteers moral support as they learned and began to practice a new skill.

After the new two-part application schedule was implemented early in the second year (appendix 1), the process changed so that the questionnaire was immediately mailed out and the client asked to fill it out. Most questions focused on background information like age, marital status, health, current homesharing arrangement, etc. Further information on Project HOME, instructions for filling out the applications, and release forms were included as part of the questionnaire packet sent to applicants. Having the client fill out the lengthy questionnaire served to educate the client about homesharing as well as to provide further evidence of the client's commitment to homesharing.

The personal interview part of the application process usually occurred after the client had filled out the questionnaire. During the interview, the volunteer interviewer or director would ask the applicant questions pertaining directly to homesharing interests and concerns. At the same time, the client could ask questions that might have been prompted by either the questions contained in the questionnaire or the information sent in the questionnaire packet.

A further modification, introduced near the end of the second year, was designed to screen out inappropriate clients and also to present the possibility of an "immediate paper match" following the interview. The modification involved arranging an interview only *after* the client had filled out and returned the application in a stamped self-addressed envelope. References could then be contacted *before* the interview. Prior to this modification, some clients had filled out the application but had not mailed them in by the time of the interview.

References supplied by candidates were now being contacted before the interview was administered but after the application had been returned. The application form thus was acting as a screening mechanism, and, according to the director, many people who had contacted HOME for help in finding a match were now deciding not to be interviewed. Such a screening device also suggested that referral agencies needed to be further educated so that they would screen even more diligently than they had been doing.

By the third year, the two-part application/interview process had become too unwieldy in the eyes of the interviewers, and, with the reluctant agreement of the researchers who would be "losing" questions, a new one-part application form was developed combining background and homesharing questions into one, smaller application questionnaire that would be administered at the time of application by the volunteer interviewer or by the director, usually in the Project HOME office after an appointment had been made. The single questionnaire application process now is the norm.

*Preliminary Agency Decisions.* As described by the second HOME director, the essence of Project HOME's service was assisting their clients to decide for themselves what to do, not making decisions for their clients:

We can't take over other peoples' problems. That is not our goal. Our goal is to assist them to solve it themselves by providing choice. But we can't make the choice for them and say, aha, this is it!

To help in that choice, a set of objective criteria with an always-present subjective component are used to arrive at potential matches for clients. The objective criteria used were basically the same for both the new and old directors of HOME with reasons for homesharing, individual interests, and personal habits such as smoking and drinking being considered. These profiles are now filled out by each volunteer interviewer after the interview and carried with them on future interviews. On occasion, a match can be suggested on the spot. More likely, this occurs back in the office. Currently, the director and her staff meet to discuss potential matches, so that personal judgments about potential matches can be used to complement the more formal information from the application schedule.

Useful in producing these personal judgments among the interviewers are questions from the application form that do more than provide information. As the second director pointed out:

> As I am talking with them and reading the application I look at what they need and are willing to accept and how much I can vary from that. I ask them what they would really like ideally and then, if appropriate, tell them so and if not, temper my response. If I do the interviewing I use it as an educational tool to point out expectations that can't be matched and need to be compromised. I try to determine how frail a person is, whether they are optimistic or pessimistic, guarded or scared and how the person approaches life. The questions asked are good because they alert people to some things they will have to deal with.

Thus, the application process, besides collecting information, provides more subjective but no less valuable information for both applicant and interviewer: It becomes a basis for educating the applicant, for discussing the whole process of homesharing with the prospective client, and for rendering a judgment about the likely compatibility of potential homesharers in staff meetings during which "matchmaking" discussions occur.

In many respects, therefore, the agency has become an important agent of resocialization for its diverse set of clients. Before involving themselves in homesharing, many clients need to consider issues they might never have thought about before, like sharing a telephone, bathroom, or kitchen with a stranger. The more the clients know about sharing and a potential sharer ahead of time, the better prepared they will be to find a suitable housemate and make their shared living arrangement successful. Problems arising in matches when such anticipatory socialization was not present are discussed in chapter 7.

*The Introduction.* During the early phases of Project Home, the director would make a paper match and then provide both the homeseeker and homeowner with basic information about each other. This would include the telephone number. However, the director soon found out that most applicants were not calling each other and arranging to get together. Thus, if a meeting was to take place, the coordinator would have to make the first introduction. Normally this first meeting was at the place of the homeowner. The potential sharer was usually driven to the site by the director, which permitted some informal preparation time before and debriefing after the introduction. During most of these introductions it was possible to separate out those matches that had no chance of working (about one third) from those in which there was common ground and the clients related well to each other. All clients were told not to make a decision to move in right away. More often than not they would simply say after a few days that they were not very interested. This led the director to conclude that many people new to the homesharing concept were just shopping around. In the early stages the seeker accounted for most of the rejections. Reasons such as "homeowner too disabled," "too far from school," "home in need of repair," or "no room for tenant's furniture" were given by some who turned down matches.

During the middle of the second year of the program, it became apparent to the director and her volunteer staff that the introduction process needed modification to facilitate clients' thinking about what they wanted from homesharing and to facilitate the actual introductions. Two changes were attempted; the first worked, the second did not. The first had to do with the greater choices for homesharers now available because of the increased pool of applicants and the more or less equal numbers of seeker and homeowner applicants in the active pool. To capitalize on the larger number of prospective sharers, the director began to continue the education process started during the application interview by giving descriptions of potential sharers to applicants she was trying to match and by encouraging the applicants to talk over issues *before* committing themselves.

> I give them a thumbnail sketch about the people available and ask them to choose whom they would like to meet. I then call up those people and give them a run down of the type of person I'm working for at that moment and if they are interested I arrange an introduction. They are encouraged to talk

about where they can complement each other. I try to bring up sticky subjects I think will be a problem and put them on the table in advance and see how they respond. I ask them to think about it overnight before they make plans and then to get back to me. I let them know a trial would be ideal. They rarely take me up on that. Everyone wants a nice quick solution. They think if they can move in all their problems will vanish. Somehow the other person will change to just what they want them to be. It's just like marriage.

While no applicant could be *forced* to follow the director's instructions about thinking through what they really wanted and about attempting a trial run, nevertheless the director and her staff had made an important organizational decision to put the responsibility for matches squarely on the shoulders of the applicants themselves while indicating that HOME was ready to help in any way it could.

Also during the middle of the second year, the staff attempted to find a way to facilitate the actual meeting of prospective sharers. At the time, sharers met in the homeowner's residence. According to the director, "Often when we would take a seeker to a person's home all they would look at is the living space instead of the person. We would end up interviewing the house instead of the person." To provide a site at which both applicants could meet on equal terms, the director applied for and received a small city grant that permitted a first introduction between potential sharers at a neutral luncheon site. This would not work for those few homeowners who were homebound, but for others it would stress the importance of the person rather than the living space. The experiment lasted only a brief time, however, as the director and her staff found that the applicants, especially the homeowners, were quite uncomfortable even at the neutral site, so that the presumed advantage gained from an introductory luncheon was, in fact, not realized.

## After the Match

The most "successful" matches have appeared to be among healthy elders or those with small infirmities and students or mid-life persons. The second director points out that "The difficult part of homesharing is when you have a very needy person who, because of isolation, over-whelms another person." Thus one distinction between homeowners and seekers that makes matching more difficult is that of space sharing versus life sharing. Says the director:

It's people who have homes who want to do life sharing with strings. They want to control the life sharing. And the people looking for housing want just space sharing but are willing to life share if that is the cost. But they may be reluctant.

Yet another major impediment to the realization of workable matches has been the unrealistic attitude of clients toward their prospective homesharers and living arrangements. Even if both sharers wanted life sharing, the expectations of each client were often at odds with one another and with what was possible, just as one finds in the early stages of many marriages.

During the process involving the application, staff discussions about potential matches, and the arrangement of introductions between prospective sharers, the director and her staff have attempted to sensitize clients to the realities of strangers sharing space (and sometimes lives). Still, many clients refused to think through problems likely to crop up or to try trial-period matches, so that the director and her staff considered additional modifications in the matchmaking process that would occur after a decision had been made by clients to homeshare.

One suggestion was to have participants in a match sign a "live-in agreement" sheet. Such a formal agreement would encourage people to make an initial commitment to stay together for at least several days so that an immediate rupture would not leave someone without time to find new living arrangements or partners. The agreement hopefully also would create a more businesslike atmosphere that might lessen the likelihood of dishonesty. For example, a smoker might be less likely to lie about a smoking habit if he or she knew there would be a commitment to homesharing for a period of time. While possibly quite useful, the live-in agreement was presented only as an option to potential sharers. Unfortunately, during the early years of the program few availed themselves of this useful device.

Another suggestion was to have a volunteer counselor visit a match shortly after it had begun to help clarify arrangements and articulate problems and solutions. The director found that in many cases "people are so anxious to get matched that they put off real discussion of arrangements" until later. In fact, volunteer interviewers and the director have from time to time been called in to help mediate problems, but there has been no organizational initiative to provide for such follow-up counseling *as a matter of course.*

What has happened, therefore, is that clients have taken the initiative in continuing contact between Project HOME and its clients. Increasingly, as the number of matches grew, the director had to devote more of her time to such postmatch counseling.

> About 90% come to you after matches have been made for help: When it has reached a crisis point and where they realize what they thought they wanted and what they got was not really what they wanted. They call me and say they don't want them to leave and they like the person but don't like what is happening and want to do something about it.

Very often the problems stemmed from misunderstandings between the sharers, which were exacerbated by the couple's inability to communicate with each other. In one instance, the homeowner wanted to be nice to the new sharer but felt the partner smoked too much and asked the director to convey that message. In another case, one member of the match was disappointed that the other didn't attend her birthday party, while the other member was upset because the first felt it was inappropriate to share a bottle of ketchup.

Thus, at first the director found herself being asked to mediate by relaying a message from one sharer to the other. During this process there was the danger of her being manipulated and appearing to be taking sides. As a result, the director instead told both sharers to sit down and discuss the problems they were having together. She argued that they should discuss options and "understand this is a natural part of a relationship. Sometimes they fight and decide to leave and then call me and give me an earful. I've had a lot of earful conversations lately." Nevertheless, the second director accepted this added responsibility for the well-being of the match and emphasized the strength of Project HOME in this respect:

> This is part of the ministry. It is not a professional placement agency. That is its strength. If they want anonymity they can go to a job service and hire a paid companion.

With increasing numbers of matches the director and her staff of volunteers have had to ask themselves what services they are capable of and should be delivering during the process of matching. They also have had to ask themselves whether there are any limits in their responsibilities to those matches already in progress. They are no longer simply providing phone numbers to potential clients as was the case in the very early stages of the program. The director's and volunteers' roles steadily expanded through increased responsibility for providing choices to applicants, for introducing the clients to each other, for ensuring some limited period of sharing, and for engaging in postmatch counseling. Interestingly, the director of RSVP had warned that it was important

> not to foster dependence. People must be educated to solve their own problems and not see us as solving problems for them. That is a trap that could be fallen into by the project. The important thing is to give responsibility to the participants and not allow us to become parent figures.

Thus far, the strategic answer given by all of the directors in their turn and by their volunteer staff has been relatively consistent: Project HOME is in existence to provide a homesharing service to its clients. The service means that the program goes beyond giving applicants telephone numbers to call and names to contact, but it also stops short of telling clients how to run their lives. While specific cases might muddy the waters somewhat, the overall strategy is based on the program's desire to be a caring service that helps but does not direct its clients.

The third director and her staff have dealt with the potential and real problems of postmatch crises in much the same way as her predecessor: They emphasize the realities of homesharing to clients when they first appear as applicants, when they are given the names of potential sharers to meet, and when sharers contact the office for help in conflicts between sharers. Specific means include giving matched applicants a sheet that discusses various stages of a relationship and what the clients can expect in the future.

To help forestall unexpected sharer conflicts, the third director began to emphasize the importance of the live-in agreement discussed above. In all cases, she and her staff now tell prospective sharers that reading and signing the agreement is required—whether the planned arrangement is one involving traditional sharing or caregiving services. Only rarely do the parties refuse to sign, and even if they do the HOME staff continues to help them (see appendix 1 for the current traditional and caregiving live-in agreements).

Another major change, discussed during the second director's tenure and finally implemented during the third director's term, is the implementation of a fee for service to both homeowner and homeseeker. The amount is nominal,[4] but broadcasts a clear signal that Project HOME indeed is offering a service beyond sharing telephone numbers and names with clients. From initial application through introductions to (if needed) postmatch counseling, the director and her volunteers attempt to balance the need for clients to be independent and make decisions on their own with the need for help in exploring all of the realistic options that exist concerning current and prospective living arrangements.

Finally, the HOME staff now have a nonliability agreement that all applicants are asked to sign (see appendix 1). Project HOME has never had to face any legal problems initiated by disgruntled sharers, but the director and her staff believe that the nonliability agreement provides both protection for the program and useful insights to applicants concerning the realities of homesharing.

Starting off as a program to give older volunteers a meaningful service experience and to help older homeowners find home sharers, Project HOME has blossomed from a very small experimental project housed in the Retired Senior Volunteer Program and focused exclusively on elders to an independent United Way agency with a cooperative arrangement of paid staff and senior volunteers who arrange a wide variety of home-sharing matches serving young and old alike. From a tentative beginning in its first year, during which fewer than a hundred applications were made and only four matches were realized, to a fifth year in which nearly three hundred applications were processed and nearly one hundred matches made, Project HOME has been an excellent case study of how a service organization grows while still retaining its initial mission.

The evolution of the program and of the match-making process in which it is engaged have been described in this chapter, but the meaning of the changes noted require a more detailed examination. Such analysis will be the focal point of the next two chapters. Chapter 3 will take a closer look at the evolving roles of the program's volunteers who made key contributions during HOME's early years. Chapter 4 will focus on the interpersonal dynamics that characterized Project HOME during its first five years and that help to explain the program's growth and success. Later, chapter 10 will evaluate the program's service delivery during its first five years and update its operation under the third director.

# 3

# Staffing Project HOME: The Significance of a Core of Executive Volunteers

As described in chapter 2, the development of Project HOME as a subunit of the larger Retired Senior Volunteer Program meant that a critical emphasis at the outset was the creation of a number of unique and meaningful assignments for a small number of older volunteers who, after a transition period overseen by a part-time director, would staff this small special project entirely on their own; that is, eventually, the volunteers would advertise, recruit, match, and administer the program without assistance from paid staff. This was a particularly good project for older volunteers, according to the RSVP director, because they "could understand the needs of homeowners and sharers to a greater degree than younger persons and thus would become effective advocates for the clients."

The volunteers themselves would be in the unique position of being *both* the recipients and the providers of services connected with HOME. To the extent that they collected and processed information necessary to match applicants for homesharing, they would be fulfilling the role of service provider. However, from the perspective of the RSVP director, their participation in this project would need to be a personally meaningful assignment. Thus, only when both the instrumental and the expressive components of the volunteers' role were present would the director's expectations for the volunteers be fully met.

As will be shown in this chapter, the role of volunteer evolved in substantial and unexpected ways that, nevertheless, were consistent with the RSVP director's initial expectations that HOME volunteers have meaningful assignments. Several years' close observation of Project HOME, in fact, suggests three different kinds of roles for volunteers since the program began. This chapter will focus on the first two: interviewers and clerks during the program's first two years and executive managers during the next three years of rapid expansion of HOME services. Chapter 10 will describe the way in which volunteers have been utilized most recently as case managers and advisory council members since the current director took over.

## INITIAL VOLUNTEER ROLES

*Early Program Stresses*

During the first six months when a staff person from the Retired Senior Volunteer Program was temporarily assigned to this project on a part-time basis to help organize and support the volunteer efforts, it became clear that much more effort and coordination would be necessary to sustain this program than was originally anticipated. Indeed, as outlined in chapter 2, eventually the growth of the program necessitated the hiring of a full-time staff person. She, in turn established Project HOME as a separate unit independent of the parent Retired Senior Volunteer Program, and, over a period of several years, the director and then her successor hired several part-time paid staff persons.

However, even with the growing centrality of the director's and (later) other staff positions, the original significance of the volunteer role did not diminish. In fact it increased at about the same time that the first full-time director began to establish Project HOME as an independent program. The parent organization could no longer assume the resource costs of a rapidly expanding service that clearly was responding to a major community need.

At this time of program expansion and independence the director's responsibilities increased substantially. Fortunately, she also had working with her a small dedicated core of volunteers who were willing to assume more of this responsibility along with her. Moreover, other volunteer personnel would also be attracted to this program including university student interns and the university researchers as consultants, evaluators, and eventually as members of the Board of Directors.

*The Expanding Role of the Volunteer*

Most of the thirteen volunteers originally recruited to serve with Project HOME only interviewed applicants for a potential match. They had a very limited role when it came to actually facilitating matches or participating in broad policy-making decisions. However, within this group of thirteen volunteers, several members expressed an interest in volunteering in an expanded way and on a more regular basis.

Evidence of the volunteers' interest concerning sustained versus sporadic involvement and expanded versus limited tasks was clearly given through their responses to questions asked by the university researchers. These questions were part of a set of open-ended interviews conducted with all the volunteers shortly after the first full-time director assumed responsibility for the program but before the program separated from the Retired Senior Volunteer Program.

The interview was designed to acquire information about the backgrounds of the volunteers as well as their preferences, satisfactions, and dissatisfactions with the program. All thirteen of the original volunteers were interviewed, in most cases in their own homes. One year after the completion of these interviews five "core" or "executive" volunteers were reinterviewed somewhat more informally. The follow-up interview was shorter and focused on their evaluation of changes in the program during the past year including their expanded role.

These volunteers, for the most part, were recently retired and had not formed new friendships and relationships outside the working environment. According to the director of Project HOME, "they indicated to me they didn't want to stay home twiddling their thumbs."

A contributing factor in their participation was the confidence the director had in the capabilities and commitment of the volunteers, which was matched only by the confidence the volunteers had in their own capabilities and commitment. They wanted to engage in activities beyond simply interviewing applicants.

In the survey of the thirteen original volunteers, more than half stated they would be willing to engage in activities besides interviewing applicants. The most popular choices were reinterviewing former applicants and working in the home office with the director. Slightly less popular were the tasks of matching people and making introductions between potential homesharers. It should be stressed that more than half the volunteers were willing to engage in *any* of the four additional activities offered to them.

In an evaluation of the importance of eight different facets of their volunteer assignment, "learning new things" was the one characteristic that all volunteers originally assigned to Project HOME believed to be "very important." All the volunteers wanted to continue to grow by increasing their learning experiences. Many of the volunteers were former teachers. Satisfaction with "helping others," "remaining active" and the presence of "flexible hours" of work were also important to a majority of the volunteers. Simply "making time pass" and "recognition for service" were less important for most of them.

Concerning commitment to the program, several responses to questions about their feelings toward their assignment suggest the willingness of the volunteers to remain with the program for relatively long intervals. Ten of the thirteen volunteers answering the question said that if the opportunity should arise they would like to work more closely with the director in the home office. Although most volunteers were satisfied with their present commitment, five of thirteen volunteers said they would like to work more hours than at present on HOME. These five volunteers were to become very important not only in providing significant assistance for the director but also in establishing and defining a new kind of volunteer position with a far greater amount of responsibility than is normally assumed by older volunteers.

## Symbiosis Between the Director and the Volunteers

The relationship between the director and the volunteers was crucial in the early success of a then fledgling program trying to establish its own unique identity in a community with a large number of services for the elderly already in place. There was very limited financial support and what little was available was of temporary duration. Fund-raising would be an immediate and pressing problem for the director, necessitating the delegation of much day-to-day responsibility to the volunteers. Working alongside the director, they appeared to accept their new responsibilities enthusiastically.

The director actively supported the volunteers by providing encouragement and also by seeking their advice. In turn she was rewarded by their loyalty and involvement. When asked on a three-response scale how helpful the director had been for them, eleven of the volunteers said "very helpful," while the remaining two said "somewhat helpful."

What seemed most important to the volunteers with regard to their relationship with the director was the amount of social interaction they had with her. Asked to discuss why they felt the director was or was not helpful to them, they said the following:

> She provides good explanations and training and takes a lot of care in helping the volunteers.
>
> S [the director] sends me the interview sheets and then talks to me when I take the interview forms to the office. I like to talk to her and she comes to talk to me.
>
> She is supportive, doesn't get defensive, is understanding, calm, enthusiastic and open to new ideas and listens.
>
> We have meetings to share what is going on; we have choices; she is easy to talk with.

The volunteers clearly enjoyed their involvement in Project HOME. And the director through her utilization and recognition of their talents was able to elicit considerable commitment and loyalty.

It was fortunate that at a time when the additional responsibility for establishing an independent agency fell on the shoulders of the director, she had a core of highly motivated enthusiastic volunteers to call on for assistance. Several other volunteers were willing to provide occasional service, mostly interviewing. According to the director:

> I experimented with the volunteers taking calls, writing news releases and doing the legwork for brochures and posters. They also indicated to me they wanted to become more involved in the matching process. They started monthly meetings and then the volunteers decided they wanted to meet more often and came up with the idea of the weekly staff meeting. It was their idea. They got together in teams on their own to put together bulletin boards and brochures. They would invite me to their meetings and I would say this is what I'm stuck on and they would volunteer to do them. It was an interactive process. Instead of me being the assigner they would say we notice these problems and what can we do about them. They increased their time in the office, did more seeker interviews. They also started doing introductions and matches and follow-ups. The only thing they didn't do was write grants.

The director's perception that the meetings performed both socioemotional and task-oriented functions was echoed by the volunteers. The meetings served to provide a time during which important information would be exchanged and during which the volunteers and director would be brought together as a cohesive unit. In the words of one volunteer, the weekly staff meetings were ways to

> come together and provide support for each other. We were all out there doing our own Project HOME thing and nobody knew what anybody else was doing.

With the meeting we didn't have to go through the director to make a match. It was also a good way to come together to find out what publicity was needed.

The weekly meeting also responded to a need of the volunteers to find out what had happened to the persons they had previously interviewed. Said one, "I would interview someone and give them some hope and it seemed to me we should get back to the people in a period of time." Another replied that previously "we had no sense of what was happening to these people." The result of these staff meetings was a greater sense of involvement. As one volunteer stated, "I guess I feel more a sense of responsibility because we meet once a week and talk about the needs of the people. We get input and feedback and I feel more responsibility and part of the program."

## Getting and Holding Human Service Volunteers

Empirical evidence on the ability of human service agencies to recruit and retain volunteer workers suggest that, from the beginning, Project HOME has been in an ideal position to do both. For instance, word of mouth is by far the most popular means by which volunteers are attracted to such organizations (Watts and Edwards 1983:13). Project HOME's early affiliation with RSVP assured both a starting pool of volunteers during the program's early period and an ongoing pipeline between current RSVP volunteers in Project HOME and RSVP volunteers who might be interested in volunteering for Project HOME. In addition, Project HOME's volunteers were themselves volunteering in other organizations as well and therefore had even more contacts to tell about Project HOME.

With respect to retaining volunteers, the most popular strategies employed by service agencies are "training, flexible scheduling, and increasing responsibility" (Watts and Edwards 1983:15). Certainly these strategies were present for Project HOME. From the early interviewer training by the university researchers to the mutual learning process that characterized the weekly meetings, the HOME volunteers were being provided training in new skills. This was welcome to volunteers who were reporting that they valued "learning new things" and wanted to continue to grow through new experiences and activities. Such motivation is consistent with the fact that many of these volunteers were former teachers who did not view retirement as a signal to stop learning and trying new experiences on.

Flexible scheduling was also provided, despite the fact that the program had no paid staff assistant to coordinate program activities during its early years. At the beginning of the program, flexibility of schedule meant the freedom to be "on call" and do intake interviews only when and where one was able to interview. During this period, the only problem of scheduling occurred when the director and university researchers attempted to get everyone—themselves and volunteers—together at the same time for the interviewer training sessions; this generally was a manageable problem. Otherwise, the volunteers made their own schedules.

During the later period in which the program was being run by the director and her small staff of "regular" volunteers (about whom more will be said in the next section), scheduling became a serious problem. This occurred because, as the program became more widely known and received increasing numbers of inquiries, the director needed continuous "staff" monitoring of the telephones. There were no paid staff, however; there were only herself and volunteers who had vacation plans, family and friendship ties, and other volunteering commitments. Balancing program needs and volunteer freedom became a difficult process, but the volunteers maintained their flexibility of scheduling to a large degree—even during these times of problematic scheduling.

Finally, as shown above, as the director's responsibilities became more diffuse, she began to shift some of the case management work to her (willing) volunteers, so that even early in the program the volunteers were given assignments involving important responsibilities. This strategy is best seen in the relationship between the director and her small core of volunteers who will be discussed in the next section and highlighted in chapter 4.

Closely related to these strategies of retaining volunteers in service agencies are three benefits the volunteers received through their work in Project HOME. If one considers the strategies as causes, then these benefits may be seen as effects. Stemming primarily from the training and increased responsibility they received, the three benefits are: camaraderie, a sense of continuity with one's earlier (work) life, and a feeling of significant accomplishment.

The benefit of camaraderie was clear to any observer present at the interviewer training sessions conducted for the volunteers. While the training itself was rather unremarkable, it was clear both before and after the sessions especially that the volunteer interviewers really appeared to enjoy one another's company, socializing and trading interviewer experiences. This benefit occurred from the beginning of the program and has continued to be a significant attraction of Project HOME for its volunteers.

The sense of continuity was seen early on for many volunteers as they were trained to conduct intake interviews. As seen above, however, the professional training and work experiences that many volunteers had meant that some Project HOME volunteers were constantly wanting to do even more. In general, many of the tasks (e.g., case management, file organization, media advertising) undertaken by volunteers during the second and third years were related to jobs and interests the volunteers had held before volunteering for Project HOME.

The third benefit, a feeling of significant accomplishment, was not immediately evident, although "helping others" was an important motivating force for volunteering at Project HOME among the original volunteers. While it is true that they were interested in the welfare of the applicants they were interviewing, there did not appear to develop among the volunteers the sense of accomplishment originally anticipated by the RSVP staff and the volunteers themselves.

Several reasons suggest themselves: First, of course, early in its existence Project HOME was hardly matching anyone because of the restrictions placed on sharer possibilities emanating from an elders-only applicant pool. Therefore, the main cause for celebration (i.e., matching applicants) occurred only rarely. When clients were matched, the sense of excitement among all concerned—RSVP director, HOME director, volunteer interviewers, and even us, the researchers—was very great, highlighting even more the large numbers of clients for whom matches were not forthcoming.

Closely related to the lack of match-making in the first year of the program was the problem of volunteer alienation from the whole matchmaking process. If one considers alienation as arising from a separation between oneself and the total work picture, somewhat like the way traditional assembly line workers have participated in only one small part of the whole production process, then it is easy to see that the volunteers' initial role in Project HOME's matchmaking was limited to their taking inquiries from, interviewing, and making recommendations regarding the potential suitability of the applicants with whom they personally have had contact.

More than once at interviewer training sessions during the first two years of the program the researchers were asked by volunteers, "Whatever happened to 'so and so'? I know she's not been matched, but she is a dear and really needs a sharer." Because the researchers were conducting follow-up interviews of applicants at the time,[1] they often could supply information to the volunteers, but the whole feedback process was rather hit or miss. Thus, initially, volunteers, instead of feeling a sense of accomplishment from their interviewer roles, were frustrated because so few clients were being matched and because they were getting little feedback on those who were not getting matched and in whom the interviewers had developed a proprietary interest.

Finally, although the camaraderie mentioned above was important, the interviewers rarely met as a group, since their work (especially during the first year) basically involved only interviewing clients. Therefore, except for the few interviewer training sessions conducted by the researchers, the volunteers usually were in contact with the office only by phone to receive the name and address of a client to interview.

Key to overcoming these difficulties was the expansion of volunteer commitment to clients. An important distinction evolving early in the program was between the occasional interviewer who was not particularly committed to HOME and the (almost) day-in-day-out worker who was taking an active interest in the welfare of the clients she was interviewing and in the general health of the program. The second director found it advantageous to recruit individuals who would provide a more ongoing commitment than the occasional volunteer who was contacted to do an intake interview because a client happened to come from her hometown or neighborhood. As she relates, "Originally volunteers were recruited with the idea they would provide sporadic service and not ongoing type services. Now we are asking them to do something else."

Opening up new tasks also provided opportunities for volunteers with different kinds of skills. Some would continue as sporadic interviewers. Others would work on a more regular basis—perhaps one day a week in the office taking phone calls, sending out packets and arranging interviews. A third assignment would be to work with homesharers in planning the financial aspects of their arrangements, since, in the words of the director, "Most people don't do detailed planning of this before they decide to live together. They are in too much of a hurry to get a match." A fourth task, that of publicizing the program, fell to one volunteer in particular who had previously worked professionally as a media consultant.

Finally, some volunteers would work with the researchers doing follow-up interviews. The advantage for the volunteers is that they would see that many who were not matched did survive without Project HOME and had either improved in personal health or had found some other housing solution. Project HOME was just one choice among a variety of solutions and was not necessarily for everyone who originally applied. In other cases the volunteers would rediscover people from an early pool of applicants, who still needed help but, perhaps because of initial problems in developing the HOME pool of applicants, had been overlooked. Their case could now be reopened. This was the beginning of what was to become an ongoing recognition of the need to develop some kind of systematic case management process for unmatched clients (and later for matched clients as well).

Remaining salient among volunteer tasks, of course, was the intake interview. The director and her volunteer staff agreed that certain modifications in the process would facilitate their ability to match applicants. Now, interviewers would fill out a short sheet detailing the major characteristics of each applicant interviewed. Each interviewer would have access to short profiles of previous interviews they and other interviewers had filled out, so they could recommend matches, in some cases, on the spot. The unique personality information one picks up while administering an interview could then be used directly to help determine compatible matches, since references would have been contacted before the interview. Having an expanded role, the volunteers would be able to see how the intake interview fit into the whole matchmaking process. The dual benefit would be a richer and more meaningful volunteer assignment plus a lessened work load for the director so she would be free for other administrative tasks such as fund-raising and, with the help of volunteer staff, publicity.

While the specific time when volunteer participation beyond interviewing became significant cannot be pinpointed, the key processes preceding this transition period are clear enough. As the program's status continued to be threatened by possible lack of funding, the director's position became threatened because of the constant simultaneous demands of client needs and organizational (especially money) needs. Without any other paid staff support, her choices were to cut back on client services, cut back on funding efforts, or shift more responsibility of service delivery to her volunteers. With the important cooperation of a

small number of willing and able volunteers, she chose the third alternative, which resulted in the evolution of a rather unique kind of service
agency worker: the executive volunteer.[2]

# THE EXECUTIVE VOLUNTEERS

## The Range of Volunteer Activities

An important thesis of this chapter is that Project HOME's small
number of core volunteers represent a relatively new, exciting direction
in the use of volunteers, especially in service organization roles. Not too
long ago, when one mentioned the word "volunteer" in a service context, the image springing to mind would be that of the "candy striper" in
the hospital or the clerical helper stuffing envelopes and answering the
phone on a sporadic basis. Indeed, these are useful services, but they by
no means suggest the range of volunteer activities undertaken.

The Retired Senior Volunteer Program in general has done much to
ensure that volunteer work undertaken by its armies of elders be meaningful to both the organizations and individuals being served by the
volunteers *and* to the volunteers themselves. Indeed, evidence has been
mounting rapidly to show that individuals of almost all ages and interests
can be enlisted to volunteer their energies in a wide variety of tasks,
many of which require learning particular skills.

Probably the most instructive suggestions as to the many kinds of tasks
for which volunteers can be trained come from the health promotion
area. Here, whether it be promoting breast self-examination (Dorwaldt
et al. 1988), doing blood pressure screening (Elder et al. 1986), or
counseling in a hypertension control program (Caraway and Van Gilder
1985), nonprofessionals of almost all ages have been to shown to be
effective learners and workers in a volunteer context requiring some
specialized skills and training. Among elders, interviewing (Havir 1986;
Seguin 1984), oral presentations to outsiders (Houghland et al. 1988),
and peer counseling (Seguin 1984) are examples of skills that volunteers
have performed well.

Less well-known is information on volunteers who, beyond the learning of specialized skills, are asked to perform managerial tasks requiring
the full range of decision-making skills one would normally associate
with paid executives. The only relevant information on such volunteers
comes from two areas: One is with respect to volunteers sitting on boards
of directors of various agencies (Conrad 1983; Miller et al. 1988; see also

the entire October-December 1985 issue of the *Journal of Voluntary Action Research*).

Boards at worst may be rubber stamps who ignorantly support or who, with equal ignorance, represent intractable obstructions to enterprising agency heads. At best, however, volunteer boards of directors may provide useful sounding boards for agency staff and at the same time relieve staff of problematic organizational duties (e.g., fund-raising). Chapter 10 will address the specific roles that Project HOME's advisory council has played since it was formed. For now, it is important only to point out that, while volunteers on boards of directors may exhibit executive skills, their commitment to the organization which they help oversee is rather sporadic, especially if they belong (as many do) to other boards of directors as well.

A second source of information comes from the managerial skills exhibited by volunteers in established and stable settings. In the provision of community-based health promotion programs, volunteers are asked to serve in a variety of roles, including those requiring planning and decision making (DePue et al. 1987). More directly relevant to the Project HOME experience, senior volunteers have been found to be effective participants in needs assessment research and service planning (Weil 1984) and as Andrus Volunteers who initiate research projects and design educational programs (Seguin 1984).

Nevertheless, even though previous research provides some insight into the importance such volunteers can have for the agencies or programs with which they are affiliated, the Project HOME case appears to be unique in that its volunteers have played a documented *active, decision-making role* in the evolution of a service. Project HOME volunteers have been given considerable authority and responsibility in the areas of policy evaluation and direction, resulting in a new kind of volunteer role during the program's rapid growth.

## Evolution of the Executive Volunteers

From the original pool of thirteen volunteers the core group of less than half that number became an important source of support for the director. Although the other volunteers continued on for a short time in their former role as interviewer, it was the commitment of her five "executive volunteers," as the director labeled them, that allowed Project HOME to prosper and grow in new directions.[3]

Further questioning of the director revealed the appropriateness of the label for this relatively unique kind of volunteer position. The "executive volunteer" can be described as a person involved in assignments characterized by the qualities of managerial responsibility, task meaningfulness, social integration, and a significant commitment of time.

With regard to the first "quality," the dictionary definition of the "executive" is a person who "controls or directs an organization" or "one who holds a position of administrative or managerial responsibility." The executive volunteer must exercise control over her work situation as well as participate in important policy decisions that impact on the whole organization or a significant part of that organization.

At the task level she must feel responsible for a large part of the product or service being processed. She will see her assigned tasks as meaningful only insofar as she clearly understands the importance of her particular assignment in the whole process. Even greater satisfaction is likely to follow from extensive participation in all or many of the tasks contributing to the final product or service.

The executive volunteer also takes pride in being a member of what she considers to be a special organization. There is a feeling of belonging to a cohesive work community where the organizational goals are understood and accepted and its members receive encouragement and support from each other.

Finally, there is the presumption that such volunteer involvement will require a fairly extensive and continuous commitment of time and energy. Although a full-time commitment would probably be undesirable for most volunteers, major responsibilities for administration and policy decision making will necessitate a fairly continuous and regular volunteer service pattern.

## Advantages of an Executive Volunteer Staff

With regard to Project HOME, the core volunteers are able to make an "executive" contribution because of the resources, talents, and skills they bring to their assignments. The five volunteers are resource-rich and do not have to expend time and energy on ordinary survival needs. All are in their sixties, have annual incomes above $15,000 and are satisfied with their present financial situation. They overwhelmingly describe their health as better than average and report they never have trouble getting around from place to place. Only one volunteer is married. All own their own home and all have at least some college education with several having advanced college degrees. All have had a long work-life history often spent in teaching or in administrative or managerial positions. All the volunteers feel that skills learned in their previous jobs are useful to them in their present volunteer assignments.

With these considerable resources and skills to draw upon, the volunteers are able to realize most of the major qualities that compose the executive volunteer role. The weekly staff meetings at which policy decisions are made *with* the director gives the volunteers opportunities to provide input at the organizational level. This direct involvement by volunteers in decision making is also appreciated by the director, for she appears to depend on them as much as they depend on her. She states:

> The volunteers are my direct feedback. I get as much satisfaction out of working with them as they get working with me. Believe me that is very mutual. They bring their own perspectives to the planning sessions just as I bring mine.

When asked whether it might not be easier simply to work with paid staff, particularly since the program was expanding so rapidly, the director said she hoped to recruit several more volunteers instead. Even one other staff member, no matter how committed, could not replace the energy and ideas that emanated from this larger group of executive volunteers. What perhaps was lost in time given to coordinating the efforts of five different people each averaging five to ten hours of service a week was more than made up for by the loyalty, enthusiasm, and creative energy these volunteers contributed to the program.

Of greatest importance to the volunteers is the much larger responsibility they have for the cases they interview. In the beginning they simply interviewed a client and their responsibility ended. Now they were involved in case management and the whole process of solving a housing problem for a particular client. The director noted that the volunteers are now often directly linked to their cases rather than being linked through her. When an applicant wants to reactivate her status she often calls the volunteer directly. The volunteers stay in contact with their clients over a long period of time referring them to other agencies when necessary and even acting as their advocate.

When the core volunteers were asked in the reinterview a year later what they found most rewarding about their participation in Project HOME, the qualities of "making a difference," social interaction and organizational integration were recurrent themes:

I guess I feel more a sense of responsibility because we meet once a week and talk about the needs of the individual cases. We get input and feedback and feel more responsible to and part of the program.

Meeting people, both associates and people I interview. Bringing people together who match happily. Hopefully helping people solve their problems.

Meeting people from all walks of life and hoping I can have some input in solving their problems of housing and everyday living. Some are so lonely; some with health and personal problems and many with financial problems.

Meeting people and being a part of P. HOME's growth and development. Providing a service that is needed. I do enjoy the volunteers and staff. They are a special and talented group whose energies can be put to good use as soon as the new directions are defined.

In addition to their greater involvement in case management and the sense of belonging to a cohesive work community, it should be noted how almost every statement of what the volunteers enjoy about Project HOME begins with the phrase "meeting people." There is a very important and valuable social and interaction component that is central to their attraction to Project HOME. This is consistent with the volunteers' work histories, which involved teaching and service experiences, all people-oriented endeavors. As former teachers, several volunteers are comfortable associating with young people. They interact frequently with university student volunteer interns, an experience that both age groups find rewarding. Three volunteers share or have recently shared their homes with young people. This affinity with young people may partially account for the rapid growth in the number of successful intergenerational matches arranged by the volunteers.

Finally, one cannot minimize the importance of the director who has an infectious enthusiasm for the program that energizes her volunteers as much as they energize her. Her willingness to delegate responsibility and assume some of the costs of coordination, which will be discussed next, is an important reason for the success of Project HOME.

## Costs of an Executive Volunteer Staff

There are few costs associated with this kind of volunteer model as reported by both the directors and the volunteers. The one frustration mentioned by the director is that "actions can't keep up with ideas." She defines herself and the volunteers as "idea people" who are frequently frustrated in efforts to secure enough funds to implement the ideas. Since funding is not stable, a considerable portion of the director's time is consumed by grant writing rather than program development. Although the volunteers have no reservations about their own roles, they do wish case management could be made even more comprehensive and systematic. Furthermore, although the volunteers are very committed to Project HOME, there have been some problems of coordination around holidays or vacation periods, during which time the director would have to assume a major share of the daily work load.

The volunteers themselves, with one exception, are all involved with other non-Project HOME activities. These range from volunteer work for the blind, girl scouts, emergency food shelter, library committee, and women helping battered women, to working a twenty-hour week as a paid receptionist. Two of the five volunteers would be interested in paid work if it became available. Although the volunteers have a strong commitment to the program and all say they could give a little more time if requested, there is some doubt as to how much of the work load the volunteers will be willing and able to assume as the program continues to expand.

The second director's answer to the need for more help was to recruit more volunteers both old and young. The current director while still retaining the core volunteers has been slowly expanding her paid staff. Student interns have been able to help out at the office as well as do interviews in rural areas that the older volunteers are reluctant or unable to do. However, student volunteers must be recruited every semester and are very difficult to obtain during the summer break. Thus, the disadvantage of using an all-volunteer staff, even a very dedicated one, is that breaks in service can occur at certain times in the year and the director or her paid assistants must then be ready to assume full responsibility for the daily functioning of the program. The demand for housing services does not necessarily slack off during holiday periods or summer recess.

On the other hand, the director did have sufficient confidence in her volunteer staff to manage the program while she herself took a two-week summer vacation. Although she carefully coordinated the time schedules of the volunteers beforehand so that someone was always available during the regular operating office hours, all decisions about the daily functioning of the program were left in the hands of the volunteer staff.

## Implications

*For Volunteers.* Older volunteers in the next century will be both more numerous and also more selective in the tasks they volunteer for. They will not only have a longer life expectancy than those elders alive today but will be likely to be less disabled, more highly educated and less impoverished. Furthermore, a greater proportion of educated elders will be engaging in or desiring to engage in volunteer service (Harris 1981).

Finally, these elders will likely include a disproportionately large number of women who will have had a more continuous work history and been involved in a wider variety of professional and managerial work roles with accompanying financial benefits than their elderly counterparts today. Such women will require and probably demand a challenging volunteer role in their later lives (see also Kaminer's [1984] observation about the volunteer profile of women now in their thirties and forties who have been inculcated with a prowork and antivolunteer ethic but who nevertheless want both).

With a growing future pool of elders characterized by high education, good health, financial adequacy, and a long history of employment it is important to ask what kinds of volunteer assignments will appeal to this population and whether society will be able to continue to benefit from the services of this important community resource. Studies by the National Council on Aging (Harris 1976, 1981) have found that, although most older people stress the "advantages" of doing volunteer work, a third of older people *agree* with the statement that "most jobs saved for volunteer workers are routine and boring and not very rewarding." An additional quarter are "not sure" whether they agree or disagree with this statement. Furthermore, the higher the incomes of the older persons the more likely are they to agree that most volunteer jobs are routine, boring, and not very rewarding. The executive volunteer positions created by Project HOME respond to this demand for challenging and meaningful assignments.

*For Agencies.* Complementary to the increasing pool of high-ability volunteers are the increasing needs of service agencies which, during these times of fiscal restraint and budget cutbacks, are scrambling to provide adequate services to their clients. Homesharing agencies in particular are finding out how useful volunteer help can be. A recent national survey reports that volunteers outnumber staff members in the shared housing area and, while over half the homesharing agencies have two or fewer paid staff, almost all use volunteers in a wide variety of ways (Shared Housing Resource Center 1988a, 1988b).

For agencies facing financial crises in the course of their development and for agencies just beginning, volunteers can fill important gaps in service provision and overall service development if only they are given the chance. While it is true that many agency professionals fear employing volunteers in any but the most trivial tasks and thus tend to underutilize them (Chambre 1987; Smith 1985), an increasingly popular view is that "Volunteering is about as far away from robots as anyone could imagine. Volunteering is service personified" (Naylor 1985). The experience of Project HOME's executive volunteers is an important practical application of this view.

Project HOME has been an extremely successful and effective program with limited paid staff and a highly dedicated small number of executive volunteers. These resource-rich volunteers brought with them to their volunteer assignments a lifetime history of meaningful work involvements. They have found through Project HOME challenges that draw on previous job-developed skills.

As the population of well-educated lifetime employed women grows in future years it will be increasingly important to provide challenging and meaningful assignments similar to those offered in Project HOME. Not only will such assignments benefit the volunteers, but the needy will gain through the reception of services that they cannot normally afford.

Hopefully experimental and challenging ventures (such as Project HOME) where the outcomes are uncertain will be particularly attractive to executive volunteers. Where funds are scarce and can be invested only in proven programs, the place of the executive volunteer may be crucial to new program development.

The women volunteers of Project HOME represent a mode of service, energy, and productivity that bodes well for society and for future generations of senior citizens. They redress the imbalance of power between young and old through their continued activity with different generations of volunteers and clients and through their continuing use of skills developed in their earlier work life.

The volunteers of Project HOME have demonstrated that older volunteers are capable of channeling a considerable amount of creative energy and assuming a great deal of responsibility. Given the likely larger cohort of well-educated, healthier, and economically better-off elderly in the future, provision of executive volunteer assignments such as the ones described here should result in both significant services to society as well as significant personally meaningful opportunities for the individual volunteers.

# 4

## Organizational Structure, Social Exchange, and Service Delivery

The description in chapter 2 of main actors and important events during Project HOME's first five years suggests that three factors especially contributed to the program's success. The first was the presence of a very flexible organizational structure. The only basic requirement for the program was that it be staffed by older volunteers who would benefit from a meaningful service commitment. Indeed, the goal of placing elders in appropriate homesharing arrangements was an important objective as well, but, as demonstrated in the second chapter, no more important than the provision of a worthwhile experience for the volunteers. Beyond this goal of satisfying volunteers' needs to do useful, fulfilling work, the program was very much left to do as it pleased. This meant that the number of volunteers and of paid staff, their duties, and their relationship with one another and the director were open to change and adjustment.

A second factor contributing to the program's success was the choice of the second director who headed the program during its second through fifth years. In retrospect, it is now clear that Project HOME required the director's role to be an entrepreneurial one that could flourish in an atmosphere of organizational flexibility. In her choice as second director, that is precisely the kind of person the RSVP director hired: a woman with vision, commitment to service, and enthusiasm for her work—in short, a person who would exploit the organization's flexible working arrangements. As a bonus, the new director brought to the program an unusually strong belief in cooperative decision making and a willingness to delegate important tasks to unpaid volunteers.

Together, the organization's structure and the personality of its second director gave rise to a third factor affecting the organization's growth and ultimate success: the principle of bartering or social exchange. Not only were clients expected to barter as they negotiated shared living arrangements with one another, but, because of its workability as an organizational principle, social exchange was the currency by which things got done within the program. This exchange involved relations between the director and her volunteer staff, between the director and the university researchers, and between the volunteer staff and the researchers.

This chapter will demonstrate how organizational flexibility, the director's personality, and social exchange affected and indeed directed the development of Project HOME during its critical first years. The first section will examine how organizational structure and the director's role affected service delivery, first by detailing the way Project HOME was organized, and second by showing how as a result service delivery improved. The second section will explain how the concept of social exchange united and motivated the organization's key actors in their mutual goal of service delivery.

# AN ENTREPRENEURIAL MODEL OF HOMESHARING SERVICE

## Social Structure and Personality

First it is important to realize how the initial structuring of Project HOME played a major role in affecting the expansion of the program's services. Two aspects of the program's initial structuring are critical in this regard: First, the volunteers, being recipients as well as givers of service, were put in positions that would give them "meaningful" experiences (i.e., interviewing) as opposed to simple clerical tasks. Second, each director in turn was given great latitude in running the program because of the RSVP director's many other, more direct concerns.

As a result of this very fluid organizational structure, the possibilities for redefining means and even ends were rather substantial. In the case of the first director (who served for only about half a year), this did not result in any significant alterations in how the program sought out, screened or attempted to match clients. Throughout the first year of its operation, Project HOME was following its mandate: On the one hand, it was providing meaningful experiences to its volunteers by having them interview homesharing applicants. On the other hand, it was attempting to provide a homesharing service to match elders with one another. In each case, it was having only limited success.

After the second director arrived at the beginning of the program's second year, it became apparent quickly that she was willing to experiment in an effort to improve the program's service delivery. In order to understand how her willingness to experiment became translated into productive action, it is necessary to examine salient characteristics of her personality. The most important of these were her commitment to service for elders and others in need, her entrepreneurial orientation, and her willingness to compromise and learn from others.

Her background as a chaplain and her later decision to enter Divinity School correctly suggest a strongly religious orientation in the director's personal makeup. Her religiosity, however, manifested itself in quite nondenominational terms. Thus, Project HOME for the director was a program with a "mission" (her word) to serve elders, disabled, and others who had serious housing needs. As a result, it was quite natural for the director to open up the client pool to nonelders shortly after she became director. Her basic commitment to service precluded her putting arbitrary limits on the recipients of that service, so a variety of clients were taken on as potential homesharers; and, for those who were inappropriately looking for homesharers (e.g., frail elders with no resources and serious physical or mental disabilities, renters wanting to use the program as an apartment-finding service), she expanded Project HOME's service to include referrals to other local agencies.[1]

Not surprisingly, the director of Project HOME was also an entrepreneur. Students of social organization draw distinctions between entrepreneurial and managerial styles of organizational leadership. The former is based on the assumption that significant changes are needed or desirable in the organization; an entrepreneurial leader will innovate to get them accomplished. The latter, on the other hand, is based on the premise that leadership is required that will maintain the organization in pretty much its present form; a managerial leader will preserve what already exists.

In the early days of Project HOME, of course, organizational norms concerning who the clientele were and how they were to be contacted, screened, and matched were, at best, loosely laid out. The organization basically was making up the rules as it went along. In the case of the second director, there were times when such flexibility ran perilously close to contradicting the original intentions of the RSVP director in furnishing RSVP volunteers to interview elders who desired to home-share with one another. For example, in expanding the pool of potential Project HOME clients to include younger applicants (both disabled and able), the director created the likelihood of nonelders being matched with nonelders. While the official HOME policy maintained that at least one of the homesharers must be sixty years old or older, in fact some few matches included no elders. Why? Simply, the director saw a potential good match and went ahead and arranged it. To be sure, the match included at least one person who was in some way incapacitated and in need of help around the house. The point to be made, however, is that the second director was willing to innovate where she saw a need to do so.

During this time, the fact that Project HOME was a subunit of RSVP and that RSVP was therefore responsible for HOME's operation did not appear to reduce the authority of the HOME director. The major reason appears to be that the RSVP director was too busy running the larger RSVP organization to provide "hands-on" direction and support to Project HOME and its director. While having considerable flexibility of direction and growth, Project HOME also had the legitimacy and security that being part of a well-established organization provided. Thus, while having both the freedom and need to articulate and carry out its own agenda in specific matters, Project HOME also was under the "umbrella" of RSVP, which provided working space, volunteers, and other in-kind support.

At the same time the HOME director was propagating ideas about the service mission of Project HOME and reaching out in new directions, she was also soliciting input from the researchers and from her volunteers. The means by which she asked for input from them is best understood in the context of the decision-making process within the Project HOME organization.

## Decision Making in Project HOME

Within the first year of its operation, Project HOME metamorphosed into an entity having the characteristics of a semidependent organization. Initially, for a short time HOME followed the "simple model" of administration in which an additional staff person is assigned from an existing agency to monitor an agency initiative. Such a procedure, point out McConnell and Usher, "runs the risk of being distracted by the priorities of the existing agency" (1980:29). Following the hiring of the first director of Project HOME, the administrative structure resembled an "intermediate model" in which a subagency is developed within an umbrella agency (i.e., RSVP). From the moment a paid director was put in charge of Project HOME, the stage was set for the subagency and umbrella agency to come into periodic conflict over resources until the point at which it was mutually agreed that Project HOME should become a separate entity from RSVP.

For its first five years, HOME operated in much the same way: The HOME director—though the only paid staff member and, thus, ultimately the only one responsible for the program's success or failure—nevertheless utilized volunteer staff and the university researchers in key roles and as general advisers during her tenure. As a result, the program was governed by informally arrived at decisions that tended to reflect consensus more times than not.

Two examples show how this decision-making process worked. The first, alluded to in the previous section, concerns the construction of the revised questionnaire shortly after the second director took over at the end of the program's first year. Herself a middle-aged homesharer, the new director already was envisioning a wider clientele for the program than just elders (most of whom were unable or unwilling to move from their homes). In her mind, the original questionnaire did not probe deeply enough about issues that would directly affect potential sharing arrangements. At the same time, despite some input into the initial application form, the researchers believed that several important background and sentiment questions needed to be added so that they could evaluate adequately how well the program served the population of area residents in need of homesharing.

After exchanging ideas over a few lunches, the director and the researchers agreed that the latter would draw up a first draft of an application schedule, get feedback from the director, and revise into a tentative final draft. The final draft would be agreed to when all parties were satisfied. While cooptation might be too strong a word to describe the director's use of the researchers (since they were receiving important cooperation from her), she nevertheless was able to achieve her goal of adding to the application form questions she deemed important through the process of *negotiation* (the result of which is in appendix 1).

A second example of the director's style of decision making is found during the critical third and fourth years when grant writing to secure outside funding was interfering more and more with the director's service to her clients. Surrounded by a number of capable volunteers who already were performing a variety of nontrivial tasks, she considered the idea of expanding the types of jobs they were doing for HOME.

> I see volunteers manning the office, taking down inquiries, sending out applications, setting up interviews and going on introductions. There is absolutely no reason why they can't be more involved. One volunteer has even had experience writing grants. She might be interested in program development.

Thus, the director was taking her cue both from what she was observing and from the possibilities these observations suggested. As described in chapter 3, the decision to expand the responsibilities was in fact a mutual decision arrived at by an opportunistic director and a group of bright, talented, and committed volunteers.

The result of the office reorganization of duties was to make Project HOME a more tightly knit, efficient service program. By the director's second year (the program's third), she was able to recollect:

> A year ago I had 12 interviewers who seldom came into the office with me. I was doing all in the office-type work and all decision making. Now I have only two to four volunteers out in the field doing interviews and have four home office volunteers who like the administrative part. So all of us are becoming involved as case workers and we are becoming more like the RSVP model where I am the director and they are like coordinators.

Thus, the director now had a functioning office staff of volunteers who, in her words, "are much more intensely involved with the program than before."

For their part, these executive volunteers were not merely reacting to suggestions by the director but rather acting on their own initiative to make suggestions themselves in what was clearly a supportive climate. For instance, the volunteers reorganized the filing system, initiated the idea that applications be returned to the office to check references before sending someone out on an interview, began meeting as a group weekly to exchange ideas, then invited the director to participate as a coequal. At one such meeting it was decided to eliminate introductory luncheons, to have a recognition get-together "for all people involved," and to do a slide presentation for a TV publicity show. With such increased responsibilities going to the volunteers and with the weekly meetings becoming the locus of group-oriented decision making, the director of HOME came to see herself more in a nurturing and supportive role vis-a-vis the executive volunteers.

On the basis of statements from volunteers, numbers and kinds of clients served, the parent RSVP's hands-off approach, and the (it seemed) always questionable financial position of the program during its early years, it now appears clear that an innovative, entrepreneurial director was an appropriate catalyst to stretch HOME's limited resources in a variety of experimental ways.[2] Far from impeding the program's development, therefore, its limited resources maximized program flexibility. Central to this flexibility was the charismatic director whose leadership style emphasized a personal enthusiasm for the program's goals, nurturing of her coworkers, and a cooperative style of decision making. In these aspects, she served not only to lead but also as an effective role model.

## Keeping Client Needs First

The flexibility within Project HOME, especially during the program's formative first four years, produced some important examples of the need for service delivery organizations to react to client needs rather than set boundaries around them. Such an approach, of course, is fraught with all kinds of dangers, not the least of which is the stretching of organizational goals beyond the ability of organizational resources to meet those goals, or a case of an organization's eyes being bigger than its stomach. In the case of Project HOME, this was a real concern voiced by the researchers to the director in the midst of the program's rapid growth during the fourth year; and, in some respects, this concern shared by the director is certainly an important reason why the organization took on an advisory board, among other things, to help with fund-raising. In the meantime, however, the director and her volunteers attempted to juggle the emotional and financial costs of expanding program services as new client needs became known. Three particular examples of the organization stretching to meet client needs will be highlighted.

*Rescuing a Moribund Program.* As was described in the descriptive history of Project HOME, the initial efforts of Project HOME staff to match elders with one another were proceeding at an agonizingly slow pace because so few elder movers could be found; almost all older clients, not surprisingly, wanted to remain at home. Also, when homesharing matches were made, the parallel physical and financial problems of the homesharers increased the likelihood of strains on the relationship between sharers.[3] Thus, by the time the second director began work at the beginning of the second year of the program, Project HOME either was going to be written off as a theoretically interesting social intervention that could not work in practice or was going to have to innovate to find ways to meet the needs of its elderly clients.

Since the elders who refused to move from their own home made up the vast majority of clients and since those few elders who said they were willing to move either had found a homesharing arrangement through Project HOME, had found some other accommodations, or themselves actually preferred staying home, in the eyes of the new director the problem was to find homesharers willing to move. Herself a homesharer, it wasn't difficult to imagine younger movers and older stayers sharing living arrangements, so pretty much on her own she decided to open up Project HOME to both young and old clients.

The infusion of "new blood" into the applicant pool had important consequences for both the program and its clients. A more diverse group of applicants willing to move (who made up the bulk of the new client pool) meant a better chance of finding an appropriate match for its elderly and sometimes frail homeowner clients. For the homeowner clients, the increased pool of possible homesharers meant more introductions with potential sharers and thus the opportunity to be more selective in choosing sharers. For Project HOME, the influx of younger applicants produced both benefits and challenges. On the plus side, it meant Project HOME had a larger pool of clients from which to put together introductions hopefully leading to homesharing matches; more clients simply gave the program a chance to do what it was in existence to do. At the same time, however, more applicants meant a greater need to screen; not everyone who applied was an appropriate candidate for Project HOME.

*Educating Clients and "Nonclients."* Early in the second director's term, it became clear to her that "now that the program has been running for awhile we should be more selective" in recruiting clients. Two kinds of potential problem clients were surfacing. The first were nonelders with a history of transient living accommodations or drug or alcohol abuse. The second, according to the director, were elders who were so frail physically that they needed to be kept under "constant observation. The best candidates are in good health but in search of financial sharing, transportation, task, and rent sharing."

With the large influx of applicants, the need to check references and to get quite detailed information about their health became paramount, so the new application form devised by the researchers and director included space for references' names, addresses, and telephone numbers and for additional health questions. With this added information, the director and her volunteer staff were better able to monitor applicants and, not surprisingly, judge the relative prospects of potential matches.

Closely related to this increased selectivity by the program was the concern by the staff that elders and others who were not appropriate candidates be given *some* direction as to what agencies, if any, in the community should be contacted. For every inquiry leading to a formal application there were at least three or four inquiries by individuals who in fact needed something other than a homesharer. Some older applicants indeed required the kind of care only a nursing home could provide, or needed the support services provided by the local Visiting Nurse Association, or needed to communicate better with their family member because their problems were best worked out in a familial context. Other applicants merely wanted roommates and so were better off advertising in the local or university newspapers, or they needed counseling for chemical dependency or the kind of housing and support the local shelters for the homeless could provide.

In fact, the hundreds upon hundreds of inquiries which the program received from individuals who received useful information from the HOME staff but who did not apply to HOME are also beneficiaries of Project HOME; it's just that the benefits they received can be inferred only from the staff's records and from anecdotal information provided by the staff.

Also important to note is the educational function performed by the application form and overall interview process. One particular example stands out in this respect: During the early months of the second director's term, she received an inquiry and partially completed application from an elderly woman who wanted to remain independent in her own home and avoid institutionalization. Her family believed, correctly (given the woman's physical condition), that their mother could not continue without the kinds of full-time services a nursing home could provide. Nothing they said would convince her to leave her home. When the woman applied to Project HOME, however, she found out *on her own* what kinds of giving as well as getting would be expected of her in a homesharing arrangement. It is hard to tell what precisely convinced her to go to a nursing home, but two facts are clear, according to the director.

First, the woman made the decision to go without any pressure being exerted on her by family or staff at HOME. Second, her decision was tied in part, at least, to the application form and interviewing process, which gave her insight as to what homesharing involved. In the case of this frail elderly woman, the application process performed an important latent function in sensitizing her to the ramifications of homesharing and giving her reason to believe that at least one better alternative existed for her. Overall, therefore, Project HOME has attempted to respond to the needs not only of "appropriate" homesharing applicants but also of those needy individuals for whom other solutions made better sense. Through its formal application process and the information its staff are able to provide callers, Project HOME has become an important clearinghouse for elders and others in need in Chittenden County. As a result, the program has become well-known itself in the human services community and even begun to receive referrals from other agencies.

*Expanding the Continuum of Care.* The first chapter outlined the idea of homesharing as a viable option to institutionalization in terms of the continuum of care ranging between complete independence and institutionalization. While this idea is not so new, the notion that a living option on the continuum of care (i.e., homesharing) might itself represent a continuum of care within the home, *is* new (see Jaffe and Howe 1988).

The need for a continuum of care within the home among its clients has clearly affected the evolution of Project HOME. Beginning in the second year of the program and during its rapid expansion, Project HOME received an increasing number of requests from frail elders and adult handicapped persons who needed a person to live with them to provide basic household assistance, twenty-four-hour protective presence in case of emergency and some personal care such as help with bathing, dressing and moving about safely. For many of these individuals, the Project HOME response of necessity was to suggest solutions other than homesharing. For others, however, the staff believed that arrangements could be made within the context of homesharing.

For frail homeowners who had enough material resources (usually money), Project HOME pioneered the recruitment and matching of paid caregivers who would provide these services for five or six days and nights each week in exchange for room, board, and a salary. These changes required that the volunteer interviewer/counselor learn assessment skills in order to determine whether the assistance the frail person requested was realistic or not.

As Project HOME began to address these caregiver needs, the program experienced tremendous growth. Not only did service statistics dramatically increase, doubling then redoubling, but the demands on staff for more in-depth counseling and education involvement also increased. Without any appreciable increase in volunteer staff, the increasing demands of personal care companion employers and caregivers stretched the resources of Project HOME personnel. At the same time, the director and her staff were committed fully to attempting to accommodate the needs of frail elders who had something to offer potential caregivers in exchange for personal care services.[4]

One important concomitant of the program's efforts to accommodate the special needs of the physically frail applicant was the willingness of the program director and her staff to act as counselors and seek out caregivers and respite workers for already matched elders whose initial good health at time of starting a match had begun to deteriorate. In many cases, the homesharer, while sympathetic, was unable to provide the caregiving services required. As a result, Project HOME interviewed applicants who would be willing to provide respite care on a regular basis to supplement the sharer's contributions. Thus, in matches involving frail elders, the number of "sharers" might include the frail homeowner, the initial homesharer, a caregiver during the weekdays, and a respite caregiver at nights and on weekends. Project HOME was now in the business of putting together not only homesharing matches but also homesharing "packages."

This service-within-a-service by Project HOME represents, along with its dependence on volunteers in key service delivery roles, one of the unique aspects of the program as it evolved during its first five years. In the case of arranging caregiver matches, Project HOME was simply following its mission to serve elders in need of homesharers. In those instances in which the homeowner had a weakened health condition and no resources to pay for caregiving, the outlook was not good and Project HOME staff were resigned only to making suggestions about other services available. In those instances in which the frail homeowner had resources to pay something for caregiving help, the staff worked overtime to find a caregiver or "package" of caregivers to help that elder remain independent at home.

Rescuing a dying program, educating clients, and expanding the concept of a continuum of care are all examples of the organization's flexibility in meeting client needs. Further, this flexible program structure combined with the leadership of an entrepreneurial director accounted for the growth and success of Project HOME during its first five years.

# A KEY TO HOMESHARING SERVICE PROVISION: SOCIAL EXCHANGE

This distinction between those who have enough to give in exchange for caregiving services and those who don't underscores the critical role which exchange plays in the entire program. Indeed, up to this point the emphasis on organizational structure and the director's personality have mostly *described* the ways in which the program grew. To be sure, the freedom allowed by a very flexible organizational structure and exploited by an entrepreneurial director provided the setting for the program's expansion of services to meet evolving client needs. Nevertheless, the dynamic of this evolution cannot be comprehended until one understands the philosophical and practical underpinnings of the relationship between program staff and clients, among program staff, and between staff and the university researchers.

The actual interactions involved in Project HOME service delivery and evaluation are best understood by focusing on the idea of social exchange, or bartering, which represents a dominant principle for all persons associated with Project HOME. While the notion of barter is obviously central to the homesharing contract between clients who desire to homeshare with one another, exchange plays a significant role also in the relations between the organization and its clients, within the organization's staff, and between the organization and the two researchers evaluating it.

## The Origins of Social Exchange in Project HOME

Before any consideration of the variety of social exchange relationships fostered by Project HOME, it is important to understand that the principle of social exchange was central to the operation of the program even before it became operational. Furthermore, once the program had begun, its flexibility and requirements for survival and growth combined to make social exchange an even more important principle.

*Project Goals.* As described in chapter 2, Project HOME was started to serve *two* groups of elders: those outside the organization in need of homesharing arrangements and RSVP volunteers within the organization who would benefit from meaningful service delivery roles such as interviewing. In addition, the researchers were brought in to produce an interview schedule to screen clients and to train the volunteers to administer it in exchange for complete access to interview data and all organization files.

Before even starting, therefore, Project HOME had already established exchange as the operating currency: Elderly homeowners would provide a place to live in exchange for the companionship, and perhaps some rent, that the home seeker would give. Volunteers would give their time and knowledge regarding other elders' needs in exchange for the psychic reward of doing meaningful service for other elders. The university researchers would donate time and expertise regarding the development and administration of interview schedules in exchange for the information from those schedules.

*Project Structure.* As described in the previous section, the very loose organizational structure in Project HOME promoted flexibility in the program's approach to service delivery on behalf of homesharing clients in two ways: First, the director received very minimal instructions from the parent RSVP organization during the time Project HOME was part of RSVP. Thus, while the RSVP coordinator provided the HOME director a continuous supply of interviewers and was sensitive to the type of creative counseling skills needed to work for HOME, and while the staff of the larger organization provided support and encouragement during the weekly RSVP staff meetings, which the HOME director attended, the second HOME director often felt alone in her position, especially after the applicant pool started to swell.

On the one hand, she highly valued the responsibility, freedom, and creativity the program demanded; on the other hand, there were attendant disadvantages of being solely in charge. As she relates it: The freedom to "implement procedures as I feel necessary" had to be balanced off by almost sole responsibility for its functioning. "I was on the creative edge by myself with other people cheering me on but not really leading me or providing me with different components I needed for my own growth." She emphasizes this aloneness with respect to the way in which fund-raising was interfering with what she believed was her primary role:

> I would liked to have had more direct interaction and supervision (from the director of RSVP)—a way for me to go in and discuss what has happened and get immediate suggestions for how to do it better. It would have helped to have someone else worry about funding because the stress of that has taken

away some of the energy I could have used to provide direct service which is
what I was hired for.

Once HOME was on its own, of course, the HOME director was both
nominally and substantively in charge.

Flexibility of structure was important in a second way, because with
minimal direction from RSVP the director was implicitly encouraged to
turn to her volunteer staff and to the university researchers for suggestions, for reactions to her initiatives, or, in her words, for "brainstorming." It is in this second instance of flexibility that the director's personality becomes important: Her sense of mission on behalf of homesharing
applicants took precedence over other considerations, so that the discussions taking place between the director and the interviewers and between
the director and the researchers were substantive and not mere formali-
ties. As will be seen below, a great many examples of social exchange
within the organization stem from the director's efforts to seek out ideas
from her staff and from the researchers.

## Social Exchange: The Currency of Project HOME

Much has been written about social exchange in the relationships
between dating and marriage partners (Vander Zanden 1984), friends
(Liebow 1967), and even large-scale organizations and societies (Blau
1977). The idea of exchange also lies at the root of Project HOME's
success in melding together various disparate groups to produce the
service that allowed the program to flourish during its early years rather
than die off as so many programs might have done under similar circumstances (i.e., shortage of funds).

The essential arguments, borrowed from Homans (1961) and Blau
(1964), boil down to the notion that people do things with and for other
people as long as there is something to be expected in return for what
one does. As a result, in such situations in which both parties are
interacting with one another on the expectation that one's giving will be
reciprocated by the other party, a *norm of reciprocity* will develop that
tends to direct the interaction between the two parties and continues as
long as the parties see benefits from the interaction. As will be demonstrated, the exchanges occurring in Project HOME involved the giving
and getting of not only material but also emotional commodities.

In the case of Project HOME, social exchange can be seen in a variety
of relationships, not the least of which are the relationships between the
program staff and the program's clients and between the homesharing

clients themselves who propose to live with one another. In this section, examples of exchange will be considered primarily in a symbolic way. That is, the emphasis will be on the exchange within the organization that reflects the exchange expected between organization and client and between client and client.

Two major relationships underscore the importance of social exchange in Project HOME, reflecting the importance the second director placed on those with whom she worked; the first is the relationship between the director and her volunteer staff, and the second is between the director and the researchers/evaluators. Each of the following discussions will emphasize the respective roles played by the main actors to indicate how social exchange was or was not taking place.

## The Program and the Volunteer Staff

*Beginnings.* During all of the first year of the program, the volunteers' major program contacts were with: first, the volunteer coordinator on loan from RSVP and, then, HOME's first director who stayed for about half a year. In each case, efforts were made by these two individuals to provide encouragement and emotional support for the volunteers, but there really was very little else that they could do. As described in the previous chapter, the volunteers' major source of accomplishment was going to have to be the fruits of their interviewing efforts: the matching of HOME applicants.

As has been seen earlier, the roles volunteers play in Project HOME have varied on the basis of where the leadership in the program lay. Initially, of course, the volunteers were seen by the RSVP director not only as service *providers* but also as key *recipients* within the program. In terms of their roles as service providers, the volunteers were perceived as doing well. The first year's turnover of about 50 percent was not considered particularly bad by the directors. There was some difficulty with two (of about fifteen) interviewers who were not collecting complete information because they failed to ask some of the more subjective life satisfaction-type questions. However, in most cases those volunteer interviewers who were most uncomfortable with the interview questions selected themselves out of this project and were assigned to other volunteer activities. In general, the directors of both HOME and RSVP were satisfied with the expertise, enthusiasm, and commitment of the volunteers.

As for being service recipients themselves, while interviewing home-sharing applicants volunteers were expected to receive the benefits from having done important work for people in need. In the language of social exchange (Homans 1961:51–82), an important requirement for the volunteers to continue to work for Project HOME was a sense of accomplishment, or reward. In this case, the reward would stem from the three sources described in the previous chapter: the ability to exercise skills that had served them well throughout their adult lives, the camaraderie involved in working with other committed volunteers, *and* the reason for their volunteering at HOME as opposed to other programs—the sense of accomplishment they received from seeing their elderly clients get matched and improve their living situations. Once the second director had developed her working relationship with the small group of executive volunteers, these rewards began to occur.

*Social Exchange and the Volunteers.* Since the third year of the program's existence, therefore, the volunteer role has grown appreciably, accompanied by important consequences for the volunteers' relationship to the program. In an ironic twist, the RSVP director's initial desire to make Project HOME be a meaningful service vehicle for RSVP volunteers has reached fruition because Project HOME volunteers themselves took the initiative to *make* their work more meaningful with the full support of a director who was willing to experiment with a reorganization of staff tasks.

At the heart of this successful exchange between program and volunteers lie two important factors. First is the goal of service delivery to clients in need. Without that important objective, it is doubtful that Project HOME could have maintained the hold that it did on its volunteer staff. Second is the HOME director who was willing to use the volunteers in a wide variety of roles making full use of their skills. The result of the program's important objective and its leadership in the hands of an entrepreneurial director was tremendous growth in a program that at one time was moribund.

## The Program and the Researchers

*The Initial Exchanges.* The researchers, like the volunteers, were operating both as service providers and recipients: The time spent in constructing and arranging for copies of the application form, training the interviewers, and acting as unpaid consultants was expected to result in

access to the completed interview application forms and enough preliminary information to make a grant application for funding of a systematic
evaluation of Project HOME feasible.

Early in the process, the evaluational component of HOME was accepted by the Director of RSVP in exchange for help in developing the
application form, which presumably would help the RSVP coordinator
on loan to HOME "make" homesharing matches. Although not at first
evident, the evaluational component of the application interview schedule would later be useful to the director as she applied to funding agencies
seeking financial support for Project HOME. Consistent with more strin-
gent requirements in times of tightened budgets, agencies were strongly
requesting evidence from outside sources of a program's viability.

The application form, therefore, was to play three roles: For RSVP
and Project HOME it was to facilitate the decision-making process concerning which applicants get introduced to each other by giving staff
important insight into each applicant's background and interests, and it
would facilitate securing grant support as the director was able to docu-
ment the program's successes and potential through "outside" evaluation.
For the researchers the application form would provide important background information, so that profiles of stayers and movers could be drawn
and the particular characteristics that help a client get matched be
isolated.

Within a year, when Andrus Foundation funding was assured and with
the encouragement and active collaboration of the second director, the
researchers made a major revision in the application instrument used to
get important information from homesharing applicants (appendix 1).
Because of its increased length it was separated into two parts, the initial
questionnaire filled out by the respondent and the interview to be administered in person after the questionnaire had been returned to the office.
The increased length made it possible for the researchers to process a
greater amount of information measuring life satisfaction and familial and
community social support. At the same time, more information was
requested concerning any disabilities of the applicant. This was in response to an expressed need felt by the HOME director to "identify more
clearly how disabled and dependent a person is."

As stated earlier, the many questions needed for the researchers' evaluation, though resulting in a lengthy instrument, were not resisted by
the director of HOME as they had been earlier by the director of RSVP
when the first, much shorter instrument was designed. In terms of the

application information to be gathered by the application questionnaire and personal interview, therefore, the HOME director and the researchers were of one mind. The only conflicts that arose had to do with question placement and wording, not content, and the few disagreements were as often as not between the researchers themselves.

In a very real sense, the initial exchanges between staff connected to Project HOME and the researchers were easily compared in an accounts receivable and accounts payable sort of way. The researchers provided: expertise in questionnaire construction; typing and reproduction of the applications (Andrus support included reproduction costs for both intake and follow-up interviews); and training of the volunteers who would be doing the application interviews. Project HOME provided: collation of the intake forms by the volunteers; volunteer interviewers; access to all client data, as long as client confidentiality was respected; and access to volunteer staff and the director for structured and unstructured interviews as part of the program evaluation.

*New Exchanges: Expanding the Evaluator Role.* From the outset, the researchers were interested in not only the client data but also the program that was providing the service delivery. As stated in their application to Andrus, the focus was to be on RSVP and how well it could deliver a homesharing service:

> Our second major objective is to evaluate RSVP's participation in this project. Specifically, we want to determine the practicability of having one small part of a medium size organization running such a program [as Project HOME] and using volunteers in various roles, particularly that of interviewer. (Fengler and Danigelis 1982)

Until the second HOME director took over in the spring of 1983, the researchers' role as evaluator was fairly clear cut and "uncontaminated." Once the researchers began to work with the new director, however, the distinction between evaluator and program volunteer became harder to maintain. The first example of the blurring relates to the roles the researchers' research assistant[5] came to play in her relationships with the program director and volunteer staff. The major ostensible roles of the assistant were to do the follow-up interviews with matched and unmatched clients of Project HOME and to record and transmit daily information concerning the work of the director and her staff to the investigators. As a result, in yet another example of exchange, the research assistant performed various clerical tasks for the Project HOME staff, attended their meetings, and generally provided the staff with any input she had on various clients whom she had interviewed for the researchers.

Although primarily responsible to the university researchers, the assistant also was often playing a role supportive of the members of the HOME organization. The director saw the student involvement as an important component of the program, because having an undergraduate student working with senior volunteers was consistent with the intergenerational focus of the homesharing matches that by then were going on. At a later date, student interns, hired through the university internship program, would become a regular part of the Project HOME staffing picture.

Each of the student assistants who worked with Project HOME had been selected on the basis of not only native intelligence and curiosity but also strong interpersonal skills. Therefore, it was not surprising that each in turn was quickly welcomed by the program staff and soon accepted as yet another volunteer in the project. At the same time, each student quickly "took" to the program and its mission and, in fact, *did* become a volunteer at the same time she was working for the researchers.

One example of the assistant's loyalty to both the researchers and the program concerns the second, two-part application, which was quite detailed and long (appendix 1). Each time the assistant would return to campus from her work with the director and volunteers, she would begin to air the interviewers' complaints about the large number of questions and the problems associated with the personal nature of questions dealing with friendships of the applicant. On the one hand, it was important for the researchers to know—whether directly or indirectly—how the volunteers who were in the field felt about the application schedule; so, in this respect, they were glad to hear their assistant's report. On the other hand, the report often carried with it the argument by their assistant that the researchers *really* ought to shorten and edit the schedule; that is, the research assistant was now a spokeswoman for Project HOME.

While this conflict concerning the assistant's role did create some difficulties, overall the fact that their assistant had become so involved with the program as to speak with its best interests in mind really gave the researchers more benefits of insight than problems. Indeed, regarding the example of the application schedule above, the volunteers' (and the student's) complaint was well-founded, and, after a year's trial, the researchers agreed to shorten it. In fact, it was their research assistant

working in conjunction with the volunteers and director who put together the working draft of the new schedule.

Thus, even the problems associated with the assistant's role conflict
often ultimately produced positive change for the program and for its
evaluators, the researchers. In the case of the application schedule change,
the volunteers became happier with the shorter, less intrusive schedule;
and, while the researchers lost some potentially useful information through
the cutting process, they retained almost all the critical background and
attitude questions and were rewarded by higher quality application data.

The second instance in which the blurring of roles occurred relates to
the way the researchers fed back information from preliminary data
analyses to the director and her staff. In the context of describing the
exchanges between herself and the researchers, the HOME director
spoke of this feedback:

> The researchers are open to my needs and the programs needs. The data has
> been valuable to me in making changes I need to make. There has been a real
> positive interchange. It has been a nice cooperative relationship. They have
> provided personal support in developing the program as well as printing and
> staff time to getting the applications done. Information is available immedi-
> ately to make alterations to serve the people.

There was an expectation, as seen in the last sentence of the previous
statement, that as information was collected it would be fed back to the
director for modification and improvement of the program. As this happened, the researchers were put in the role of consultants as well as
evaluators. Such a process was a necessary part of the healthy cooperative
relationship established between service provider and researcher, but it
did lessen the impartiality and nonintrusiveness of the research evaluation. Thus, as the program evolved it was at least in a small way a result
of the participation of the researchers as volunteer consultants.

A final way in which the researchers' roles became blurred stems from
actual volunteer work the researchers did for the program. This does not
refer to the initial agreement to exchange their expertise and resources
for information, although such an exchange helped develop the norm of
reciprocity that characterized the ongoing relationship between the researchers and the director. Rather, it refers to the actual publicizing and
promoting of the program.

This occurred in three ways. First, starting in the summer of 1983,
only a few months after the second director had begun working for

Project HOME, the researchers began to present at professional meetings papers describing: the applicants to this homesharing program, the kinds of characteristics that facilitated applicant success in finding sharers, the differences the program made to those who homeshared, the special qualities of volunteer-based service delivery programs, and the unique emphasis of Project HOME's contribution to the continuum of care within the home.

While the researchers' objective was merely to present dispassionate descriptions of how Project HOME worked and whom it served, it became very clear from the first meeting that large numbers of service providers were in attendance who were seeking information on "how to do a homesharing program." As a result, in describing whom the program served and how it operated, the researchers were promulgating the program.

A second way in which they acted as volunteers occurred during the program's second year when the director decided to seek funding from the city to finance introductory luncheons for clients who were to be introduced to each other. The director had found that introductions in the stayer's home was very uncomfortable for both clients—the stayer because he or she felt as if the other person were scrutinizing and appraising the home and all its furnishings and the mover because he or she was on the other person's "turf."

One of the researchers at the time was on an advisory council to the mayor of the city and automatically offered to write a letter of support for the project. Whether the letter had any bearing on the final outcome or not,[6] the important thing is that the researcher who wrote the letter of support felt it was not only appropriate but even important to do so. Again research and evaluation was taking a back seat to the volunteer role which the researchers were at times slipping into.

Similarly, one of the researchers accompanied the director on several occasions when she appeared before various local funding organizations. His role was to testify as to the efficacy of Project HOME. In addition, both researchers supplied the director with valuable documentation to support her petitions to various local and state granting agencies. Both also appeared on a regional radio talk show with the director to advertise the concept of homesharing in general and the virtues of Project HOME in particular. In another instance of cooperative effort, both researchers and the director made a joint presentation before an international symposium on the aged and disabled.

Another way in which both researchers acted as volunteers stems from the time Project HOME became intergenerational. In more than one of their classes, the researchers advertised the program, telling their students about the opportunities of homesharing with elders. In at least two instances, students of the researchers did apply to (and eventually find a homesharer through) Project HOME. One of the researchers continues to show the videotape of Project HOME before hundreds of students each semester in his classes on aging and on family. On a broader scale, such advertising also indirectly reached the parents and grandparents of in-state students who heard about Project HOME in their classes. By advertising the program, the researchers had again played the role of volunteers, rather than researchers and evaluators.

In one final way, the roles of researchers and volunteers were potentially set in opposition to one another. This occurred near the end of the second director's tenure when she was putting together the advisory board for Project HOME. Nothing seemed more natural to her (or to the researchers) than putting both senior volunteers and the researcher volunteers on the board. So the researchers accepted, with the understanding that their primary roles would focus on planning and evaluation. Again, during the board meetings, in committee with other board members, and on the selection committee to choose the new director, the researchers were clearly in the position of being spokespersons for Project HOME. Their goals were not only consistent with Project HOME's goals; in the case of our Planning and Evaluation Committee work, the researchers helped articulate what the stated mission of Project HOME was.

The above role blurring actually *facilitated* evaluation of the program in two ways. First, the researchers' relationship with the director was strengthened, because they were volunteering their services. As the director relates:

> I'm delighted with the relationship back and forth. I feel we are colleagues. We work well together and have complementary goals and there is a lot of feedback that is valuable. That friendliness and openness of wanting the program to work and evaluating it to improve it instead of calling to task and blaming things on it has been a wonderful ambience to work in. Our files have been completely open to you and you have been open to us while maintaining clients' anonymity at the same time. That is the kind of relationship there ought to be.

Without this openness and trust, the kinds of insights the director gave the researchers concerning homesharing couples, volunteer commitment and the like would not have been forthcoming. There would not have been the sorts of brainstorming sessions described earlier that gave fruit to these, often spontaneously arrived at, insights. In a related way, the researchers themselves would not have developed the sorts of insights expressed in this chapter concerning the workings of the organization without the many informal conversations they had with the director.

This open relationship between the evaluators and the evaluated was, in fact, a natural result of the desire by both groups to see the program work well. Early on, the researchers began feeding back information to the program concerning, for example, imbalances in the applicant stayer:mover ratio and the particular problems of hearing-impaired stayer applicants. Such results were reported in the paper presentations alluded to earlier, but the researchers' concern as evaluators was also to provide direct feedback to the program staff so that problems in the program could be addressed. Because of the open relationship with the director, they felt no restraints in providing feedback—whether it was positive *or* negative; in each case, the feedback was given in hopes of strengthening the program.

A second, equally important advantage of the researchers taking on the role of volunteers was that it represented a natural extension of the idea of social exchange that permeated the program. The director and the researchers now were exchanging ideas concerning such things as the role of evaluation in service delivery and the imperatives facing a volunteer-based organization, so that the social exchange that had begun as a fairly impartial *quid pro quo* was now unconsciously proceeding because each of the parties cared both about each other's roles and about the program. In contrast to much of what has been said in criticism of the too rational basis of social exchange theory, what was occurring in Project HOME was social exchange of a more altruistic nature. In the context of the way the program was structured, with everyone involved giving of themselves for the benefit of the clients, it was easy, in fact, to work for with the director and her staff for the good of the program and its clients.

## Changing of the Guard

In an appropriate epilogue to this discussion of the social exchange relationships in Project HOME, it is interesting to note that the core volunteers (the senior volunteers who have been a mainstay of Project

HOME since its inception) have remained a critical element of the program, while the peripheral volunteers (the researchers who were involved with the program in one way or another from its inception) have begun to disengage. As described in an earlier chapter, the volunteers now have taken over the task of revising the application schedule. After the researchers' assistant modified the early two-part form, the researchers' role in questionnaire construction steadily declined with the tacit agreement of all parties (more on this in chapters 10 and 11, which consider the costs of evaluator-service provider collaborations).

Similarly, as the volunteers began to take on more varied tasks in the office as well as in the field, the director began to rely on them more than on the researchers for emotional support. This is not to say that relations became strained between the researchers and the director; rather, they simply changed as the program staff became more self-sufficient in its human and material resources and as priorities of the researchers shifted to other projects. From the point of view of the program staff, the donation of needed expertise and material (training of interviewers, supplying typing and paper, etc.) were not needed any more, and the major evaluational work that could benefit the program directly had been accomplished during the first five years. From the point of view of the researchers, the most important information for the overall analysis of the program, its staff, and its clients had been accomplished, and time was now needed to distance themselves from the program to do a comprehensive analysis and write-up of findings.

In an unexpected but very instructive way, Project HOME evolved from being a service arm of the area Retired Senior Volunteer Program, whose aim was to serve elder clients and service providers alike, into a much larger, independent service agency that remained faithful to these original twin goals through the process of social exchange. Critical to Project HOME's successful growth were flexible organizational structure promoted by the parent RSVP agency and the hiring of an entrepreneurial director who was left to structure the program as she saw fit.

Keeping as a central objective the idea of serving as many of their clients' needs as possible, through expansion and redirection of program initiatives if necessary, the director and her staff molded their organizational machinery in the image of the clients whom they were serving: They remained faithful to the idea of bartering, or social exchange, as the main currency by which the program would run. In the relationships between client and client and between program and clients, but most critically among the director, her staff and the university researchers, Project HOME demonstrated that a service program with limited material resources *can* succeed. Instrumental in this program's evolution, social exchange provided a viable set of substitutes for the material resources the program lacked during its early years and produced a framework that supports the program to this very day.

The next four chapters shift away from an emphasis on the Project HOME organization to consider in detail the clients whom Project HOME serves, beginning with a description of who Project HOME's clients are.

# 5
## Who Wants to Homeshare and Why

Chapters 5 through 8 examine the Project HOME clients in detail. This chapter and the next consider the whole range of clients, including those who did not find homesharers through the program. The focus in these chapters, therefore, will be on the individual characteristics possessed by all applicants and the *unit of analysis* the *individual client*. In chapters 7 and 8, emphasis will turn to those clients who have found a homesharer. There the focus will be on the interaction between sharers and their thoughts about one another and the *unit of analysis* the *homesharing match*, which includes two (and sometimes more) clients.

In all four chapters, it will be useful to remember the major assumptions of exchange theory discussed in chapter 4 with reference to the organization. Just as surely as exchange helped the program through its early stages, so too do the principles of social exchange underlie the whole idea of homesharing itself. In this chapter and the next, characteristics of stayers and movers will be contrasted with an eye toward measuring the potential "fit" between them in prospective shared housing arrangements. The nature of actual exchanges will be developed in detail in chapters 7 and 8.

The evidence available from previous studies is quite limited regarding homesharing clients in general, since most focus only on clients who have found sharers (e.g., Jaffe 1989b; Jaffe and Howe 1988; Jaffe and

Wellin 1989; Pynoos and June 1989; Schreter 1986; Thuras 1989). An exception is the early work of Pritchard (1983), which found a sample of older San Diego adults interested in homesharing to be predominantly female, widowed or divorced, and desiring to have someone move in with them rather than move into someone else's home.

The changes in leadership and the administrative structure described in the previous three chapters have obviously had an important impact on the type of client whom Project HOME serves. In particular, the hiring of an entrepreneurial director who gave her staff substantial free-dom in decision making has resulted in two significant changes in the applicant pool: First, the program began to accept applications from adults of all ages, not just elders, after the first year. Second, a little later, the range of homesharing arrangements supported was expanded from just renter payment to include homeowner payment in cases where the homeowner is frail and in need of caregiving help.

Based on the detailed application form and interview schedule used by the program (see appendix 1), this chapter describes the variegated applicant pool during the first four years of the program, shows how the pool has changed, and contrasts the differences among the major groups of clients served by the program. Throughout the analysis, emphasis will be placed on the degree of complementarity of characteristics between stayers and movers. Further examination will also show critical differ-ences between stayers who need extensive personal care services and those who do not, and critical differences between movers who are willing to provide these services and those who are not.

The application interview information used in this chapter is divided into five logical clusters: background, income and health, home, home-sharing profile, and homesharing expectations. The first three clusters should distinguish applicants who want to stay put from those who are willing to move, while the last two should provide insights into the common characteristics all applicants share.

Although much of the information that follows is based on single questions, several items (e.g., physical capacity, housing problems, atti-tude toward sharer's lifestyle, household services) represent indices con-structed from two or more questions.[1] In the following section, charac-teristics of stayers and movers are compared and major changes in each group's composition over time are described (tables 5.1–5.5).[2]

# STAYERS AND MOVERS

## Background

*Stayer/Mover Differences.* In table 5.1 only gender is distributed similarly within the two groups, as approximately three-quarters of both stayers and movers are women. As expected, the home provider who chooses to stay is generally much older than the home seeker who is willing to move. This age difference, in turn, accounts for many other contrasts between the two groups. For example, even though both groups

TABLE 5.1

*Percent Selected Background Characteristics of Project HOME Applicants by Stayer/ Mover Status and Time, April 1982–March 1986*

| | Stayers | | | Movers | | | |
|---|---|---|---|---|---|---|---|
| | Total (N = 247) | Year 1 (N = 54) | Year 4 (N = 86) | Total (N = 369) | Year 1 (N = 29) | Year 4 (N = 199) | Difference[a] |
| **Gender** | | | | | | | |
| male | 23.7 | | | 27.6 | | | |
| female | 76.3 | no change | | 72.4 | no change | | d = +.04 ns |
| **Age** | | | | | | | |
| under 30 | 6.1 | | | 41.3 | 17.2 | 43.4 | |
| 30–49 | 13.8 | | | 30.6 | 17.2 | 34.2 | |
| 50–69 | 24.7 | | | 20.2 | 37.9 | 17.9 | |
| 70 and over | 55.5 | no change | | 7.9 | 27.6 | 4.6 | d = +.65*** |
| **Marital status** | | | | | | | |
| married | 16.0 | | | 6.1 | 7.1 | 8.8 | |
| widowed | 58.6 | | | 14.2 | 39.3 | 11.9 | |
| divorced/ | | | | | | | |
| separated | 15.2 | | | 25.3 | 21.4 | 23.7 | |
| never married | 10.2 | no change | | 54.3 | 32.1 | 55.7 | chi² = 187.*** |
| **Education** | | | | | | | |
| less than h.s. | 33.1 | | | 15.0 | | | |
| h.s. graduate | 23.3 | | | 32.1 | | | |
| some college | 21.2 | | | 31.6 | | | |
| college graduate | 22.5 | no change | | 21.3 | no change | | d = −.14** |
| **Work status[b]** | | | | | | | |
| working for pay | 24.5 | 76.9 | 15.3 | 39.0 | 70.0 | 42.7 | |
| retired | 51.0 | 0.0 | 68.2 | 8.7 | 10.0 | 7.5 | |
| unemployed | 4.5 | 0.0 | 4.7 | 35.5 | 10.0 | 36.2 | |
| other | 20.0 | 23.1 | 11.8 | 16.8 | 10.0 | 13.6 | chi² = 153.*** |

NOTE: Some percentage totals do not equal 100.0 due to rounding error.

[a]Somers' d is used for ordinal level variables and chi² for nominal level variables.

[b]Many respondents are missing data for year 1, so differences between years 1 and 4 need to be interpreted with caution.

ns p > .05
* p ≤ .05
** p ≤ .01
*** p ≤ .001

are not married, the stayers are most likely to be widowed, while the movers are most likely never to have been married. Consistent with being an older population, the stayers are also slightly less educated and much more likely to be retired than the movers, who are likely to be either working for pay or unemployed.

*The Intergenerational Emphasis.* The decision by Project HOME to expand the applicant pool from only elders to anyone interested is clearly reflected by significant increases after the first year in the proportion of mover applicants who are young, never married, and either working for pay or unemployed. During this time, the stayer pool remains relatively unchanged, with the exception of work status. The drop in employed and increase in retired suggests a less active, but not older, stayer pool in later years. This change likely reflects the program's efforts to respond to the needs of frail and disabled elders.

## Income and Health

*Stayer/Mover Differences.* In order to determine the relative economic well-being of the stayers and movers, three indicators of financial well-being were used: actual income, which has been trichotomized for statistical convenience, perception of expenses relative to living situation, and relative income satisfaction. Consistent with the background comparisons, table 5.2 shows that older stayers have significantly higher incomes and are significantly more likely to be satisfied with their income than the younger movers. At the same time, there is no overall difference in how the two groups perceive expenses relative to living situation, since only a little more than one-third of both stayers and movers believe their current living situation to be too expensive.

Health is measured by a physical capacity scale based on the number of everyday chores a person is able to do without help, and four questions asking about the applicant's perceptions regarding health. In addition, because of the large numbers of elder applicants, a scale measuring use of senior services is included. Table 5.2 shows significant differences between stayers and movers consistent with the relative ages of the two groups. For instance, while over half of the stayers are incapacitated in at least one area, less than one in ten of the movers is. Perception of vision, hearing, and mobility all show the same kinds of differences, but overall assessment of health does not show as great a difference. Finally, almost half of the stayers but only about one in twenty movers use at least one senior service.

Table 5.2
*Percent Income and Health Characteristics of Applicants by Stayer/Mover Status and Time*

| | Stayers | | | Movers | | | |
|---|---|---|---|---|---|---|---|
| | Total (N = 247) | Year 1 (N = 54) | Year 4 (N = 86) | Total (N = 369) | Year 1 (N = 29) | Year 4 (N = 199) | Difference[a] |
| Income | | | | | | | |
| under $5,000 | 15.2 | | | 53.3 | | | |
| $5,000–6,999 | 22.6 | | | 24.5 | | | |
| $7,000 plus | 62.1 | no change | | 22.3 | no change | | d = +.48*** |
| Living situation | | | | | | | |
| too expensive | 38.3 | 45.3 | 35.1 | 38.8 | 23.1 | 41.1 | |
| not too expensive | 61.7 | 54.7 | 64.9 | 61.2 | 76.9 | 58.9 | d = +.00 ns |
| Income satisfaction[b] | | | | | | | |
| not at all | 19.6 | | | 54.4 | 34.5 | 61.4 | |
| more or less | 28.2 | | | 33.0 | 34.5 | 28.6 | |
| pretty well | 52.2 | no change | | 12.6 | 31.0 | 10.0 | d = +.48*** |
| Physical capacity | | | | | | | |
| low | 59.6 | | | 7.9 | 24.1 | 2.5 | |
| high | 40.4 | no change | | 92.1 | 75.9 | 97.5 | d = +.52*** |
| Perception of vision | | | | | | | |
| poor | 27.3 | | | 4.4 | 13.8 | 2.6 | |
| good | 53.5 | | | 52.2 | 58.6 | 51.0 | |
| excellent | 19.2 | no change | | 43.4 | 27.6 | 46.4 | d = +.36*** |
| Perception of hearing | | | | | | | |
| poor | 17.8 | | | 3.3 | | | |
| good | 56.2 | | | 36.3 | | | |
| excellent | 26.0 | no change | | 60.4 | no change | | d = +.39*** |
| Perception of mobility | | | | | | | |
| poor | 36.0 | 28.3 | 43.5 | 3.0 | | | |
| good | 38.4 | 43.4 | 38.8 | 33.5 | | | |
| excellent | 25.6 | 28.3 | 17.6 | 63.5 | no change | | d = +.49*** |
| Perception of health[b] | | | | | | | |
| worse than average | 14.3 | | | 3.4 | | | |
| about average | 48.8 | | | 51.9 | | | |
| better than average | 36.9 | no change | | 44.8 | no change | | d = +.14** |
| Senior service used[c] | | | | | | | |
| none | 54.1 | 46.7 | 57.1 | 95.7 | 84.4 | 97.5 | |
| at least one | 45.9 | 53.3 | 42.9 | 4.3 | 15.6 | 2.5 | d = +.42*** |

NOTE: for [a], [b], ns, *, **, ***, see table 5.1 notes.
[c] Information is not available for year 1; year 2 is used as base year instead.

*Exchanging Money for Health Care?* When major changes in income and health among stayers and movers are considered, some patterns become evident in table 5.2. For example, later stayers have more disposable income, are less mobile, and have less experience with senior services than earlier stayers. This is consistent with background changes in work status observed, and it strongly suggests that the program increasingly began to emphasize service to frail homeowners who have the resources to pay for the kinds of services that a strict barter or rental arrangement could not induce. These frailer applicants, therefore, appear to be in a better bargaining situation than their predecessors when negotiating with potential homesharers.

On the other hand, there is a clear increase in the proportion of movers who perceive themselves as having financial problems but who also have no physical limitations. To the extent that these younger, healthier applicants have expertise and interest in providing extended services, they too are likely to be in a better bargaining situation. In any event, the "new" types of stayer and mover applicants suggest the possibility of homesharing arrangements different from those in which the stayer provides shelter in exchange for rent or services or a combination of the two. Where the stayer is quite frail but has financial resources and the mover is healthy but in financial need there is the potential for the stayer to *pay* the mover for services. These differences suggest that such clients experience different kinds of exchanges in actual matches, as will be shown in chapter 7.

## Living Situation

*Stayer/Mover Differences.* Serving as a connecting link between general background and income and health characteristics and issues directly pertaining to homesharing are questions about current home arrangements, neighborhood, and transportation. Concerning home, several clear differences emerge between stayers and movers (table 5.3): For one thing, stayers, who are more likely to be older and widowed, are much more likely to own their own homes and live alone. Also, as measured by a scale that reflects problems with upkeep, isolation, and fear of crime, stayers are almost four times as likely as movers to be concerned about at least two of these problems.

With respect to neighborhood, while stayers are more likely to have friends in the neighborhood, the differences between stayers and movers are weak. Perception of neighborhood problems, as measured by a two-item scale focusing on location and on neighborhood issues in general, shows a larger difference between the more satisfied stayers and the less satisfied movers.

Transportation issues distinguish stayers and movers with respect to means but not ends: On the one hand, only a little over one-half of the stayers can drive a car without help, while four-fifths of the movers can. On the other hand, stayers appear to be at no disadvantage, because at

TABLE 5.3

*Percent Living Situation Characteristics of Applicants by Stayer/Mover Status and Time*

| | Stayers | | | Movers | | | |
|---|---|---|---|---|---|---|---|
| | Total (N = 247) | Year 1 (N = 54) | Year 4 (N = 86) | Total (N = 369) | Year 1 (N = 29) | Year 4 (N = 199) | Difference[a] |
| Home status | | | | | | | |
| rent | 28.6 | 18.9 | 34.9 | 88.8 | | | |
| own | 71.4 | 81.1 | 65.1 | 11.2 | no change | | $d = +.60$*** |
| Home population | | | | | | | |
| by self | 55.2 | 69.2 | 56.0 | 26.3 | 34.5 | 19.5 | |
| with other(s) | 44.8 | 30.8 | 44.0 | 73.7 | 65.5 | 80.5 | $d = -.29$*** |
| Housing problems[b] | | | | | | | |
| 2 or 3 prob. | 44.4 | 57.7 | 41.1 | 11.5 | | | |
| 1 problem | 34.5 | 32.7 | 35.6 | 31.4 | | | |
| no problems | 21.1 | 9.6 | 23.3 | 57.1 | no change | | $d = -.46$*** |
| Friends in neighborhood[b] | | | | | | | |
| none | 16.2 | | | 19.6 | | | |
| a few | 40.9 | | | 41.3 | | | |
| most | 27.8 | | | 34.3 | | | |
| all | 15.2 | no change | | 4.8 | no change | | $d = +.09$* |
| Neighborhood problems[b] | | | | | | | |
| 1 or 2 prob. | 11.4 | 17.0 | 5.5 | 33.0 | | | |
| no problems | 88.6 | 83.0 | 94.5 | 67.0 | no change | | $d = +.22$*** |
| Drive car | | | | | | | |
| no; need help | 56.7 | | | 18.4 | 41.4 | 7.1 | |
| yes, w/o help | 43.3 | no change | | 81.6 | 58.6 | 92.9 | $d = -.38$*** |
| Transportation problems[b] | | | | | | | |
| always | 6.9 | | | 2.5 | 6.9 | 1.9 | |
| often | 8.4 | | | 6.5 | 13.8 | 6.4 | |
| sometimes | 26.2 | | | 38.4 | 34.5 | 33.8 | |
| never | 58.4 | no change | | 52.6 | 44.8 | 58.0 | $d = +.02$ ns |

NOTE: for [a,b], ns, *, **, ***, see table 5.1 notes.

least half of them report no problem in getting to where they want to go —about the same proportion as movers.

*Home, Neighborhood and the Resources to Cope.* For reasons that can be attributed only partially to background, income, and health profile changes, Project HOME applicants during the fourth year of the program appear to have fewer problems related to home and neighborhood than first-year applicants. For stayers, it may be that the increased number of renters and applicants living with others enhances support systems to counter housing, neighborhood, and transportation problems. This is especially likely in the case of transportation: While over half the stayers can't drive a car, only one in seven always or often has transportation problems. Clearly, others—whether it is family or friends—are providing transportation assistance to some extent.

For movers, the increases in drivers and those living with others and the decrease in transportation problems are probably due directly to the influx of younger applicants after the first year. Younger renters are more likely to be living with roommates (this is especially true of students) and to have access to a vehicle or be able to walk to their destinations. Overall, while differences in home, neighborhood, and transportation distinguish stayers from movers, the trend over time within both groups is toward individuals who are living with others. This suggests the possibility that stayers and movers during the fourth year are much more likely than their predecessors to have individuals to whom they can turn for help. The importance of such potential support groups for applicants who do get matched will be explored in greater detail in chapters 7 and 8.

## Homesharing Profiles

*Stayer/Mover Differences.* In this section and the next, issues directly related to homesharing are considered. Table 5.4 describes lifestyles, attitudes toward sharer's lifestyles, and a series of questions pertaining to homesharing experiences. Initially, it was expected that homesharing profiles would be somewhat similar between the two groups because of their mutual interest in homesharing.

With respect to lifestyle, there are, in fact, some small but significant differences between stayers and movers: Stayers are less likely to smoke and drink alcohol but more likely to own pets and have overnight company. The largest of these differences is in pet ownership, which makes sense since most movers tend to be renters and renters are often not allowed pets.

Attitudes toward sharer's lifestyle show even larger differences between the two groups. When it comes to considering a sharer who smokes, drinks alcohol, has a pet, or has overnight company, two-thirds of the stayers object to anyone having two or more of these traits, while only about one sixth of the movers so object. Stayers are also more likely to object to a sharer who uses a cane, walker, or wheelchair and sharing with students or children, and more likely to give a gender preference for sharer. These differences are consistent with the fact that stayers are offering space in *their own* home to a stranger.

Finally, stayers and movers are distinguishable on the basis of their previous homesharing experiences and their expectations for future homesharing. While a majority in each group has had homesharing experience, movers have had more. Not unrelated to experience, stayers are

TABLE 5.4

*Percent Homesharing Profiles for Applicants by Stayer/Mover Status and Time*

| | Stayers | | | Movers | | | |
|---|---|---|---|---|---|---|---|
| | Total (N = 247) | Year 1 (N = 54) | Year 4 (N = 86) | Total (N = 369) | Year 1 (N = 29) | Year 4 (N = 199) | Difference[a] |
| **Lifestyle** | | | | | | | |
| smokes | 24.0 | 31.5 | 18.8 | 31.9 | no change | | d = −.08* |
| drinks | 34.8 | no change | | 45.5 | no change | | d = −.11** |
| owns pet(s) | 40.2 | no change | | 17.9 | no change | | d = +.22*** |
| has overnight company | 50.2 | 29.6 | 61.9 | 40.6 | 13.8 | 42.4 | d = +.10*** |
| **Attitude toward sharer's lifestyle[b]** | | | | | | | |
| objects to ≥ 2 | 66.0 | | | 17.2 | | | |
| objects only to 1 | 22.5 | | | 29.6 | | | |
| objects to none | 11.5 | no change | | 53.2 | no change | | d = −.57*** |
| **Attitude toward disabled sharer** | | | | | | | |
| objects to any | 49.1 | | | 7.5 | | | |
| distinguishes | 33.8 | | | 11.6 | | | |
| objects to none | 17.1 | no change | | 80.9 | no change | | d = −.67*** |
| **Attitude toward sharing with student/children[b,c]** | | | | | | | |
| objects to both | 51.6 | | | 33.9 | 25.6 | 42.7 | |
| objects to 1 | 36.5 | | | 26.8 | 25.6 | 27.4 | |
| objects to neither | 11.9 | no change | | 39.3 | 48.8 | 29.9 | d = −.29*** |
| **Gender preference of sharer** | | | | | | | |
| gender matters | 77.7 | | | 39.9 | 50.0 | 35.4 | |
| gender doesn't matter | 22.3 | no change | | 60.1 | 50.0 | 64.6 | d = −.38*** |
| **Experience sharing[c]** | | | | | | | |
| no | 43.3 | 38.2 | 48.8 | 28.1 | 38.3 | 25.8 | |
| yes | 56.7 | 61.8 | 51.2 | 71.9 | 61.7 | 74.2 | d = −.15*** |
| **How long want to homeshare[b,c]** | | | | | | | |
| finite period | 31.9 | 37.0 | 23.7 | 64.7 | | | |
| infinitely | 68.1 | 63.0 | 76.3 | 35.3 | no change | | d = +.33*** |
| **Employing other means to find homesharer[b,c]** | | | | | | | |
| no | 65.4 | 62.5 | 81.4 | 65.6 | | | |
| yes | 34.6 | 37.5 | 18.6 | 34.4 | no change | | d = +.00 ns |

NOTE: for [a],[b], ns, *, **, ***, see table 5.1 notes.

   [c] See table 5.2 note.

much more likely to want their homesharing arrangement to be indefinite or permanent. After all, the vast majority are in their own or a relative's home and not in some transition dwelling, so they are not as mobile as younger mover applicants—many of whom in the program's fourth year are students (a particularly transient group).

*Restrictive Stayers and Flexible Movers?* Table 5.4 shows some strong differences between movers and stayers that over time either remain relatively constant or increase in magnitude. Of particular importance is the difference in flexibility, as represented by answers to questions concerning the lifestyle, disability, age, and gender of one's potential sharer: Stayers are *much* more restrictive. Again, one is looking at people who live in their own home and who do not want to relinquish any more authority than is absolutely necessary.

Equally noteworthy are the differences in homesharing experience and expectation concerning duration of prospective matches: Movers, with more experience in homesharing and also answering with respect to the unknown (place as well as sharer), are significantly more likely than stayers to specify a time limit on possible homesharing arrangements. In addition, many movers are in a period of transition: Either they are looking for inexpensive lodging as they go through some crisis in their life or as they attend school or (as is the case with those who would provide services for income) they are looking for a "job" that will be of finite duration (see Jaffe's analysis of young sharer applicants' status passages [1989b:42ff.]).

Finally, a majority of both groups have come to Project HOME apparently as a last resort, because they are employing no other means of finding homesharers. Given the critical situation in which many applicants find themselves, the various restrictions stayers place on potential arrangements, and the limited homesharing experiences of many of the stayers, what is it that applicants expect to give to and get from each other?

## Homesharing Expectations

*Stayer/Mover Differences.* Some partial answers are in table 5.5, which, consistent with the principle of social exchange, shows stayers and movers to complement one another in critical areas related to homesharing expectations. For example, stayers are much more likely to need and movers much more likely to provide housework, laundry, and cooking services (household service scale) and nursing and health care services (nursing service scale). Nevertheless, based on an examination of the percentages in the "need," "cooperate," and "provide" categories for each group, it appears that stayers and movers are each composed of two subgroups: stayers who need services and stayers who don't but also won't provide any, and movers who are willing to provide services and movers who won't provide but also don't need services. The key distinctions regarding services will be explored in more detail in the following sections.

The remaining items listed in table 5.5 are a combination of scales

TABLE 5.5
Percent Homesharing Expectations for Applicants by Stayer/Mover Status and Time

| | Stayers | | | Movers | | | |
|---|---|---|---|---|---|---|---|
| | Total (N = 247) | Year 1 (N = 54) | Year 4 (N = 86) | Total (N = 369) | Year 1 (N = 29) | Year 4 (N = 199) | Difference[a] |
| Household services[c] | | | | | | | |
| need | 57.5 | | | 6.3 | 25.5 | 4.1 | |
| cooperate | 35.9 | | | 28.1 | 25.5 | 24.0 | |
| provide | 6.6 | no change | | 65.6 | 48.9 | 71.9 | d = −.73*** |
| Nursing services[c] | | | | | | | |
| need | 42.0 | 37.9 | 49.4 | 3.4 | 6.5 | 3.6 | |
| cooperate | 48.9 | 55.2 | 44.4 | 41.6 | 67.4 | 32.5 | |
| provide | 9.2 | 6.9 | 6.2 | 55.0 | 26.1 | 63.9 | d = −.62*** |
| Importance of money matters[b] | | | | | | | |
| low | 40.5 | 28.0 | 45.2 | 4.8 | | | |
| medium | 39.0 | 48.0 | 37.1 | 58.6 | | | |
| high | 20.5 | 24.0 | 17.7 | 36.6 | no change | | d = −.38*** |
| Importance of helping each other | | | | | | | |
| low | 7.5 | | | 32.6 | 10.3 | 36.2 | |
| medium | 31.9 | | | 46.4 | 48.3 | 47.6 | |
| high | 60.6 | no change | | 21.0 | 41.4 | 16.2 | d = +.46*** |
| Importance of sharing companionship | | | | | | | |
| low | 12.9 | 7.5 | 13.0 | 13.5 | | | |
| medium | 26.7 | 13.2 | 27.3 | 30.4 | | | |
| high | 60.3 | 79.2 | 59.7 | 56.1 | no change | | d = +.04 ns |
| Compatability concerns | | | | | | | |
| low | 29.9 | 19.6 | 32.9 | 29.9 | 6.9 | 35.5 | |
| medium | 56.7 | 66.7 | 53.4 | 53.0 | 58.6 | 51.1 | |
| high | 13.4 | 13.7 | 13.7 | 17.1 | 34.5 | 13.4 | d = −.03 ns |
| Giving more than getting concerns | | | | | | | |
| low | 62.6 | 48.0 | 63.3 | 62.3 | 41.4 | 70.2 | |
| medium | 17.2 | 20.0 | 20.0 | 25.5 | 48.3 | 18.6 | |
| high | 20.2 | 32.0 | 16.7 | 12.2 | 10.3 | 11.2 | d = +.03 ns |
| Keeping own things concerns[b] | | | | | | | |
| low | 59.4 | 46.9 | 66.1 | 72.0 | | | |
| medium | 13.7 | 10.2 | 15.3 | 14.9 | | | |
| high | 26.9 | 42.9 | 18.6 | 13.1 | no change | | d = +.15*** |
| Importance of sharing driving | | | | | | | |
| low | 51.8 | | | 66.5 | 55.6 | 71.4 | |
| medium | 22.6 | | | 20.6 | 25.9 | 15.9 | |
| high | 25.7 | no change | | 12.9 | 18.5 | 12.7 | d = +.17*** |

NOTE: for [a], [b], ns, *, **, ***, see table 5.1 notes.
[c] See table 5.2 note.

and single questions that speak to homesharing issues the applicants feel are important or about which they have serious concerns. The items that most distinguish stayers and movers involve helping one another, which stayers emphasize, and money, which movers emphasize. Despite the complementarity between stayers and movers regarding services, this differential emphasis each group places on finances and helping one another suggests potential conflicts in matches if there is not agreement on what those services are worth.

Interestingly, emphases on companionship, compatibility, and being taken advantage of are equally shared by both groups. Thus, while each group may emphasize different aspects of potential homesharing arrangements (money vs. helping one another), substantial segments of both stayers and movers appear to understand the importance of being compatible with one's sharer.

*The Evolution of New Homesharing Forms.* Changes over the first four years of the program in homesharing expectations highlight the increased diversity of both stayers and movers. Basically, these changes are directly attributable to the increase in the numbers of frail stayers and caregiver movers.

Among stayers, there are two kinds of changes: Later applicants are more task-oriented and less concerned with the sorts of problems that tend to creep into interpersonal relationships. For example, consistent with the deteriorating mobility noted in table 5.2, later stayers are somewhat more likely to require nursing services. At the same time, they are less likely to stress the importance of money and companionship and are less concerned over compatibility, giving more than getting, and keeping one's own things than are early stayers. The largest change is in the area of keeping one's own things, as the percent highly concerned drops by one half. The increasing numbers of frail homeowners are apparently willing to compromise more in order to receive services that will allow them to remain at home.

Among movers, three kinds of changes occur: First, and most dramatic, is the increase in the proportion of movers who are willing to provide both household and nursing services. Second, later movers are also much less likely than their earlier counterparts to stress the importance of helping each other and of sharing driving. At first glance, this might appear to contradict the increase in the proportion of movers willing to provide services. On the other hand, it is likely that the two trends together suggest an increase in the number of movers who expect to provide services for their sharers, not in exchange for other services the sharer will provide, but rather for money, given the financial concerns voiced by later movers in table 5.2. Finally, as in the case of stayers, later movers are also less likely to be concerned about compatibility and giving more than getting.

The tendencies for stayers and movers alike to become less concerned over time with interpersonal compatibility and to emphasize more the need for (stayers) or willingness to provide (movers) services are consistent with the two kinds of homesharing arrangements described in chapter 2. Both involve key kinds of social exchanges, as will be seen in chapter 7, but differ as to the kind of resources exchanged. The first, more traditional, one is represented by applicants who expect to cooperate in an exchange of services, with the mover perhaps also paying rent or partial rent. Within this arrangement, of course, there is a wide range of relationships possible: As described in chapter 1, both material and emotional space may be shared to varying degrees, so that one arrangement may involve nothing more than a renter paying for a room, while another may represent a truly cooperative homesharing in which sharers spend time together cooking, gardening, talking, etc., and share chores with the mover paying token or no rent.

The second kind of homesharing arrangement, indicated especially by the data in table 5.5 but also by the income and health changes observed from table 5.2, appears to be characterized by the situation in which the healthy and able mover provides particular services for the frail stayer. Given the relative financial standing of the two groups, especially after the program's first two years, it is unlikely that the mover also pays rent or partial rent; rather, it is more likely that the stayer will pay something for those services.

## Who Are Project HOME's Clients?

The empirical evidence on homesharing applicants from the first four years of Project HOME's existence suggest two generalizations about the characteristics of the applicant pool. First, of course, the overall picture of stayers and movers is quite different in fundamental ways: The former group is older, more likely to be in frail health but also more likely to be better off financially and more satisfied with their finances than is the latter group. Furthermore, stayers are more likely to be living alone and in their own home and, not surprisingly, more concerned with problems centered around the home. Finally, stayers are more restrictive regarding the kinds of people they will let into their home, much more in need of services, and much more likely to emphasize sharers helping one another (while movers stress money issues).

These clear distinctions between stayers notwithstanding, the data also show sufficiently large changes over time in the makeup of both the stayer and the mover pools of applicants to suggest the need to distinguish different types of stayers and movers. For example, the stayer pool becomes, on average, frailer but less concerned with living expenses and more concerned with receiving nursing services between years one and four. The mover pool shows even greater change, starting with the critical decision by the second director to open the doors to nonelderly applicants. Movers, by year four, are generally more likely to be younger and never married than early mover applicants. In addition, later movers are more concerned about finances but in better health, less restrictive regarding potential sharers, and more willing to provide both household and nursing services than are early movers. This distinction concerning services is fundamental to understanding the four different kinds of applicants to Project HOME.

## FOUR TYPES OF APPLICANTS

Altogether, these basic differences between stayers and movers and the change over time in the make-up of each group closely relate to two major organizational initiatives and program responses described in the previous three chapters. Directly after assuming leadership of the program at the beginning of its second year, the new director opened applications to nonelders, creating an influx of younger, healthier, more mobile, but still financially poor movers. During the second and third years of the program, the director and her staff, seeing the increasingly obvious needs of stayers who required both a homesharer and caregiver, began to seek out movers who would be willing to provide not only a presence but also expanded services for frail homeowners.

As a result, it is useful to distinguish *kinds* of stayers and *kinds* of movers. The central distinctions used by Project HOME are whether services are provided by the mover for the stayer and whether the mover receives payment for those services. In cases where services are provided by the mover and money goes from the stayer to the mover, the arrangement is labeled a caregiving or personal care companion one; all other cases are labeled traditional homesharing.[3] Therefore, from now on, stayers and movers will be subdivided into traditional homesharer applicants and what will be called caregiving or personal care companion (PCC) applicants, distinguishing four kinds of applicants (tables 5.6–5.10). Rather than proceed through a description of differences for each kind of applicant by characteristic, however, the following discussion will summarize the major differences among the subgroups for all five types of characteristics at once.[4]

TABLE 5.6
Background Characteristics By Four Types of Applicants

| | Providers (N = 146) | Employers (N = 101) | Lodgers (N = 204) | Caregivers (N = 165) | Differences[a] |
|---|---|---|---|---|---|
| Gender | | | | | |
| male | 21.9 | 26.3 | 37.3 | 15.8 | |
| female | 78.1 | 73.7 | 62.7 | 84.2 | ••• |
| Age | | | | | |
| under 30 | 6.2 | 5.9 | 41.9 | 40.5 | |
| 30–49 | 18.5 | 6.9 | 30.5 | 30.7 | |
| 50–69 | 28.1 | 19.8 | 17.2 | 23.9 | |
| 70 and over | 47.3 | 67.3 | 10.3 | 4.9 | ••• |
| Marital status | | | | | |
| married | 13.9 | 19.0 | 5.4 | 7.0 | |
| widowed | 56.9 | 61.0 | 14.9 | 13.4 | |
| divorced, separated | 21.5 | 6.0 | 24.3 | 26.8 | |
| never married | 7.6 | 14.0 | 55.4 | 52.9 | ••• |
| Education | | | | | |
| less than h.s. | 30.3 | 37.2 | 14.6 | 15.4 | |
| h.s. graduate | 21.1 | 26.6 | 25.1 | 40.7 | |
| some college | 23.2 | 18.1 | 35.7 | 26.5 | |
| college graduate | 25.4 | 18.1 | 24.6 | 17.3 | ••• |
| Work status | | | | | |
| working for pay | 37.1 | 10.5 | 44.6 | 32.5 | |
| retired | 34.3 | 69.5 | 10.9 | 6.2 | |
| unemployed | 3.8 | 5.3 | 23.4 | 49.4 | |
| other | 24.8 | 14.7 | 21.2 | 11.7 | ••• |

NOTE: Some percentage totals do not equal 100.0 due to rounding error.
[a] Chi$^2$ test used to contrast four types of applicants.

ns p > .05
• p ≤ .05
•• p ≤ .01
••• p ≤ .001

## (Home) Providers: Stayers Who Want to Share

According to Project HOME staff, the prototypic stayer was initially envisaged to be an elderly homeowner, probably widowed, who needed someone to provide companionship, some help around the house, and some small payment in exchange for a place to live in a kind of family-like setting. The traditional stayer applicant comes closest to this original ideal. From now on, consistent with a major characteristic of this group, they will be referred to as "home providers" or more simply "providers."

Based on qualities that characterize the majority of them, the following profile of home providers emerges: They are generally likely to be females, at least fifty years old, widowed, with no more than a high school degree, and either working for pay or retired. Further, most have incomes in excess of $7,000, no physical impairment in everyday activities, and

TABLE 5.7
*Income and Health Characteristics By Four Types of Applicants*

|  | Providers (N = 146) | Employers (N = 101) | Lodgers (N = 204) | Caregivers (N = 165) | Differences[a] |
|---|---|---|---|---|---|
| Income |  |  |  |  |  |
| under $5,000 | 17.4 | 12.1 | 46.5 | 61.7 |  |
| $5,000–6,999 | 22.2 | 23.2 | 25.2 | 23.5 |  |
| $7,000 plus | 60.4 | 64.6 | 28.2 | 14.8 | ••• |
| Living situation |  |  |  |  |  |
| too expensive | 49.0 | 20.7 | 37.2 | 40.7 |  |
| not too expensive | 51.0 | 79.3 | 62.8 | 59.3 | ••• |
| Income satisfaction |  |  |  |  |  |
| not at all | 20.6 | 17.8 | 44.3 | 66.2 |  |
| more or less | 30.9 | 23.3 | 38.9 | 26.1 |  |
| pretty well | 48.5 | 58.9 | 16.8 | 7.7 | ••• |
| Physical capacity |  |  |  |  |  |
| low | 44.2 | 83.3 | 11.8 | 3.1 |  |
| high | 55.8 | 16.7 | 88.2 | 96.1 | ••• |
| Perception of vision |  |  |  |  |  |
| poor | 23.4 | 33.0 | 6.0 | 2.4 |  |
| good | 52.4 | 55.0 | 51.5 | 53.0 |  |
| excellent | 24.1 | 12.0 | 42.5 | 44.5 | ••• |
| Perception of hearing |  |  |  |  |  |
| poor | 11.9 | 26.3 | 4.0 | 2.4 |  |
| good | 53.8 | 59.6 | 36.5 | 36.0 |  |
| excellent | 34.3 | 14.1 | 59.5 | 61.6 | ••• |
| Perception of mobility |  |  |  |  |  |
| poor | 23.6 | 54.1 | 4.0 | 1.8 |  |
| good | 39.6 | 36.7 | 32.3 | 35.0 |  |
| excellent | 36.8 | 9.2 | 63.7 | 63.2 | ••• |
| Perception of health |  |  |  |  |  |
| below average | 13.8 | 15.2 | 5.7 | 0.7 |  |
| average | 47.1 | 51.9 | 49.4 | 54.7 |  |
| above average | 39.1 | 32.9 | 44.8 | 44.7 | ••• |
| Senior service used |  |  |  |  |  |
| none | 65.1 | 43.8 | 94.9 | 96.7 |  |
| at least one | 34.9 | 56.2 | 5.1 | 3.3 | ••• |

NOTE: for [a], ns, •, ••, •••, see table 5.6 notes.

do not use senior services. Most own their own homes, live alone, and perceive no neighborhood problems; in addition, the majority can drive without help and never have transportation problems.

Regarding homesharing, the vast majority are nonsmokers, and they would restrict their choice of sharers in terms of lifestyle, disability, students or children, and gender; over half have shared before, want an indefinite or permanent homesharing arrangement, and are seeking homesharers only through Project HOME. Most provider applicants wish to do their own household and nursing services or cooperate with their

TABLE 5.8
Living Situation Characteristics By Four Types of Applicants

| | Providers (N = 146) | Employers (N = 101) | Lodgers (N = 204) | Caregivers (N = 165) | Differences[a] |
|---|---|---|---|---|---|
| Home status | | | | | |
| rent | 23.6 | 35.6 | 90.6 | 86.5 | |
| own | 76.4 | 64.4 | 9.4 | 13.5 | ••• |
| Home population | | | | | |
| by self | 54.9 | 55.7 | 29.5 | 22.4 | |
| with other(s) | 45.1 | 44.3 | 70.5 | 77.6 | ••• |
| Housing problems | | | | | |
| 2 or 3 problems | 43.2 | 46.4 | 15.3 | 6.9 | |
| 1 problem | 34.5 | 34.5 | 29.9 | 33.1 | |
| no problems | 22.3 | 19.0 | 54.8 | 60.0 | ••• |
| Friends in neighborhood | | | | | |
| none | 16.4 | 15.7 | 20.0 | 19.0 | |
| a few | 38.3 | 45.7 | 44.0 | 38.0 | |
| most | 28.1 | 27.1 | 32.0 | 37.2 | |
| all | 17.2 | 11.4 | 4.0 | 5.8 | •• |
| Neighborhood problems | | | | | |
| 1 or 2 problems | 10.6 | 12.8 | 34.8 | 30.8 | |
| no problems | 89.4 | 87.2 | 65.2 | 69.2 | ••• |
| Drive car | | | | | |
| no; need help | 40.6 | 81.1 | 20.2 | 16.0 | |
| Yes, w/o help | 59.4 | 18.9 | 79.8 | 84.0 | ••• |
| Transportation problems | | | | | |
| always | 5.4 | 9.6 | 2.8 | 2.1 | |
| often | 7.0 | 11.0 | 9.0 | 3.4 | |
| sometimes | 24.8 | 28.8 | 39.5 | 37.0 | |
| never | 62.8 | 50.7 | 48.6 | 57.5 | ••• |

NOTE: for [a], ns, •, ••, •••, see table 5.6 notes.

sharer, and they place great importance on helping each other and sharing companionship. At the same time, they give low priority to concerns over giving more than getting and keeping one's own things and to the importance of sharing driving.

The emerging picture portrays home providers as older women in reasonably good health who want to share materially and interpersonally with someone for an indefinite period of time. In contrast to the other three groups, they generally are seeking an arrangement in which service delivery is either a two-way street or "closed to traffic" (both sharers go their own way, taking care of their own needs).

## Lodgers: Movers Who Want to Share

Movers who want to homeshare in the prototypic arrangement tend to be looking primarily for a place to stay in exchange for providing some

TABLE 5.9

*Homesharing Profiles By Four Types of Applicants*

| | Providers (N = 146) | Employers (N = 101) | Lodgers (N = 204) | Caregivers (N = 165) | Differences[a] |
|---|---|---|---|---|---|
| Lifestyle | | | | | |
| smokes | 29.5 | 16.0 | 26.5 | 38.2 | ••• |
| drinks | 40.7 | 26.3 | 47.7 | 42.7 | ••• |
| owns pet(s) | 47.3 | 29.6 | 15.9 | 20.4 | ••• |
| has overnight company | 48.6 | 52.6 | 44.9 | 35.1 | ••• |
| Attitude toward sharer's lifestyle; objects to: | | | | | |
| at least 2 | 66.4 | 65.5 | 17.2 | 17.2 | |
| only to 1 | 22.1 | 23.0 | 33.1 | 25.5 | |
| none | 11.5 | 11.5 | 49.7 | 57.2 | ••• |
| Attitude toward disabled sharer | | | | | |
| objects to any | 46.4 | 53.6 | 8.3 | 6.5 | |
| distinguishes | 39.9 | 23.8 | 14.1 | 8.5 | |
| objects to none | 13.8 | 22.6 | 77.6 | 85.0 | ••• |
| Attitude toward sharing with student/children; objects to: | | | | | |
| both | 46.4 | 57.3 | 28.9 | 39.8 | |
| 1 | 45.2 | 26.7 | 29.6 | 23.4 | |
| neither | 8.3 | 16.0 | 41.4 | 36.7 | ••• |
| Gender preference of sharer | | | | | |
| matters | 75.5 | 80.8 | 39.2 | 40.7 | |
| doesn't matter | 24.5 | 19.2 | 60.8 | 59.3 | ••• |
| Experience sharing | | | | | |
| no | 41.8 | 44.9 | 31.8 | 23.9 | |
| yes | 58.2 | 55.1 | 68.2 | 76.1 | ••• |
| How long want to homeshare | | | | | |
| finite period | 35.0 | 28.8 | 67.3 | 61.7 | |
| infinitely | 65.0 | 71.3 | 32.7 | 38.3 | ••• |
| Employing other means to find homesharer | | | | | |
| no | 59.3 | 72.0 | 61.1 | 71.2 | |
| yes | 40.7 | 28.0 | 38.9 | 28.8 | ns |

NOTE: for [a], ns, •, ••, •••, see table 5.6 notes.

combination of money and services. While many of these applicants are more than paying lodgers, the term "lodger" will be used to emphasize the exchange of money for housing.

The majority of lodgers are female, under fifty years old (almost half are under thirty), have never been married, and are in college, have had some college, or have graduated from college; almost half of them are working for pay. Most lodgers are earning less than $7,000 but don't see their current living situation as too expensive; the majority also have no physical limitations, perceive their hearing and mobility to be excellent, and, given their age and health, do not use senior services. The vast majority of lodgers currently rent and live with at least one other person, and most perceive no problems in housing or neighborhood, and can drive without help.

TABLE 5.10

*Homesharing Expectations By Four Types of Applicants*

| | Providers (N = 146) | Employers (N = 101) | Lodgers (N = 204) | Caregivers (N = 165) | Differences[a] |
|---|---|---|---|---|---|
| Household services | | | | | |
| need | 39.6 | 75.6 | 9.7 | 2.6 | |
| cooperate | 52.7 | 18.9 | 38.6 | 16.1 | |
| provide | 7.7 | 5.6 | 51.7 | 81.3 | ••• |
| Nursing services | | | | | |
| need | 23.5 | 59.6 | 4.2 | 2.6 | |
| cooperate | 64.7 | 33.7 | 54.2 | 27.9 | |
| provide | 11.8 | 6.7 | 41.7 | 69.5 | ••• |
| Importance of money matters | | | | | |
| low | 26.2 | 65.3 | 5.2 | 4.2 | |
| medium | 44.6 | 29.3 | 59.7 | 57.0 | |
| high | 29.2 | 5.3 | 35.1 | 38.7 | ••• |
| Importance of helping each other | | | | | |
| low | 10.9 | 2.2 | 27.5 | 39.0 | |
| medium | 38.0 | 22.5 | 47.7 | 44.8 | |
| high | 51.1 | 75.3 | 24.9 | 16.2 | ••• |
| Importance of sharing companionship | | | | | |
| low | 14.1 | 11.1 | 15.8 | 10.7 | |
| medium | 26.8 | 26.7 | 31.1 | 29.6 | |
| high | 59.2 | 62.2 | 53.1 | 59.7 | ns |
| Compatability concerns | | | | | |
| low | 28.7 | 31.8 | 26.2 | 34.6 | |
| medium | 56.6 | 56.8 | 54.9 | 50.6 | |
| high | 14.7 | 11.4 | 19.0 | 14.7 | ns |
| Giving more than getting concerns | | | | | |
| low | 56.9 | 72.6 | 54.6 | 72.0 | |
| medium | 16.9 | 17.8 | 30.1 | 19.7 | |
| high | 26.2 | 9.6 | 15.3 | 8.3 | ••• |
| Keeping own things concerns | | | | | |
| low | 55.8 | 64.9 | 71.1 | 73.1 | |
| medium | 12.5 | 15.6 | 14.4 | 15.4 | |
| high | 31.7 | 19.5 | 14.4 | 11.5 | ••• |
| Importance of sharing driving | | | | | |
| low | 56.4 | 44.2 | 66.8 | 66.0 | |
| medium | 25.0 | 18.6 | 20.7 | 20.5 | |
| high | 18.6 | 37.2 | 12.4 | 13.5 | ••• |

NOTE: for [a], ns, •, ••, •••, see table 5.6 notes.

A great majority do not smoke or own pets, and almost half have no objection to sharing with smokers, drinkers, pet owners, or providers who have overnight guests. Most are willing to share with someone whose mobility is impaired and requires crutches, walker, or wheelchair and don't care whether their sharer is male or female. Most have had experience sharing, want a limited homesharing arrangement, and are seeking a homesharer only through Project HOME. Finally, most lodgers are willing to provide some household services but prefer to cooperate on nursing or let each sharer be responsible for her or his own personal care needs; most place high importance on sharing companionship and are not concerned about giving more than getting or keeping one's own things; and most place a low priority on shared driving.

The typical lodger applicant, therefore, tends to be a young working or unemployed female with low income but in very good health who wants to share materially and interpersonally—for a limited period of time.

Lodger applicants differ significantly from the other three groups in two major background characteristics: First, while likely to be female, their ranks contain a significantly high minority of males, and, second, lodgers include a larger proportion of college students and college graduates than any of the other groups. Based only on the gender and education mix of the lodgers, one is tempted to argue that lodger applicants generally are characterized by the kinds of needs most young people in their position exhibit: a place to stay which costs little and a sharing arrangement with few strings attached.

## Employers: Stayers Who Need Caregiver Services

Differing in certain key respects from traditional home providers are those stayers who offer both a place to stay and a stipend in exchange for services from their homesharer; because they are paying for services received, they will be designated as employers or service recipients.

Based on their most significant characteristics, the following profile applies generally to these personal care companion employers: They are females who are at least seventy years of age and widowed, have had no more than a high school degree, and have retired from work. Additionally, most have an income over $7,000, see their living situation expenses as reasonable and are pretty well satisfied with their income; however, they are hampered in doing one or more daily activities and perceive their mobility to be poor, probably accounting for their greater likelihood of using one or more senior services. Most own their own homes and live by themselves and tend to have one or more housing problems but no neighborhood problems. While the vast majority cannot drive a car or need help to do so, half never have transportation problems.

The vast majority of employers do not smoke, drink alcohol, or own pets; a little over half do have overnight company. Most have serious objections to lifestyle incompatibilities, disabled sharers, and students or children, and for most of them gender of sharer does matter; most have shared before, want an indefinite or permanent arrangement, and are dependent only on Project HOME for finding a sharer.

The majority of employers need household and nursing services, and place a low priority on money matters but a high one on helping each other and sharing companionship. Finally, most are not concerned over giving more than getting and keeping one's own things.

Typically, therefore, applicants in need of and willing to pay for caregiver services are women in their seventies, satisfied with their income but in frail health, and who need both household and nursing services for an indefinite period.

Most strikingly different about employers is their age, with two-thirds being seventy or over; by contrast, slightly less than half of the providers are seventy or older. Related to their age, this group that wishes to employ caregivers in their own home is out of the work force, experiencing health problems, and needing household and (to a lesser extent) nursing services. In counterpoint to their frail health, these stayer applicants, while not appearing to have any more money than providers, nevertheless are significantly less concerned over present living expenses and in general more satisfied with their income than any of the other applicant groups.

While not traditional in the sense of early Project HOME staff expectations about who their stayer clients would be, employers nevertheless represent traditional bartering in every respect, given that they are willing to barter money and a place to stay in exchange for a caregiver's help in retaining a degree of independence.

## Caregivers: Movers Who Are Willing to Provide Caregiving

The last group of applicants are movers who offer to provide care for their sharers. Since caregiving is preeminent in their profile, they will be labeled as caregivers. Most caregivers are female, under fifty (although one-quarter are between fifty and sixty-nine), have a high school degree or less, and are working for pay or unemployed. About two-thirds have incomes below $5,000 and are dissatisfied with their income, but over half aren't concerned with their living expenses. Regarding health, almost all have no physical limitations, and most perceive their hearing and mobility to be excellent; almost none use senior services. Most caregiver applicants are renters and live with at least one other person.

The majority perceive no housing or neighborhood problems, drive without help and never have transportation problems.

With respect to homesharing issues, most caregivers do not smoke, drink alcohol, or have pets or overnight company. The majority are willing to share with people who do smoke, drink, etc., and who are disabled and require help in getting around, and most caregiver applicants do not care about their sharer's gender. Similar to lodger applicants, caregivers have homeshared before, want to share for a limited time, and are seeking a sharer only through Project HOME. Consistent with their status, caregiver applicants are generally willing to provide household and nursing services. Also, they place a high priority on sharing companionship, have little concern over giving more than getting and keeping one's own things, and deemphasize the importance of sharing driving.

In summary, caregiver applicants appear to be women covering a wide range of ages, having a low income with which they are not satisfied, and willing to provide both household and nursing services in a limited term arrangement.

These movers who say they are willing to provide services for a fee and a place to live are also distinguishable from the other three groups in a variety of ways. One has to do with finances: They are significantly more likely than any of the other groups of applicants to be unemployed and earn less than $5,000 per year. As a result, they not surprisingly are most likely to be dissatisfied with their income.

While very similar to lodgers in living situation characteristics, caregivers do differ on some homesharing issues—not only from lodgers but also from both types of stayers. For example, they are least likely to have overnight company and to emphasize the importance of homesharers' helping each other. Most significant, of course, is that caregivers are the group most willing to provide both household and nursing services for their sharer. Certainly in terms of complementarity of needs and abilities, employers and caregivers appear to be made for each other.

This chapter has been concerned with describing the wide range of applicants to Project HOME during the program's critical first four years. Initially, distinctions were drawn between applicants who wished to remain at home and those who were willing to move into someone else's home. Stemming primarily from large age and home ownership differences, significant contrasts have been drawn with respect to income and health, concerns over housing and neighborhood, flexibility over type of homesharer desired, homesharing experience, and expectations. Specifically, stayers can be described as older homeowners who have more money but poorer health than movers, who are less flexible than movers over the kind of homesharer they will accept, who emphasize helping one another more than do movers, and who will need a variety of household and nursing services, which movers are more willing to provide.

The first four years of Project HOME are characterized simultaneously by rapid change and increasing stability. The evolution of the program's mission, described in chapter 2, has resulted, therefore, in not two but rather four types of applicants: home providers, lodgers, employers, and caregivers. Home providers and lodgers represent the traditional bartering arrangement in which the provider gives a place to stay in exchange for rent, or rent and services, or services. In no case does the provider pay money to the lodger. The "new" format in homesharing involves an individual who employs someone to provide care in the employer's home. In this instance, money does go from the stayer to the mover, as the caregiver becomes an employee working in someone else's home.

Comparisons of the four groups of applicants show that, while both groups of stayers tend to share many of the stayer characteristics described above, the relatively frailer health and better *perceived* financial situation of employers sets them apart from home providers in several significant ways. Similarly, while applicants who move are similar to each other in many ways, caregivers are distinguished by their greater financial need and willingness to provide a variety of services. In many respects, therefore, the applicants to Project HOME appear to fall into two groups— sharer and personal care companion applicants, each of which has a good "fit" between movers and stayers. How good is the fit? Some answers will be found in chapter 6.

# 6

# Who Gets Matched and Who Doesn't

Now that the four major groups of applicants to Project HOME have been described, several issues arise. Foremost, of course, are concerns about what characteristics of applicants affect the likelihood of their getting matched. Four questions are particularly important: How does each group fare in its desire to find a suitable homesharer? Has there been any change over time in the ability of Project HOME to find suitable matches for its applicants? What characteristics in general facilitate the ability of each type of applicant to find someone with whom to share housing? What characteristics hinder applicants? Knowing the answers to these questions will help to clarify how well Project HOME has served its diverse clientele and whether there are particular client characteristics on which this organization and other service agencies need to focus their attention more closely.[1]

As pointed out at the beginning of the previous chapter, despite much recent research on the nature of homesharing matches and how they fare (e.g., Jaffe 1989b; Pritchard 1983; Pynoos and June 1989; Thuras 1989), until now comprehensive data have been lacking as to who the typical homesharing stayer and mover applicants are. Unfortunately, data are also lacking as to what facilitates applicants finding sharers through agency intervention. While the results in this chapter speak to the experience of one homesharing program's clientele, major conclusions regarding factors that affect applicants' chances nevertheless should be generalizable to other programs.

# WHO GETS MATCHED?

## A Historical Overview

To establish a point of departure, it is useful to examine how many Project HOME clients have been matched during the first five years of the program's existence. Table 6.1 describes the overall percentage of matched clients by client type (provider, lodger, employer, caregiver) and, for each client type, by year. Examination of the totals on the right shows that, while about one third of all the program's 867 applicants were matched, personal care companion (PCC) applicants are matched at a rate almost twice that of sharer applicants (44.5% vs. 24.1% respectively). Among the four types of applicants, the frail employers are most likely to be matched (54.2%), while the least likely to be matched are the lodgers, whose success rate of 23.4 percent is only slightly worse than the rate for providers.

Overall, therefore, it appears that either there is something positive that PCC applicants have and sharer applicants do not have or the program has emphasized the needs of PCC applicants over those of sharer applicants or some combination of the two reasons. In subsequent analyses, it will be clear that a combination of the two reasons is closest to the truth. At the same time Project HOME was pushing hard to find caregivers for frail homeowners who were in serious need of human resources to help them to continue to live at home, these frail elders were willing to pay money for the care, something home providers in a traditional sharing arrangement were not able or willing to do.

Changes from year to year are both substantial and informative generally and with respect to each type of applicant. An examination of the bottom totals shows a curvilinear relationship between time and proportion of matches: Flanked by the very low percentage of successful matches in the first year and the somewhat higher ones of years four and five, the second and third years' percentages represent a high mark for the program. The low early percentage is understandable because of the program's early problems with a limited and unbalanced pool of applicants, but the later drop from the second and third boom years needs further exploration. Is it part of a natural settling-in period that all service programs undergo, or does it stem from some combination of applicant pool size (too big) and agency personnel (too few)? Part of the answer comes from a separate examination of the success rates of each type of applicant.

For *providers*, the first year was the worst, then matters got much better in the second year, dropped off in the third and fourth, and reached a high point in the fifth. During this time, the numbers of provider applicants fluctuated only slightly, dropping from a high in year one to a low in year two, but generally stabilizing during the third through fifth years.

The match rate picture for *lodgers* is similar, but does not show the sort of rebounding power exhibited in the case of providers. In the first year, the success rate was low, then more than doubled during the second year, dropped off in the third and fourth year, and rebounded in the fifth. Unlike the consistent or slightly decreasing numbers of providers over time, the rate of lodger applicants steadily increased during the first three

TABLE 6.1
*Percent Project HOME Applicants Matched by Type of Applicant and Year*

| | Year | | | | | |
|---|---|---|---|---|---|---|
| | 1 | 2 | 3 | 4 | 5 | Total |
| Traditional arrangements | | | | | | |
| providers | 12.5% | 32.1% | 26.3% | 21.9% | 46.7% | 26.1% |
| | (48) | (28) | (38) | (32) | (30) | (176) |
| lodgers | 17.4% | 36.7% | 30.6% | 15.7% | 25.7% | 23.4% |
| | (23) | (30) | (49) | (102) | (74) | (278) |
| traditional | 14.1% | 34.5% | 28.7% | 17.2% | 31.7% | 24.4% |
| subtotal | (71) | (58) | (87) | (134) | (104) | (454) |
| Personal care companion (PCC) arrangements | | | | | | |
| employers | 66.7% | 100.0% | 61.3% | 49.1% | 43.9% | 54.6% |
| | (6) | (10) | (31) | (53) | (41) | (141) |
| caregivers | 66.7% | 55.6% | 50.0% | 43.9% | 25.0% | 40.2% |
| | (6) | (18) | (44) | (98) | (80) | (246) |
| PCC | 66.7% | 71.4% | 54.7% | 45.7% | 31.4% | 45.5% |
| subtotal | (12) | (28) | (75) | (151) | (121) | (387) |
| Total | 21.7% | 46.5% | 40.7% | 32.3% | 31.6% | 34.1% |
| | (83) | (86) | (162) | (285) | (225) | (841) |

NOTE: Each number in parentheses indicates number of applicants specific to year and applicant group. Period covered for each year includes twelve months from April 1 through March 31 of following calendar year: April 1, 1982–March 31, 1983; April 1, 1983–March 31, 1984; April 1, 1984–March 31, 1985; April 1, 1985–March 31, 1986; and April 1, 1986–March 31, 1987. Figures for the first four years are based on applicants who filled out application forms and for whom we have substantial intake data. A few applicants during this time became matched without having filled out forms. Percent matched for these years, therefore, may slightly underrepresent those matched. Figures for the fifth year are taken directly from the application and match logs used by the Project HOME staff.

years, then more than doubled in the fourth year before declining in the fifth year.

Therefore, table 6.1 portrays three major kinds of differences between providers and lodgers: differences in numbers of applicants, differences in patterns of numbers of applicants over time, and differences in patterns of match rates over time. In short, the probability of providers getting matched appears to have increased at the same time the numbers of lodger applicants has increased, while the relatively steady numbers of provider applicants have done nothing to improve the chances of lodgers getting matched.

Based on what is known about the program in its early period, it is relatively easy to account for the low rates of sharer matches during the first year. First, Project HOME was a new program. As a new initiative not only locally but nationally, a homesharing service in the early 1980s was truly a place where staff learned on the job. Particularly difficult were the problems staff would have in discovering criteria upon which to make match recommendations during the first months of the program. This difficulty would depress the overall rate of match-making and thus result in low success rates for both provider and lodger applicants (who together accounted for over three-quarters of the applicant pool during the first year).

The second reason for the low success rates among sharer applicants during the first year is the numerical imbalance in the sharer applicant pool: There was a better than two-to-one ratio of providers to lodgers. Particularly hard hit would be the provider applicants who were in the majority and whose 12.5 percent success rate attests to the general failure of this group to be matched.

Closely related is the third reason for poor success rates for both provider and lodger applicants: As shown in the previous chapter, the early lodger pool contained many frail elders. Being frail, many were unable or unwilling to perform the expected duties of a lodger. For those providers needing help with chores and the like, someone as old and frail as oneself would not make an ideal homesharer. Streib (1978) found this very problem was a significant contributor to the demise of the Miami homesharing program mentioned in chapter 1.

It is possible that the higher success rates during the second through fifth years stem from the reverse of the three problems just described. For one thing Project HOME staff now had more experience in matching clients. For another, aware of the imbalance in numbers between provider and lodger applicants, the director made a conscious effort and succeeded in redressing the imbalance by recruiting more lodger applicants. Finally, as a way to increase the pool of *matchable* lodger applicants, the director opened up the program to younger clients, thereby attracting lodger applicants who would be able to provide services for home providers in exchange for a place to stay.[2] Clearly, organizational initiatives were instrumental in determining the relative success rates of providers and lodgers getting matched after the first year.

Examination of the later starting personal care companion aspect of Project HOME produces yet another set of trends. In particular, the handful of *employer* applicants at the start of the program were better than even money to get matched, including a perfect ten for ten in the second year, but, as time went on and the numbers of frail homeowners needing a caregiver increased, the likelihood of their being matched steadily declined to a low point during the fifth year. It should be noted, however, that the "low point" shows a 43.9 percent match rate, which is about the same as the best rate for providers and better than the best year for lodgers.

The *caregiver* picture is similar to that for the employers but, in a sense, more extreme. From a high of 66.7 percent match rate during the first year, when there were only six caregiver applicants, the success rate for matching caregivers declined steadily through the fifth year, at which time only one-quarter of the caregiver applicants were matched. Especially noteworthy is that this dramatic decline occurred at the same time as an equally dramatic increase in the numbers of caregiver applicants from year one (6) to year five (80).

The large increases in numbers of both kinds of personal care companion applicants suggest, however indirectly, that there might be something about later applicants, in particular caregivers, which produces obstacles to getting matched. For example, the large increase in caregiver applicants may have been in name rather than in fact; that is, later applicants may have said they wanted be caregivers simply because they needed the money even though they did not have the caregiving skills and interest required.[3] In fact, when the match rates for each subgroup are broken down by characteristic, it will be clear that this explanation is reasonable.

Overall, therefore, it appears that important factors affecting the likelihood of traditional sharers getting matched stem from the organization itself. From early tentative fumbling to the decision to make the program intergenerational, the reasons for fluctuation over time in the success rates of provider and lodger applicants appear to have a primarily organizational source, rather than anything peculiar to the applicants themselves. On the other hand, while the influx of caregiver applicants during the second and third years was an organizational initiative and surely affected match-making rates for employers and caregivers alike, it is likely that particular characteristics of the caregiver applicants especially had an effect on the decreasing rate at which they became matched over time. This and other individual-level explanations are explored next, as the five groups of characteristics discussed in the previous chapter are examined separately for clues as to what qualities help and what qualities hinder each type of applicant.

## Background

As table 6.2 shows, among *provider* applicants, gender, age, marital status, education, and work status are all irrelevant in predicting who gets matched and who does not. These findings have important implications: First, no particular type of applicant appears to be "discriminated" against. Although females and the married and widowed stand a better chance than males and the never married, the numbers of applicants in the latter groups are so small that the differences observed are not statistically significant. Second, the lack of importance of background suggests that either it is completely irrelevant or Project HOME staff are taking it into account when proposing matches and there is enough heterogeneity in the lodger applicant pool to accommodate the applicants of diverse background among the providers.

Interestingly, two background characteristics do matter for *lodgers*. Gender is important in that, contrary to the suggested pattern for providers, male lodgers have twice as good a chance as female lodgers of getting matched. The obvious explanation is that male lodgers may be more likely to offer services needed by providers, like snow shoveling, fixing things around the house, and providing a deterrent to neighborhood crime.

Again, contrary to the pattern for providers, the never married and widowed lodger applicants are significantly more likely than the married to get matched. A possible reason is that the widowed or never married applicant represents a difficult but manageable sharer with whom to negotiate rights and duties, while a married applicant brings with him- or herself at least one significant other whose needs and desires need to

TABLE 6.2
*Percent Applicants Matched by Background Characteristics and Applicant Group*

| | Traditional | | PCC | |
|---|---|---|---|---|
| Predictor[a] | Provider | Lodgers | Employer | Caregivers |
| **Gender** | | | | |
| male | 12.5 (32) | 32.9 (76) | 57.7 (26) | 42.3 (26) |
| female | 24.6 (114) | 16.4 (128) | 61.6 (73) | 48.2 (139) |
| d | +.12 ns | −.16** | +.04 ns | +.06 ns |
| **Age** | | | | |
| under 30 | 22.2 (9) | 24.7 (85) | 66.7 (6) | 28.8 (66) |
| 30–49 | 18.5 (27) | 25.8 (62) | 71.4 (7) | 44.0 (50) |
| 50–69 | 26.8 (41) | 17.1 (35) | 65.0 (20) | 74.4 (39) |
| 70 and over | 20.3 (69) | 14.3 (21) | 55.9 (68) | 87.5 (8) |
| d | −.01 ns | −.05 ns | −.10 ns | +.31*** |
| **Marital status** | | | | |
| married | 30.0 (20) | 0.0 (11) | 36.8 (19) | 63.6 (11) |
| widowed | 22.0 (82) | 23.3 (30) | 62.3 (61) | 81.0 (21) |
| divorced, separated | 22.6 (31) | 12.2 (49) | 83.3 (6) | 52.4 (42) |
| never married | 9.1 (11) | 28.6 (112) | 64.3 (14) | 33.7 (83) |
| chi[2] | 1.80 ns | 8.58* | 5.76 ns | 17.29*** |
| **Education** | | | | |
| less than h.s. | 23.3 (43) | 20.7 (29) | 54.3 (35) | 64.0 (25) |
| h.s. graduate | 23.3 (30) | 16.0 (50) | 72.0 (25) | 45.5 (66) |
| some college | 12.1 (33) | 26.8 (71) | 52.9 (17) | 46.5 (43) |
| college graduate | 27.8 (36) | 26.5 (49) | 58.8 (17) | 35.7 (28) |
| d | +.00 ns | +.05 ns | +.02 ns | −.10* |
| **Work status[b]** | | | | |
| working for pay | 30.8 (39) | 23.2 (82) | 50.0 (10) | 35.8 (53) |
| retired | 19.4 (36) | 20.0 (20) | 59.1 (66) | 70.0 (10) |
| unemployed | 25.0 (4) | 20.9 (43) | 80.0 (5) | 49.4 (80) |
| other | 26.9 (26) | 28.2 (39) | 57.1 (14) | 52.6 (19) |
| chi[2] | 1.28 ns | 0.78 ns | 1.27 ns | 5.09 ns |

NOTE: First number in each row refers to percent of applicants with that particular characteristic who were matched with a homesharer. Second number (in parenthesis) is the total number of applicants, matched and unmatched, who have the particular characteristic. Thus, e.g., 12.5% of the 32 male home providers were matched.

[a] For each predictor, significant differences between/among categories are based on Somer's d for ordinal level variables and chi[2] for nominal level variables.

[b] Many respondents are missing data, so totals for each group of applicants will be less than for other variables.

ns p > .05
* p ≤ .05
** p ≤ .01
*** p ≤ .001

be taken into account. The prospect of opening one's home to a "team" of sharers is one that may threaten home provider applicants with more problems than prompted them to seek a homesharer in the first place. Also, it is possible that married lodger applicants are less needy than unmarried lodger applicants and therefore more choosy themselves.

Among personal care companion applicants, the chances of *employers* getting matched is, as with providers, unaffected by gender, age, marital status, education, or work status. The largest difference among the statistically insignificant ones found is that between married and all unmarried employer applicants. Those applicants who already have someone living with them are much less likely to find a caregiver than those who are not married, probably because either the partner is already providing care and the employer applicant can afford to be very choosy or the partner is also frail and needs looking after and the caregiver applicants are unwilling to sign up for double caregiving.

For *caregivers*, three interrelated background characteristics make a great deal of difference as to who gets matched and who doesn't. Most compelling and instructive are the data for age: The older one is, the better one's chances of getting matched. It is not surprising, therefore, to see that widowed applicants and applicants with less than a high school degree are significantly more likely to get matched than their younger never married and college educated counterparts.[4] These findings suggest that important differences exist among caregiver applicants, and that these differences are somehow related to one's age. Analysis of subsequent tables will show that the reasons are found primarily in the willingness of successful caregiver applicants to play the caregiver role. Somewhat important too is the preference that frail elders have for older caregivers, although there are notable exceptions to this tendency as will be seen in chapters 7 and 8.

In terms of previously stated assumptions about the relative importance of organizational initiative and individual applicant characteristics, it appears that modifications are in order regarding the latter. Contrary to expectation, some individual background characteristics are important predictors for lodgers but not for employers. Originally, it was predicted that the sharer applicants' success rates in getting matched would not depend on applicant characteristics but that the rates of PCC applicants would. The importance of gender and marital status for lodger and of age for caregiver applicants and the lack of any background predictor for provider and employer applicants suggest a revised argument: Based on background characteristics at least, stayers appear to be treated the same no matter what their background, while certain background characteristics of movers do differentiate that group, regardless of whether one is a traditional sharer or PCC applicant.

## Income and Health

Data on income tend to corroborate the finding that background does not affect *provider* applicants' chances of getting matched, as shown in the income and income perception comparisons in table 6.3. At the same time, health, as measured by a variety of indicators, *does*. For example, providers without limitations are almost three times more likely to get matched than those with some limitation; and providers who perceive their mobility to be excellent are ten times more likely to be matched than those whose self-described mobility is poor.

These results relative to health are both illuminating and disturbing. For service providers and clients alike, it is important to know that poor health is a barrier to home providers being able to find a lodger willing to share accommodations in a traditional homesharing arrangement. At the same time, it is distressing to note that frail homeowners who need services around the house and are unable to pay for them (and who therefore can't afford the personal care companion arrangement) may be slipping through the cracks of Project HOME.

For *lodgers*, income and health are not significantly correlated with the probability of getting matched. With respect to income, the lack of association is real. In the case of health, however, those lodgers in better health appear to have an advantage, but the number of lodger applicants in poor health is so small that the results are statistically nonsignificant. Thus, while income does not affect the chances of either providers or lodgers, the likelihood of each type of sharer applicant getting matched is enhanced by good health—especially in the case of home providers. Apparently very few homesharing applicants want to get involved with someone in frail health.

Among the personal care companion applicants for whom a frail individual is central to the homesharing arrangement, income and health both appear to be irrelevant in predicting who gets matched and who does not. Among *employers*, whose income is presumably sufficient to pay for a caregiver, income variation does not correlate with likelihood of getting matched. While those who perceive their living situation to be

TABLE 6.3

*Percent Applicants Matched by Income and Health Characteristics and Applicant Group*

| | Traditional | | PCC | |
|---|---|---|---|---|
| Predictor[a] | Provider | Lodgers | Employer | Caregivers |
| **Income** | | | | |
| under $5,000 | 28.0  (25) | 24.5  (94) | 58.3  (12) | 47.0  (100) |
| $5,000–6,999 | 21.9  (32) | 21.6  (51) | 69.6  (23) | 55.3  (38) |
| $7,000 plus | 20.7  (87) | 21.1  (57) | 56.3  (64) | 33.3  (24) |
| d | − .04 ns | − .03 ns | − .08 ns | − .03 ns |
| **Living situation**[b] | | | | |
| too expensive | 18.6  (70) | 26.2  (61) | 50.0  (18) | 50.9  (55) |
| not too expensive | 24.7  (73) | 22.3  (103) | 63.8  (69) | 38.8  (80) |
| d | + .06 ns | − .04 ns | + .14 ns | − .12 ns |
| **Income satisfaction**[b] | | | | |
| not at all | 21.4  (28) | 17.6  (74) | 61.5  (13) | 48.9  (94) |
| more or Less | 28.6  (42) | 32.3  (65) | 52.9  (17) | 37.8  (37) |
| pretty well | 18.2  (66) | 21.4  (28) | 67.4  (43) | 54.5  (11) |
| d | − .05 ns | + .07 ns | + .08 ns | + .05 ns |
| **Physical capacity** | | | | |
| low | 12.3  (57) | 12.5  (24) | 55.7  (70) | 60.0  (5) |
| high | 33.3  (72) | 24.0  (179) | 64.3  (14) | 46.8  (158) |
| d | + .21** | + .12 ns | + .09 ns | − .13 ns |
| **Perception of vision** | | | | |
| poor | 11.8  (34) | 16.7  (12) | 57.6  (33) | 50.0  (4) |
| good | 21.1  (76) | 25.2  (103) | 61.8  (55) | 55.2  (87) |
| excellent | 34.3  (35) | 20.0  (85) | 50.0  (12) | 37.0  (73) |
| d | + .13* | − .03 ns | − .01 ns | − .17* |
| **Perception of hearing** | | | | |
| poor | 17.6  (17) | 12.5  (8) | 61.5  (26) | 25.0  (4) |
| good | 15.6  (77) | 26.0  (73) | 59.3  (59) | 55.9  (59) |
| excellent | 32.7  (49) | 21.0  (119) | 57.1  (14) | 42.6  (101) |
| d | + .13* | − .03 ns | − .01 ns | − .11 ns |
| **Perception of mobility** | | | | |
| poor | 2.9  (34) | 12.5  (8) | 52.8  (53) | 33.3  (3) |
| good | 21.1  (57) | 21.5  (65) | 66.7  (36) | 49.1  (57) |
| excellent | 34.0  (53) | 24.2  (128) | 66.7  (9) | 45.6  (103) |
| d | + .19*** | + .04 ns | + .12 ns | − .02 ns |
| **Perception of health**[b] | | | | |
| worse than average | 0.0  (19) | 20.0  (10) | 41.7  (12) | 0.0  (1) |
| about average | 23.1  (65) | 26.7  (86) | 65.9  (41) | 48.8  (82) |
| better than average | 29.6  (54) | 23.1  (78) | 65.4  (26) | 41.8  (67) |
| d | + .14* | − .02 ns | + .10 ns | − .06 ns |
| **Senior service used**[c] | | | | |
| none | 31.5  (54) | 22.9  (166) | 71.8  (39) | 45.9  (148) |
| at least one | 20.7  (29) | 33.3  (9) | 48.0  (50) | 60.0  (5) |
| d | − .11 ns | + .10 ns | − .24* | + .14 ns |

NOTE: for [a], [b], ns, *, **, ***, see table 6.2 notes.

[c] Information is not available for year 1; therefore, group totals may be less than for other predictors.

too expensive are less likely to be matched than those who aren't concerned with current living expenses, the number of potential employers
who are worried about expenses is too small for the difference to be
statistically significant. With respect to health, a commodity in short
supply among employer applicants, variability again is not correlated
with success rate in being matched; and, again, much of the reason
appears to be the paucity of employer applicants in the better health
categories.

One interesting finding for the employer applicants is that those with
no senior service experience are significantly more likely to be matched
than those with some experience. One possible reason is that those
connected to senior services have more resources on which to depend
and are, therefore, more likely to be choosy when considering caregivers.
Another possible explanation is that the Project HOME staff are more
sensitive to the problems of employer applicants who are not "plugged in"
to the network of senior services.

Finally, money and health apparently have no predictive ability concerning likelihood of getting matched among *caregiver* applicants either.
For all but one predictor, there is no significant correlation and no
pattern to the data. Vision, alone among the health predictors, does
significantly correlate with chance of getting matched, but in a negative
sense: Those with poor or good vision are *more* likely to be matched than
those with excellent vision. Most likely, this finding derives from the
earlier (table 6.2) results, which show that older caregiver applicants are
more likely to be matched than younger ones, who generally have better
eyesight than their elders.

While income and health do not have significant effects on the likelihood of lodgers, employers, and caregivers getting matched, poor health
is an extremely important inhibitor of providers' chances of getting
matched. This finding has important policy implications, as it indicates
a potentially serious weakness in the program's efforts to service needy
homesharing applicants.

If these frail homeowners could pay for health care services they would
be in the PCC applicant pool, but, as shown in the previous chapter,
their financial concerns are greater than those of employer applicants
and so payment seems an unlikely solution. Therefore, they are in the
traditional sharer pool and dependent on trading space in their home for
someone to provide a presence and perhaps some services. Unfortunately
for many frail provider applicants, the poor success rates for the frail in

that group indicates there are too few lodger applicants are willing to make the trade.

## Living Situation

For all four groups of applicants, living situation overall appears to have no appreciable effect on who gets matched and who doesn't (table 6.4). At the same time, one characteristic of their living situation is

TABLE 6.4

*Percent Applicants Matched by Living Situation Characteristics and Applicant Group*

| | Traditional | | PCC | |
|---|---|---|---|---|
| Predictor[a] | Provider | Lodgers | Employer | Caregivers |
| **Home status** | | | | |
| rent | 23.5  (34) | 21.7  (184) | 55.6  (36) | 46.8  (141) |
| own | 20.9  (110) | 31.6  (19) | 61.5  (65) | 54.5  (22) |
| d | −.03 ns | +.10 ns | +.06 ns | +.08 ns |
| **Home population** | | | | |
| by self | 22.8  (79) | 16.1  (56) | 66.7  (54) | 60.0  (35) |
| with other(s) | 21.5  (65) | 24.6  (134) | 46.5  (43) | 44.6  (121) |
| d | −.01 ns | +.09 ns | −.20* | −.16 ns |
| **Housing problems[b]** | | | | |
| 2 or 3 prob. | 18.3  (60) | 16.7  (24) | 69.2  (39) | 44.4  (9) |
| 1 problem | 27.1  (48) | 25.5  (47) | 58.6  (29) | 41.9  (43) |
| no problems | 22.6  (31) | 24.4  (86) | 56.3  (16) | 41.0  (78) |
| d | +.04 ns | +.03 ns | −.11 ns | −.01 ns |
| **Friends in neighborhood[b]** | | | | |
| none | 23.8  (21) | 11.4  (35) | 81.8  (11) | 61.5  (26) |
| a few | 28.6  (49) | 23.4  (77) | 65.6  (32) | 32.7  (52) |
| most | 22.2  (36) | 33.9  (56) | 52.6  (19) | 52.9  (51) |
| all | 9.1  (22) | 14.3  (7) | 75.0  (8) | 75.0  (8) |
| d | −.08 ns | +.11* | −.09 ns | +.05 ns |
| **Neighborhood problems[b]** | | | | |
| 1 or 2 problems | 6.7  (15) | 26.8  (56) | 72.7  (11) | 34.1  (41) |
| no problems | 23.6  (127) | 21.9  (105) | 58.7  (75) | 44.6  (92) |
| d | +.17 ns | −.05 ns | −.14 ns | +.10 ns |
| **Drive car** | | | | |
| no; need help | 17.2  (58) | 19.5  (41) | 57.1  (77) | 65.4  (26) |
| yes; without help | 25.9  (85) | 23.5  (162) | 66.7  (18) | 44.1  (136) |
| d | +.09 ns | +.04 ns | +.10 ns | +.22* |
| **Transportation problems[b]** | | | | |
| always | 0.0  (7) | 20.0  (5) | 57.1  (7) | 66.7  (3) |
| often | 0.0  (9) | 12.5  (16) | 62.5  (8) | 60.0  (5) |
| sometimes | 18.8  (32) | 25.7  (70) | 61.9  (21) | 50.0  (54) |
| never | 28.4  (81) | 26.7  (86) | 67.6  (37) | 41.7  (84) |
| d | +.16** | +.05 ns | +.06 ns | −.10 ns |

NOTE: for [a], [b], ns, *, **, ***, see table 6.2 notes.

significant for each type of applicant, but it is a different one for each type. For home *providers*, those with no transportation problems have the best chance of getting matched. Sadly, none of the sixteen provider applicants who have transportation problems "always" or "often" was matched. Consistent with this result is the tendency for drivers to have a better chance of being matched, although this finding is not statistically significant. Insofar as transportation problems are related to health and physical capacity limitations, it is not surprising to see that the less mobile are at a disadvantage yet again.

Among *lodger* applicants, the more friends one has, the better are one's chances of getting matched. One might expect that the opposite would be true, that those with friends in their neighborhood would be more likely to be choosy about leaving, more inclined to stay near friends. It may be that having many friends nearby is a source of strength for the lodger applicant and indicates someone who would be attractive to a home provider. In any event, the finding does not appear to represent a particularly important predictor of being matched.

Among potential *employers*, the only significant predictor of getting matched or not is whether one lives alone. Those who live alone have about a 20 percent better chance of getting matched than those who already are living with someone. This is consistent with the table 6.2 result, which shows that married applicants are at a disadvantage in the employer pool, and the table 6.3 result, which shows that those employer applicants who are unconnected to senior services are at an advantage. It may be that both the employer applicant and Project HOME staff are more committed to finding a caregiver when the employer applicant is living alone than when he or she has resources in the form of people living in the household or agencies providing services. To the extent that these explanations are true, the program is filling an important gap in services for frail and disabled homeowners who need and can pay for caregiver services.

Among *caregiver* applicants, those who can drive a car without help are about 20 percent *less* likely to get matched than those who cannot drive or who need help to drive. On the face of it this doesn't make sense, until one realizes that ability to drive decreases with increasing age, both as a function of many older people not having learned to drive and as a result of increasing physical limitations, especially problems with one's eyes. In this light, the result is consistent with the earlier findings in table 6.2 regarding age and table 6.3 regarding vision, which underscore the advantage older applicants, with presumably inferior vision, have relative to younger applicants.

The results regarding living situation characteristics shed additional light on the interplay between organizational initiative and applicant characteristics in one important way. For provider applicants, the key mobility indicator measuring trouble with transportation reinforces the point made earlier that there are needy provider applicants who are not being matched. To the extent that provider applicants who have trouble with transportation also have health problems, they are indeed hampered in finding prospective sharers from the lodger pool.

## Homesharing Profiles

Results concerning homesharing profiles substantially advance an understanding of why some homesharing applicants get matched and others do not, not so much because of the numbers of qualities predicting success rate but because of the particular qualities involved (table 6.5). Among *providers*, for example, two qualities appear to matter: a certain degree of flexibility and a realistic attitude toward homesharing. Concerning flexibility, those who don't care about their sharer's gender are more than twice as likely to get matched as those who do care.

Related to flexibility is the question of how realistic the provider applicant is regarding the homesharing arrangement he or she envisions. In this respect, it is suggestive, although the results are not quite statistically significant, that previous experience in homesharing and placement of a finite time limit on the homesharing arrangement appear to characterize provider applicants who have the best chance of getting matched.

For *lodgers*, the results are similar, though not identical. For one thing, flexibility is important here too, but with respect to attitude toward the disabled, students, and children as sharers, rather than concern over the sharer's gender. Those lodgers who don't care whether they share with someone who is disabled, a student, or a family with children are significantly more likely to get matched than those who do care. At the same time, being choosy about gender is not a predictor of match success rate for lodgers, as it was for providers.

Realistic expectations are even more clearly important for lodgers than for providers in two respects: First, those experienced in sharing are nearly twice as likely to be matched as those who are not experienced.

TABLE 6.5
*Percent Applicants Matched by Homesharing Profiles and Applicant Group*

| Predictor[a] | Traditional | | PCC | |
|---|---|---|---|---|
| | Provider | Lodgers | Employer | Caregivers |
| smoker | 20.9 (43) | 20.8 (53) | 62.5 (16) | 42.9 (63) |
| nonsmoker | 22.3 (103) | 23.8 (147) | 59.5 (84) | 50.5 (101) |
| d | +.01 ns | +.03 ns | −.03 ns | +.08 ns |
| drinker | 16.9 (59) | 24.2 (95) | 61.5 (26) | 50.0 (70) |
| nondrinker | 25.6 (86) | 22.1 (104) | 58.9 (73) | 45.7 (94) |
| d | +.09 ns | −.02 ns | −.03 ns | −.04 ns |
| pet owner | 24.6 (69) | 12.5 (32) | 41.4 (29) | 51.5 (33) |
| nonpet owner | 19.5 (77) | 24.9 (169) | 68.1 (69) | 46.5 (129) |
| d | −.05 ns | +.12 ns | +.26** | −.05 ns |
| overnight company | 25.0 (68) | 23.9 (88) | 60.0 (50) | 44.4 (54) |
| no overnight company | 20.8 (72) | 21.3 (108) | 60.0 (45) | 49.0 (100) |
| d | −.04 ns | −.03 ns | +.00 ns | +.05 ns |
| **Attitude toward sharer's lifestyle[b]** | | | | |
| objects to 2 or 3 | 24.7 (81) | 24.1 (29) | 59.6 (57) | 32.0 (25) |
| objects only to 1 | 33.3 (27) | 25.0 (56) | 60.0 (20) | 48.6 (37) |
| objects to none | 0.0 (14) | 22.6 (84) | 60.0 (10) | 50.6 (83) |
| d | −.06 ns | −.02 ns | +.00 ns | +.10 ns |
| **Attitude toward disabled sharer** | | | | |
| objects to any | 17.2 (64) | 0.0 (16) | 53.3 (45) | 20.0 (10) |
| distinguishes | 27.3 (55) | 18.5 (27) | 65.0 (20) | 46.2 (13) |
| objects to none | 26.3 (19) | 25.5 (149) | 68.4 (19) | 50.8 (130) |
| d | +.08 ns | −.14* | +.12 ns | +.16 ns |
| **Attitude toward sharing with student/children[b,c]** | | | | |
| objects to both | 20.5 (39) | 11.4 (44) | 51.2 (43) | 49.0 (51) |
| objects to one | 34.2 (38) | 15.6 (45) | 80.0 (20) | 46.7 (30) |
| objects to neither | 28.6 (7) | 34.9 (63) | 75.0 (12) | 38.3 (47) |
| d | +.10 ns | +.17** | +.22* | −.08 ns |
| **Gender preference of sharer** | | | | |
| matters | 16.7 (108) | 20.0 (80) | 61.3 (80) | 50.0 (66) |
| doesn't matter | 37.1 (35) | 24.2 (124) | 57.9 (19) | 44.8 (96) |
| d | +.20** | +.04 ns | −.03 ns | −.05 ns |
| **Experience sharing[c]** | | | | |
| no | 18.4 (38) | 14.0 (57) | 57.5 (40) | 51.4 (37) |
| yes | 32.1 (53) | 26.2 (122) | 63.3 (49) | 44.1 (118) |
| d | +.14 ns | +.12* | +.05 ns | −.07 ns |
| **How long want to homeshare[b,c]** | | | | |
| finite period | 32.1 (28) | 27.1 (107) | 47.8 (23) | 41.4 (87) |
| infinitely | 21.2 (52) | 9.6 (52) | 63.2 (57) | 55.6 (54) |
| d | −.11 ns | −.17** | +.15 ns | +.14 ns |
| **Employing other means to find homesharer[b,c]** | | | | |
| no | 22.9 (48) | 26.2 (61) | 59.3 (54) | 44.4 (36) |
| yes | 30.3 (33) | 20.8 (96) | 61.9 (21) | 46.1 (89) |
| d | +.07 ns | −.05 ns | +.03 ns | +.02 ns |

NOTE: for [a], [b], ns, *, **, ***, see table 6.2 notes.

[c] See table 6.3 note.

Second, those lodger applicants who anticipate a homesharing arrangement of a finite period are nearly three times more likely to get matched as those who prefer an indefinite or permanent arrangement.

Both of these findings, significant for lodgers but not for providers, underscore the importance of a realistic outlook as an asset for lodgers in finding a home. Lodgers with prior experiences know first-hand what sharing can be like; furthermore, they realize that sharing arrangements are relatively fragile agreements that, for the most part, are useful for limited periods of time and therefore quite different from ideal permanent linkages, like marriage.

Among frail or disabled applicants who would stay at home and be *employers* to a caregiving homesharer, two profile indicators significantly predict success at getting matched. First, employer applicants who do not have pets are over 25 percent more likely to find a caregiver than are pet owners. This large difference, evident here but not among home providers in the traditional homesharing arrangement, is somewhat perplexing. It doesn't appear that the choosiness of caregiver applicants is the reason, because well over half of them object to none of the possibly hindering lifestyle indicators: smoking, drinking, overnight guests, *and* pets. Possibly, having a pet makes the employer applicant more choosy about who will live and work in the same home as the pet; it may be that "Fido" or "Boots" has been given veto power that often gets exercised. Possibly one's pet provides important emotional support for employer applicants, analogous to some of the same support provided by another person living in the same household. At any rate, the ownership of a pet *is* an inhibiting factor to getting matched among employers.

The second predictor of success for employers is nearly as strong and more easily explained. Employer applicants who object both to student caregivers and caregivers with children have a 20 percent *lower* chance of getting matched than those who object to one or the other or to neither. Flexibility would appear to be important to this group of applicants as well. Interestingly, the sharer applicants who most nearly resemble the employer in this sense are the lodgers, rather than the providers. Perhaps it is the idea of paying money out (which both employers and many lodgers do) which makes these two groups kindred spirits in this case.

*Caregiver* applicants, unlike the other three groups, show no statistically significant homesharer profile predictor of match success. Nonsignificant findings that nonetheless appear to reflect patterns are important in two respects. First, those who object the least to a sharer's lifestyle and disability are most likely to get matched, again pointing out the importance of flexibility. In the case of caregivers, however, the findings are not statistically significant in part because the majority of caregiver applicants have no objections regarding a sharer's lifestyle or disability. It is probably the role of caregiver that best accounts both for the pattern found and for its nonsignificance.

A second pattern among caregivers, while also not statistically significant, is important because it parallels a (similarly nonsignificant) pattern among employer applicants. Contrary to sharer applicants who profit from wanting a homesharing arrangement of limited duration, both types of personal care companion applicants appear to be helped by wanting an arrangement of greater permanence. This contrast suggests that traditional and personal care companion arrangements are based on very different philosophies. In the former, the emphasis is on temporary respite through an arrangement that has a definite concluding point, while, in the latter, it is perceived by both parties as an arrangement of relatively long duration, presumably because of the long-term needs of the frail and disabled person needing care.

Here, more than with any of the previous sets of characteristics, individual applicant characteristics matter for each of the four groups of homesharers. The importance of flexibility for all four subgroups and of realistic expectations for lodgers underscores the sort of mind set one needs to compete successfully for homesharers, no matter what the type of arrangement being sought. At the same time, the tentative findings regarding desired permanence in a sharing arrangement do differentiate sharer and PCC applicants.

## Homesharing Expectations

Table 6.6 shows that many of the explanations earlier offered about the success rates of the four types of applicants are probably accurate, but it also produces some unexpected results. For *providers,* four predictors are statistically significant, and they all point out the advisability of providers' anticipating their homesharing arrangement along the lines of landlord-renter rather than friends or family. How well the actual arrangements coincide with the expectation is another matter and will be considered in detail in chapters 7 and 8, but the plain fact is that providers who expect little from their sharer have a better chance of getting matched than those who expect a lot.

TABLE 6.6
Percent Applicants Matched by Homesharing Expectations and Applicant Group

| | Traditional | | PCC | |
|---|---|---|---|---|
| Predictor[a] | Provider | Lodgers | Employer | Caregivers |
| **Household services[c]** | | | | |
| need | 16.7  (36) | 23.5  (17) | 58.8  (68) | 25.0  (4) |
| cooperate | 31.3  (48) | 26.5  (68) | 58.8  (17) | 32.0  (25) |
| provide | 42.9  (7) | 22.0  (91) | 80.0  (5) | 50.0  (126) |
| d | +.15* | −.03 ns | +.06 ns | +.19* |
| **Nursing services[c]** | | | | |
| need | 15.0  (20) | 0.0  (7) | 52.8  (53) | 25.0  (4) |
| cooperate | 30.9  (55) | 27.5  (91) | 66.7  (30) | 48.8  (43) |
| provide | 30.0  (10) | 21.4  (70) | 66.7  (6) | 46.7  (107) |
| d | +.11 ns | −.01 ns | +.13 ns | +.01 ns |
| **Importance of money matters[b]** | | | | |
| low | 17.6  (34) | 0.0  (10) | 67.3  (49) | 33.3  (6) |
| medium | 24.1  (58) | 26.3  (114) | 45.5  (22) | 35.8  (81) |
| high | 23.7  (38) | 22.4  (67) | 100.0  (4) | 54.5  (55) |
| d | +.04 ns | +.02 ns | −.09 ns | +.17* |
| **Importance of helping each other** | | | | |
| low | 53.3  (15) | 18.9  (53) | 0.0  (2) | 50.0  (60) |
| medium | 23.1  (52) | 22.8  (92) | 45.0  (20) | 43.5  (69) |
| high | 14.3  (70) | 25.0  (48) | 62.7  (67) | 36.0  (25) |
| d | −.18** | +.04 ns | +.22* | −.08 ns |
| **Importance of sharing companionship** | | | | |
| low | 20.0  (20) | 16.1  (31) | 50.0  (10) | 58.8  (17) |
| medium | 28.9  (38) | 24.6  (61) | 58.3  (24) | 44.7  (47) |
| high | 20.2  (84) | 23.1  (104) | 58.9  (56) | 44.2  (95) |
| d | −.04 ns | +.03 ns | +.04 ns | −.05 ns |
| **Compatability concerns** | | | | |
| low | 17.9  (39) | 23.5  (51) | 35.7  (28) | 42.6  (54) |
| medium | 26.0  (77) | 22.4  (107) | 66.0  (50) | 44.3  (79) |
| high | 20.0  (20) | 18.9  (37) | 80.0  (10) | 56.5  (23) |
| d | +.03 ns | −.03 ns | +.28** | +.06 ns |
| **Giving more than getting concerns** | | | | |
| low | 17.6  (74) | 19.6  (107) | 50.9  (53) | 44.2  (113) |
| medium | 22.7  (22) | 27.1  (59) | 69.2  (13) | 45.2  (31) |
| high | 32.4  (34) | 23.3  (30) | 71.4  (7) | 53.8  (13) |
| d | +.11* | +.05 ns | +.18 ns | +.04 ns |
| **Keeping own things concerns[b]** | | | | |
| low | 19.4  (67) | 23.2  (138) | 54.0  (50) | 48.2  (114) |
| medium | 40.0  (15) | 25.0  (28) | 66.7  (12) | 41.7  (24) |
| high | 18.4  (38) | 17.9  (28) | 66.7  (15) | 33.3  (18) |
| d | +.01 ns | −.02 ns | +.10 ns | −.10 ns |
| **Importance of sharing driving** | | | | |
| low | 27.8  (79) | 24.8  (129) | 52.6  (38) | 46.6  (103) |
| medium | 14.3  (35) | 17.5  (40) | 50.0  (16) | 53.1  (32) |
| high | 11.5  (26) | 16.7  (24) | 71.9  (32) | 33.3  (21) |
| d | −.13* | −.07 ns | +.14 ns | −.03 ns |

NOTE: for [a], [b], ns, *, **, ***, see table 6.2 notes.

[c] See table 6.3 note.

For example, provider applicants wishing to provide or cooperate with respect to household and nursing services are twice as likely to get matched as those who need such services; and this household effect is statistically significant. Those who place little emphasis on sharers' helping each other are three times more likely to get matched than those who value helping, while those who are very concerned about giving too much are almost twice as likely to get matched as those who are not so concerned. Finally, those provider applicants who deemphasize shared driving are over twice as likely to get matched as those who emphasize shared driving. Thus, the provider applicants who express a desire to live separate lives and who don't want to give too much in the sharing arrangement have a distinct advantage in finding homesharers.

Interestingly, none of the homesharing expectations significantly predict whether *lodgers* will get matched. While it is not entirely clear why, the distribution of homesharing expectations of lodgers themselves are at least partially responsible. Of particular importance is the question of nursing services. Table 6.6 shows that *none* of the lodger applicants who needed them got matched. At the same time, the finding is statistically insignificant because of the skewed distribution for the nursing services scale: Only seven lodger applicants needed nursing services.

Contrary to provider applicants, potential *employers* appear to benefit from wanting involvement with their caregiver. For example, almost two-thirds of those placing a high value on helping one another, but less than half of those placing a medium value, and none of the two who say helping one another is unimportant were matched. Even more striking are the results concerning compatibility: Over twice as many of those employer applicants who emphasized compatibility were matched as opposed to applicants who deemphasized it. Not significant but showing the same pattern are the results concerning sharing companionship, underscoring the conclusion that would-be employers increase their chances of getting matched as they increase their commitment to what would appear to be a highly personal, rather than business, relationship with their caregiver.

The success of *caregiver* applicants, on the other hand, appears to be dependent on whether they are willing to provide services and how much they emphasize money matters. Very few caregiver applicants require services, but as one goes from needing to cooperating to providing, the chances of getting matched increases—significantly with respect to household services but not significantly with respect to nursing services.

At the same time, those caregiver applicants who place a high value on money matters are 20 percent more likely to get matched than those who place a low value on money, and the difference is significant.

As in the case of homesharer profiles, expectations distinguish successful providers, employers, and caregivers from unsuccessful ones. As a provider applicant, one is better off not needing services and keeping the proposed relationship with the sharer one that maximizes each sharer's privacy. As an employer applicant, success at getting matched comes to those wanting to *maximize* a personal rather than business arrangement with sharer, while successful caregiver applicants tend to be those who emphasize the business end of the relationship (providing service, money matters).

Basically, therefore, the different homesharing expectations characterizing matched providers and employers highlight a fundamental distinction between the two types of homesharing arrangements. In the former, where the homeowner has only space to offer in exchange for money or money and services, one is best off expecting a business relationship between landlord and tenant.[5] In the latter, where it is the homeowner who is going to pay for services, it is not only reasonable but advisable to expect a more personal relationship with one's caregiver.[6]

## Four Keys for Successful Applicants

The previous discussion has demonstrated that both organizational initiative and individual applicant characteristics have predictive power in determining who gets matched and who doesn't. The last section of this chapter will consider the organization and how it serves individual applicants, but first key applicant qualities need to be emphasized.

Of central importance is the fact that those qualities enhancing one type of applicant's chances in getting matched may have little or no effect on any of the other three types of applicants. In fact, one may summarize the major findings from tables 6.2 through 6.6 by arguing that different characteristics appear to stand out for each group. Among *providers*, the most important predictor of success is good health, as measured by a variety of indicators: The better a provider's health, the better will be her or his chances of getting matched. The second most important predictor is the willingness to deemphasize a personal relationship with one's sharer, as measured by the household services, helping each other, and concern over giving more than getting indicators: Provider applicants who prefer to keep household duties separate or share in

them equally, who deemphasize helping each other, and who are concerned over giving too much stand a better chance of getting matched.
Thus, the successful provider applicant is one who most closely resembles
a healthy landlord in the sort of minimum shared space scenario described in chapter 1.

The most successful *lodgers*, on the other hand, are flexible regarding
sharing arrangements, as measured by their willingness to share with
disabled sharers, student sharers, or sharers with children, and by their
desire for a limited-time sharing arrangement. Further suggestive of this
flexibility is the advantage enjoyed by males and by widows and the
never married. It is possible that males and the widowed and never
married have fewer demands on them that would interfere with any
homesharing arrangement (phone calls, family visiting, etc.). Thus,
lodgers who are successful at finding sharers are likely to have been
flexible in their choice of sharers, have had limited goals regarding
homesharing, and themselves had few interpersonal or other emotional
ties to interfere with a homesharing arrangement.

If lodgers are hampered by restrictive ties in their search for providers,
then *employers* "suffer" from a similar limitation: Employer applicants
who live with at least one other person or who own pets are all at a
disadvantage in finding caregivers, compared to employers who live alone
or own no pets. The fact that employers who are using senior services are
also at a disadvantage in getting matched suggests the possibility that
support systems are already in place for many unmatched employer applicants. The other person(s) in the home with the applicant may already
be doing some caregiving or one's pet may be providing needed companionship and emotional care in the same way that senior services are
providing useful amenities; therefore, the employer applicant with one or
more of these resources at her or his disposal is more likely to be choosy
about caregivers and not be easily satisfied. Also helping employers get
matched is an emphasis on sharers helping each other and on compatibility. Overall, successful employer applicants are characterized by having
few interpersonal (and animal) resources and by a concern over the
interpersonal relationship they will have with their caregiver.

Finally, *caregivers* who get matched tend to be older, widowed, willing
to provide services and concerned over money matters. Together these
predictors paint the picture of a person with experience in caregiving
who understands what providing care involves and who wants very much
to have a job using those caregiving skills. As will be argued in chapter

10, however, some caregiver applicants actually prefer a job that does not involve personal care, and as employment opportunities expand in the community they are likely to turn away from homesharing.

In the case of personal care companion applicants, therefore, the key to getting matched appears to reside in knowing that the relationship between employer and caregiver is both an intensely personal one and one that is nevertheless based on fee for services. Both employers and caregivers profit from understanding these basic facts, at least before getting matched. With respect to sharers, on the other hand, it is not so much understanding as having the "right" characteristics that matters: Providers should be healthy, and lodgers should have few complicating ties with others. At the same time, there is a sense in which understanding comes into play in the traditional homesharing arrangement: Providers, unlike employers, should understand that the arrangement is one for the purpose primarily of sharing material, rather than emotional, space; and lodgers, for their part, should be flexible with respect to the kinds of sharers with whom they would be willing to live. In sum, traditional and personal care companion homesharing arrangements are different from one another, not only because of the different characteristics of each kind of applicant but also because of the differences in those characteristics that best predict who gets matched.

## THE PROJECT "HOME" MISSION AS PROCESS

In chapter 2, the brief history of Project HOME vividly described how much the organization changed during its first five years. Much of this change was both a reaction to the needs of the program's clientele and a cause of modifications in the make-up of that clientele. Thus, the extent to which applicants are successful in getting matched with homesharers is inextricably tied both to the individual characteristics those applicants possess and to the goals and structure of the organization that attempts to serve them.

### Organizational Goals and Structure

Regarding program goals, it is clear that the trend results support the notion that Project HOME's primary concern is the homesharing needs of its provider and employer applicants. For one thing, even though the overall success rate figures in table 6.1 show only employer applicants to have a better than even chance of getting matched, in the latest year in the series provider and employer applicants are nearly twice as successful as lodger and caregiver applicants. The greater success rate of the two stayer groups does not appear to be due to any particular characteristics helping providers and employers rather than lodgers and caregivers, so one conclusion is that an important part of the reason must be found in the program's efforts on behalf of its primary clientele.

The analysis of length of time between application and match (appendix 2) is relevant here. It also suggests that Project HOME focuses primarily on stayer applicants, because the two stayer groups, especially provider applicants, take much longer to match than the other two groups. Thus, Project HOME keeps on file and attempts to serve applicants for whom it apparently is difficult to find sharers. Employer applicants are not in quite the same vulnerable position as provider applicants, because they bring an important resource with them (money), while providers are in the position of having to barter or request rent.

Finally, the comparison by groups of multiple match (serial or concurrent) applicants (appendix 2) shows, again, differences between stayer and mover applicants. Providers and employers are much more likely to have shared more than once. In those cases in which an applicant has had two or more sharers, one could argue that the applicant possesses negative traits that make it difficult to stay with a sharer; but then one has to ask what it is that at the same time makes this unattractive sharer attractive to others.

While the data examined so far do not allow a comprehensive solution to this apparent paradox, it is quite likely that part of the answer lies in the fact that people who may look good "on paper" because they possess various important resources (e.g., large home, convenient location, money) may have trouble keeping sharers because of emotional or health needs that become apparent only after the homesharing has begun. Another part of the explanation is that people with attractive qualities lose sharers through no fault of their own but because of changes in the circumstances of their sharers. Students finishing up school and unemployed sharers finding work in another region are such examples of "mobility without blame." In the next two chapters, these individual trait explanations will be explored.

Another explanation lies within the organization's goals and structure. When providers and employers have been matched and, for whatever reason, become "unmatched," then the Project HOME director and her staff are faced with the responsibility of taking care of someone who, in most cases, still needs their services. Lodgers move on to new jobs, to new relationships, and, in many cases, to new cities. Caregivers have a ready-made service that is in constant demand. Providers and employers, however, are tied down to their homes and often are in frail health. Thus, after Project HOME staff have met, arranged a match for, and followed up on a stayer client who has come to the program, in many cases as a last resort, it is not surprising, after a match involving the still-needy stayer client is dissolved, that the staff feel a special sense of obligation to find a sharer for that client.

This obligation is consistent with the case management philosophy espoused by the volunteers who, from the inception of Project HOME, have wanted to be kept informed about "their" applicants' well-being. Even more important in a policy context, the obligation felt by the director and her volunteers is in line with the notion of a continuum of care within the home that implies, at least theoretically, that as client circumstances change, their needs regarding homesharing will change also. Therefore, when some provider and employer clients find their matches dissolve because their health is failing, Project HOME has tried to help the client put together a sharing arrangement or set of arrangements that can help the client stay at home despite declining health (see chapter 8).

## Individual Applicant Characteristics

While there are organizational patterns common to both groups of stayers and that distinguish them from movers, individual characteristics both separate out and tie together all four groups of applicants. As described earlier in this chapter, successful provider applicants are characterized by being in good health and expecting to share on the basis of a landlord-tenant relationship, lodgers by flexibility in their expectations, employers by being alone and depending on their financial resources, and caregivers by experience, willingness to provide service, and a concern over financial arrangements (tables 6.2–6.6).

Each of these sets of characteristics, while appearing to be unique to one and only one group, nevertheless highlight the complementarity of the two traditional homesharing applicants and of the personal care companion applicants. In the former arrangement, the need to find a compatible middle space between many providers' desire for "instant family" to fill in their lonely hours and many lodgers' desire for a "no-strings attached" landlord-renter relationship is highlighted. In the latter arrangement, the need for services among employers who have no human (or animal) resources and the willingness to provide services among caretakers mesh perfectly.

In summary, the data on success rates for matches underscores the importance of both organization mission and individual applicant characteristics. With respect to the former, the unimportance of background characteristics in predicting stayer matches highlights the primary mission of Project HOME, the program: to help elders and other frail homeowners stay at home in relative independence, no matter the age, gender, education, or marital or work status of the applicant.

Despite the efforts of program staff, there are important applicant characteristics that have predicted whether one gets matched or not. In particular, successful applicants must have some positive characteristic that attracts a sharer, whether it be good health (providers), flexibility (lodgers), money (employers), or a willingness to provide services for money (caregivers). Those most vulnerable and with little to offer have had the greatest problem getting matched, as has been the case of frail homeowners with transportation problems who want a traditional sharing arrangement.

The next two chapters describe what happens to those clients who do get matched. The emphasis first will be on the distinctiveness of the two sharing arrangements with respect to social exchange (chapter 7), and then on the continuum of care within the home and the special case of employer-caregiver relationships (chapter 8).

# 7

# Homesharing Arrangements and the Continuum of Care

Until now, the question of what happens once applicants are matched has only been implied (by the analyses offered in the previous two chapters on who wants to homeshare and who is successful in finding a homesharer) or addressed theoretically (by the speculations offered in chapter 1). This chapter empirically examines the different kinds of homesharing matches, paying particular attention to the distinction between traditional sharing matches and matches involving paid personal care companions, or caregivers.

Throughout this chapter, a guiding principle will be the idea that all homesharing matches taken together illuminate the importance of viewing homesharing along a continuum of care. Today, a home provider may need only a lodger to be a companion and perform a few chores in exchange for a place to stay. Tomorrow, this same home provider may need to become an employer of a caregiver because of deteriorating health. Theoretically, therefore, it is possible for an individual to be supported at home from a time of minimal need (e.g., someone for company) to a time of maximum need (e.g., 24–hour care; terminal care).

In order to understand the ways in which traditional and personal care companion living arrangements are both similar to and different from each other, two major questions are addressed in this chapter: first, what are the fundamental exchanges that occur in traditional and caregiving matches that produce overall satisfaction among participants? second, what are the unexpected exchanges that also affect sharer satisfaction? At the end, the idea of a continuum of care will be reconsidered in order to place the findings in perspective.

# FUNDAMENTAL HOMESHARING EXCHANGES

To evaluate the nature of the exchange within homesharing matches among the 216 clients who were matched during the program's first four years, a representative sample was selected for intensive follow-up. The sample consists of 14 providers, 18 lodgers, 22 employers, and 20 caregivers (a total of 74 sharers). A series of open- and close-ended questions were used to elicit specifics about the kinds of exchanges made, satisfaction with living arrangement and exchange of services, adjustments made and problems encountered, and the sources of both satisfaction and dissatisfaction in the arrangement. (See appendix 3 for the interview schedule used and appendix 4 for detailed information about the characteristics of the clients interviewed.)

## Social Exchange Theory and Homesharing

Recent work in the application of social exchange theory to gerontology has concentrated on the relative lack of resources possessed by the elderly (Bengtson and Dowd 1981; Dowd 1975, 1980a, 1980b). The experiences of homesharers, however, suggest that social exchange between elders and others in particular contexts may very well be a relationship between equals. Despite Dowd's (1980a:599ff.) reasonable assertion that elders are likely to run into serious conflicts in relationships with younger individuals, homesharing actually appears to maximize the possibility of mutual satisfaction between elders and their younger sharers.

Indeed, the majority of each type of homesharer—provider, lodger, employer, and caregiver—indicated to us a general satisfaction with their homesharing arrangement, and the remainder of this section will describe the basic exchanges that make these arrangements satisfactory.

The nature of the exchange in homesharing is greatly contingent on whether one is referring to traditional homesharing or personal care companion arrangements. In the case of traditional homesharing matches, the older home provider has a living environment to exchange with the lodger for rental income and usually some limited service and/or companionship. In the caregiving arrangement, the commitment and responsibilities of the person who moves in are so extensive that it is not enough for the homeowner to provide shelter; she or he must also provide a stipend as well as shelter to the caregiver. There are also instances in which no money is exchanged: when the services provided are greater than in the typical homesharing situation yet less than is common where a personal care companion is present. Since no money is provided the caregiver, this will be treated as a special type of traditional homesharing. Let us consider the two key resources in homesharing exchanges: money and services (particularly health services).

## The Significance of the Financial Incentive

*When Money Goes from Lodger to Provider.* The most obvious asset of exchange for owners is their home. All but one of the providers in the follow-up sample own their own homes. (About three quarters of employers in the sample also own their own homes.) In contrast, very few movers own a home. Those that do are usually satisfied with visiting their homes weekends or on days off. Another key difference between provider and lodger is money. As shown in chapter 5, stayers in both traditional homesharing and in personal care companion matches have more money and fewer financial concerns than movers.

In the traditional sharing arrangements studied, lodgers pay between $80 and $200 a month for rent. About a third pay the home providers less than $100, another third between $100 and $199, and the final third $200. For providers, the financial incentive actually does not appear to be central, although several do mention that the added money is a welcome supplement to their income, especially in light of high home maintenance costs. Says one homeowner, "With increased taxes this money really helps me pay my bills." A more typical response is that "it helps out but it wasn't a major part in the original decision." For most home providers, while the added money is desirable, it is not the most important reason for sharing.

For most lodgers, money *is* given as the major or even sole reason why they are homesharing. For example, a widow prefers living alone but, having a bill of over $5,000 from her husband's death to pay off, lives with a home provider to reduce her expenses while she attempts to pay her debt. In other cases, students need inexpensive places to stay while attending college, because many simply cannot afford the going rate of rents in what has become a landlord's market. In another instance, a visiting professor lodges to reduce the financial burden entailed by his family living in another state.

*No Money Exchange Between Providers and Lodgers.* There are also a half dozen matches in the follow-up sample in which no money is exchanged. These sharers are assigned to the traditional homesharing category, because the services provided in lieu of payment are usually fairly minimal or shared equally between homeowner and home mover. Also, Project HOME classifies a match as a personal care companion arrangement only if a stipend is paid by the stayer to the mover.

Examples of sharing arrangements in which no money is exchanged again include a variety of situations. In one, an 89-year-old woman felt lonely and wanted to be around people and so has invited a married couple to live with her. No rent is paid. However, they help with some of the heavy chores such as household cleaning and mowing the lawn. Also, the wife is a nurse, which further reassures the older homeowner. In another case where no money is exchanged, a 92-year-old woman needs someone to be in the house every night in case something unforeseen should happen to her and so has a nonpaying lodger. She also has someone else who comes in five days a week to do the housekeeping, so the homesharing arrangement actually involves no exchange of tangible services.

In still another case, a college student, in exchange for free shelter, is committed to cooking one meal a day for an elderly married couple who tend to get quite tired late in the day. As he describes it, "At 4:30 they tell me what to make for dinner. They had already shopped for the ingredients and they are waiting for me. She sometimes helps with the cooking but has no energy to clean up afterwards. She likes to be useful. She still cooks breakfast and lunch, but I do dinner more and more as her health is declining." In addition, he takes out the trash and provides some conversation as he shares the evening meal with them and cleans up afterward.

A final example in which no money is exchanged involves a young married couple trying to save enough money for a down payment on a home of their own who lodge with an older woman and help her with some basic household cleaning tasks. The wife also helps the older woman in home maintenance tasks by washing windows, putting up screens, checking the boiler and mowing the lawn.

There is no formula specifying how much a given quantity or quality of service is worth. Each partner in a match must work out what he or she feels is equitable, although the staff of Project HOME is available as a "sounding board." In one case a lodger may agree to pay a stipend for spending nights in an elder's home, while in another case the same situation will result in no exchange of money. And, as shown by the case of the 92-year-old woman who wants someone available "in case," some arrangements require no exchange of services.

*When Money Goes from Employer to Caregiver.* In the personal care companion sharing arrangement, the homeowner pays a stipend to the live-in caregiver in exchange for a considerable amount of care and a major commitment of time. Usually this is a full-time job for most caregivers, in contrast to the lodgers who have studies or employment that take them away from the home for major portions of each day. Frequently, in personal care companion matches, a paid respite caregiver is found who substitutes for the primary caregiver for one or two days during the week to give the primary caregiver time off from work.

Because caregivers are engaging in full-time work, the income stipend is quite important for most of them, as suggested in chapter 5 by the dissatisfaction with their own income that they report. In addition to free room and board, caregivers receive between $60 and $200 a week; the majority earn between $150 and $175 a week. Most caregivers are very attracted to this work because of their need for a paying job, while most employers are grateful the service is available and willing to pay for it.

Nevertheless, because of the nature of the demands on them, only a few caregivers mention the financial incentive alone; indeed, for some it is definitely a secondary reason for homesharing. As a group, caregivers are very devoted to their homesharers. One widowed caregiver, for example, took care of her parents until they died and then lived with her son. She describes the motivating force in her becoming a caregiver by recalling that she wanted "to do something on my own—to do something other than live at my son's not doing anything. I wanted to help someone so I decided to try homesharing for awhile." Another woman has always wanted to be a nurse, likes old people, and, after her husband died, began doing housekeeping and caring for others.

For some caregivers, there is a spiritual or learning component attached to their job. One woman says that the Lord told her to take this job. She receives such messages through dreams and finds great satisfaction in taking care of someone else. In another case, a young married couple is caring for a dying woman suffering from dementia. The husband is practicing his training as a certified nurse's assistant, but they both emphasize the way in which caregiving is providing them with an important learning experience: "We're learning about death, compassion and about how a human being changes into a person no longer able to care for herself."

About one quarter of the caregivers, like most lodgers, give money or geographical location as their main reason to share. For example, a couple with an infant are caring for a paraplegic so they can save for their own future home. A woman caregives because she "needed a place to live that wouldn't be expensive." She also wants "to experience another geographical area." Still another caregiver reports that she is "desperate for work again" after a divorce. Caregiving, therefore, is one avenue of employment for displaced homemakers. A college student working four days a week finds that caregiving is a "good way to make and save money and it has provided me with free study time." The woman she is caring for suffers from advanced Alzheimer's but is immobile enough and sleeps often enough to allow the student caregiver study time.

Not a single employer expresses any concern about the financial cost of a caregiver. One homeowner, reflecting on his time in a nursing home, complains about how much it cost him while he was there, but not about the cost of paying his caregiver, which is substantially less. For many employers, money is not a salient issue, because they are not even aware of the monetary arrangements that frequently are handled by younger relatives. Instead, these elders are concerned about health care, domestic task support, and companionship needs that must be met if they are to live in reasonable comfort in their own homes.

*The Importance of Money.* For some traditional homesharing arrangements, money is unimportant in the sense that none is exchanged and thus neither sharer is financially beholden to the other. For other traditional homesharing arrangements and for all caregiving arrangements, money is exchanged, but its importance varies greatly, depending, it would appear, more on the attitude of the sharer toward money than on the amount of money involved or the need by the sharer for money (although these are not trivial matters).

While both kinds of matches tend to involve exchanges based on money (with the exception of the few straight barter traditional matches described above), there are important differences between them. First, obviously the money exchange is in the opposite direction: Homeowners *receive* money in most traditional matches but *give* money in all caregiving matches. Second, despite this difference, money seems to be a more important motivator for the home seeker in both arrangements. Third, the need for money among caregivers, the "neediest" of the four groups, is nevertheless tempered by the social obligation they feel in their roles and the affection they have for their employers.

## Responding to the Health Needs and Disabilities of Stayers

*Providers and Lodgers.* Traditional homesharing matches ostensibly do not involve significant personal care, but, in fact, about a third of the lodgers matched *are* willing to provide such services. This is important for those like the relatively independent 92-year-old woman who wants someone around to notify the hospital if she should pass out. Instead of *paying* $65 a night for a nurse to be with her as happened when she first came home from the hospital, she is now *receiving* between $80 and $100 a month from a succession of college students who share her home and provide her with the minimal services she requires.

In another case, a homeowner is just barely able to manage at home by himself. Earlier, he was seriously considering moving to a group home, "but I felt it would be better to stay here because I was familiar with this house. I'd only move if it got so bad that I had to stay in a hospital." His sight is very poor, and he is quite lonely because his wife is in a nursing home. He remarks that were it not for his homesharer, a 77-year-old woman, "I probably would have been here living alone letting housework slide and being very lonely." She cooks, cleans and spends much time talking with him. They also watch TV together. In addition she pays him $150 a month to live in his home.

There are also several cases of traditional sharing arrangements in which the very slight exchange of services make the relationship seem like one between landlord and tenant. Since it is in the private home of the owner where space is frequently shared, however, some form of exchanging services usually develops. In one case, an older woman shares her home with two men for financial reasons and because "I also don't like living alone. I live in a big house out here in the country, so I felt better having others living here with me." Her lodgers pay her between $125 and $200 a month for their rooms and for use of her house. All three homesharers, including the older homeowner, have their own cars and drive from the country some ten miles to the city almost every day. Both lodgers are responsible for cleaning up the kitchen and their own rooms, but a cleaning lady comes once a week to do a thorough cleaning of the house. Outside professionals, directed by the owner's nephew, provide home maintenance services when needed.

Despite this seeming independence from each other, there is considerable interaction among the three homesharers. For example, one lodger puts drops in the homeowner's eyes each morning and evening "because it's difficult to do with only one hand." In addition, although all three keep their own food and follow their own meal schedules, the owner reports that they frequently "take turns cooking and sometimes we share the food." Finally, the older homeowner spends considerable time with one of her sharers in conversation; they go out to movies, dinner, and church, and even meet each other's friends. In addition to receiving income and companionship, she feels secure knowing she is not alone at night. It is important to her to "know someone is coming in and out so if I'm sick or if I fall someone is there to see I'm all right."

In another case, a young homesharer pays $140 a month to share a trailer with an older man who had always lived alone. Since his health had deteriorated his doctor wanted him to have someone stay with him. A brother lives about five miles away and helps him with groceries and doctor's appointments. However, the lodger helps keep track of the furnace, and shares responsibility for cleaning and minor home maintenance chores. Although cooking separate meals frequently, they almost always eat together. They also share an interest in maintaining a small garden. Each has daily medication to take and they monitor each other's consumption. As the homeowner says, "If I noticed he hasn't taken his medication I'll remind him. He'll do the same for me with my medication. We check on each other."

*Employers and Caregivers.* In contrast to lodgers, nine out of ten of all matched caregivers indicated a willingness to provide household services and seven out of ten a willingness to provide nursing services. Complementarily, the major needs of homeowners who request personal care companions are health maintenance, domestic task assistance, and companionship. Home maintenance with its occasional demand for assistance can readily be responded to by a relative or friendly neighbor: A grandchild cuts the lawn, and a son makes sure the roof is repaired and the house painted by arranging for the services from local contractors.

Tasks of daily living, however, require ongoing assistance usually pro- vided by the live-in personal care companion and respite workers.

In one of the caregiver matches, a quadriplegic is almost totally depen- dent on a married couple for her survival. She cannot even feed herself. She needs a dressing changed on a daily basis, and occasionally her "rosebud" (a tube and bag for urinating) must also be changed whenever accidents occur or the visiting nurse is not available. In addition, the live-in couple is responsible for all the housework, cooking, and much of the home maintenance, although the children of the homeowner are available for help with the latter.

In another match, an elderly man has a woman caregiver whose presence prevents him from having to live in a nursing home, because she is available to care for him twenty-four hours a day. When a previous match dissolved after five weeks, he had to return to the hospital. His caregiver, who has been with him for over two years, helps him with bathing, changes his dressing, and "sees that I take my medication." She does "everything that is necessary to run a house such as housecleaning, cooking, ironing, washing clothes and doing dishes." For home mainte- nance, "I usually call in a plumber or whatever is needed."

Finally, a woman who was in the hospital for a month following two heart attacks has been unable to do anything on her own. Her personal care companion takes care of her personal needs in addition to doing the housework, cooking and even keeping a garden going. The caregiver also fulfills a social need for her employer. "I would be very lonely if she wasn't here. On Sundays when she isn't here too much I get lonely."

These examples of employers with personal care companions are typi- cal. Personal and domestic care is quite comprehensive and continuous. Without the presence of a personal care companion, most of these homeowners would be either in institutions or living with family mem- bers. The personal care companion homesharing arrangement allows frail older and handicapped people to remain in their own homes basically independent of their children.

*The Importance of Services.* Traditional and caregiving matches, as expected, are also distinguishable with respect to service provision. In exchange for the money they receive, caregivers provide extensive ser- vices for their homeowners and thus may be said to be fully employed by their living arrangement. Despite the greater prevalence of household and personal care services in caregiving matches, however, an impressive minority of traditional matches also have been found to include service provision of one kind or another by the lodger.

## The Continuum of Care within the Home

The homesharing arrangements described above demonstrate the existence of a significantly broad continuum of care, interdependence, and support ranging from traditional homesharers who lead very independent lives similar to a boarder-landlord arrangement to the kind of comprehensive in-house care required by very frail elders and provided by personal care companions. In some cases, no money is exchanged and a moderate level of care is provided for free shelter. However, there is no fixed monetary figure attached to specific levels of services and the financial arrangement is negotiated by each participant in the match.

With regard to providers, the additional income brought in by a lodger is valued, but frequently not as much as the companionship of the lodger and the relationship that ensues. In other traditional arrangements, some limited services are valued. For the lodger, on the other hand, the homesharing arrangement is basically a cost-saving means of obtaining shelter. However, because the lodgers live in private homes with many shared spaces there are frequent opportunities for shared verbal interaction and the performance of helpful tasks, especially around mealtime.

For some lodgers this presents pleasant unanticipated opportunities for fellowship, and, indeed, many lodgers have found their hosts fascinating and historically knowledgeable. However, as will be described later, where there are major differences in expectations for verbal intimacy and companionship between providers and lodgers, there can be feelings of guilt, obligation, and dissatisfaction.

With regard to employers, their home is a major financial asset. They are generally grateful to their caregivers for services that assist them to remain at home. There is little evidence that payment to the caregiver is a major financial burden, although some bargaining about the actual stipend often existed at the time of the original homesharing placement.

For the caregiver, theirs is usually a full-time job, so that the stipend plus free food and shelter are very important to them. In addition, the caregivers are part of a unique arrangement in which their job and living situation exist in the same physical space. One does not go home at five o'clock in the afternoon after a day's work, and few caregivers see their living situation as only a job. Such intense and continuous interaction with one person almost always leads to bonds of affection and interdependency. Several caregivers are motivated by strong humanitarian or spiritual values of care and service. Although serving as caregiver is their livelihood, it also is a very satisfying way to implement a kind of religious mission or utilize the nurturing skills developed earlier in life while rearing a family.

On the other hand, the constant demands for attention and service can become overwhelming for some caregivers who would then seek respite help through Project HOME or assistance from their employer's family. Without such help, they are likely to experience considerable anxiety and dissatisfaction. Locating the major sources of satisfaction and dissatisfaction for sharers will be explored next.

## UNANTICIPATED CONSEQUENCES IN HOMESHARING EXCHANGES

While money and services are important exchange resources in home-sharing arrangements, they aren't the only ones. There are other resources that initially seem not to have been anticipated by either the sharers or the homesharing agency but which sharers mentioned in response to the follow-up questions about the specific sources of their feelings about sharing. As already indicated, most sharers are happy with their shared living situation;[1] yet, even among the happy sharers there are irritants and problems threatening the arrangement. Practically, some of these concerns predominate in traditional matches and others in caregiving matches. Analytically, they underscore two aspects of exchange theory: the "norm of reciprocity" and the "rule of distributive justice."

### The Norm of Reciprocity in Traditional Sharing

The norm of reciprocity says that good deeds inspire good deeds. As Bengtson and Dowd (1981:63–64) put it, "The basic principle, then, which underlies much of social interaction is the fact that an individual who supplies rewarding services to another obligates him." In traditional matches, after the financial and (where applicable) limited service exchanges are agreed upon, money and services tend not to be a problem. Still, difficulties can arise in three other areas: lifestyle, social interaction, and access.

*Lifestyle.* When two people begin to live together, even if they plan to retain separate lifestyles and keep living spaces distinct, there are bound to be adjustments. In homesharing, in contrast to the courtship period usually preceding a marriage, there is rarely a trial period during which personal habits and idiosyncracies can be discovered and accepted. So in a homesharing arrangement many of these discoveries must be made as the couple actually begins to live together. When the overall lifestyles of the sharers are compatible or interaction so minimal that lifestyle is relatively unimportant, then the relationship between sharers is balanced and relatively reciprocal. When lifestyles conflict, the balance in the relationship is tipped.

One of the worst situations involves a lodger whose responsibility is to be available at night in case the female homeowner has a seizure. The lodger hadn't been told about this condition and "would have liked to have known what to do" in case a seizure did occur. The lack of parking and the dirty condition of the house were also unexpected. Furthermore, the lodger reports that the homeowner "goes to the bathroom all over her bed and on the floors and she's living in an unsanitary environment." According to the lodger, the homeowner's daughter is "blind to her mother's condition" and has no sympathy for the lodger. Because the homeowner turns off the heat and opens the windows in cold weather, the lodger also complains about being cold all the time. Obviously, there has been a serious lack of communication between homesharers as well as between the agency staff and the homesharers, but this case fortunately is an exception.

In another case, a female lodger has had to adjust to *not* doing the housework that she actually enjoys doing. Of greater concern to her is getting used to having a dog in the house. She doesn't like pets and "the dog poops and pees all over the house. I make sure she cleans it up—not me." Of lesser concern, though still problematic, is the fact that the owner expects the lodger to wait up for her if she goes out, but when the lodger goes out the owner makes a fuss about being left alone. In spite of all these issues, the lodger surprisingly says she is "very satisfied" with the arrangement. She is happy because she doesn't "have to account to anyone and I have usage of the entire house." She has few responsibilities toward her home provider.

This particular case suggests two interesting conclusions about lifestyle conflicts between sharers: First, specific application questions about issues that might create problems (e.g., pet ownership), even though asked, do not necessarily cause the prospective sharers to clarify their positions ahead of time. Second, an articulated list of grievances do not always produce a general negative evaluation of a homesharing arrangement. Actual problems, though real to the sharer, may be relatively less important in that individual's mind than the benefits gained from the arrangement and therefore misleading if described in a vacuum.

*Social Interaction.* In spite of often large differences in age, there is little evidence of conflict because of a "generation gap" between sharers. Most homeowners want companionship from their lodgers, and are satisfied when they receive it. Typical of their desires are comments like: "I like company—I don't like being alone," "I like to have people around," "Mainly I need someone here at night," "The house is too big to live alone," and "I enjoy people. It's too lonely living alone." The benefits they receive from interacting with their lodgers are also clear. Common observations from satisfied providers are "I like my present homesharer because he doesn't hibernate in his room all the time," "Our communication is open," and "The major benefit of homesharing is companionship."

For their part, many lodgers also get satisfaction from interaction with their home providers. For example, a graduate student living in the home of a relatively independent older woman views homesharing as basically an enjoyable learning experience, despite some constraints because of his busy work schedule: "I am learning a lot about living with an older person, and it helps me because my father is sixty-seven. It sensitizes me to the problems of older people."

In another match, a young lodger remarks that he would be distraught if he had to live alone.

> That is a nice thing when somebody needs somebody and someone needs it themselves—When you leave we'll probably sit down and talk about this meeting and he'll probably remind me of my doctor's appointment. We help each other. I know the telephone number in case of an emergency and I know CPR. We entertain each other. He tells me a lot of stories about when he was younger. I love to hear him talk about his young wild years.

His home provider describes himself as a "loner" who had always lived by himself. Yet he considers his arrangement with his lodger as very satisfying. "We share everything and have respect for each other." The older man's one concern is that because he uses the bathroom a lot at night he might wake up his lodger.

In a final example, a pair of students at two different times have lived with the reasonably independent 92-year-old woman who needs someone home at night in case she falls. She thoroughly enjoys the stimulation that each of the four students sharing her home has been bringing into her household. The students themselves (we interviewed the most recent pair) are equally enthusiastic about their sharer who is seventy years their senior. In the first case, a 20-year-old college student is amazed at the vitality and breadth of historical knowledge of her home provider.

> When I first met her at 91 I figured she'd be crippled, couldn't hear and couldn't defend herself. She walks all over Burlington and has her nose in many things from state government to her church. It was nice to be around her. It was funny to see people come to the house and meet her for the first time. They'd try to help her up the stairs or help her get up out of the chair. We'd sort of chuckle to each other and she'd just say "I'm O.K. I'm not as old as I am." I learned to have a better understanding for some old folks. They're not all the same.

The homeowner herself fosters this closeness by encouraging the students "to feel like this is their home." They don't spend a lot of time here but when they do they have free run of the place."

In some arrangements interaction is minimal; but this is acceptable to both parties, including those few providers who are content to let their lodgers lead independent lives. "I didn't have to make any compromises, because we both could do what we wanted. We came and went as we pleased," recalls one provider. The lodger is rarely there during the day and, when she is, she is in her room listening to music. This is sufficient for the homeowner, since "just knowing she's here is a comfort."

For the couple who have a student prepare their evening meal, social interaction with their lodger is not important, since they have each other for conversation and companionship. The student has his circle of friends and has no desire to become more involved in their lives, and so all are satisfied with their limited social interaction.

Although most of the traditional matches observed are working well, others are not because of the conflicting social interaction needs of each sharer. For example, an elderly woman owner wants someone who can cook meals and act as a mealtime companion, since she dislikes eating alone. Instead, she has a lodger who stays in her room "with the door closed most of the time and, if not that, she was out walking the streets. As far as a companion goes, forget it."

Another homeowner wants to have someone living in her home primarily in case she falls, but she also desires companionship. Unfortunately, her overall satisfaction with the relationship is tempered by not getting the companionship she wants. As the provider remarks, "it really wasn't a mutual companionship because I always talked but [my sharer] was not willing to be more than a babysitter."

Some lodgers too are discontented because of their perceived social obligation to the homeowner. Typical is the case of the lodger who complains, "I found myself not going out, because she [the provider] made me feel guilty for going out." In the beginning, the lodger felt free to come and go as she pleased, but, after a while, she complains

> [The provider] started hinting about being afraid of the dark and being alone so I started to be with her more. I always felt like I had to talk to her. I felt like I couldn't go up to my room to relax after a day of work. She would sleep all day and stay up late and I'd stay up with her. I couldn't sleep at night. I never had private time either.

The lodger also does several errands like grocery shopping for the provider, but the key source of dissatisfaction is the social expectation, a need not originally anticipated by the lodger when the match was made.

Whether the homeowner was aware of her own need for companionship at the time of application is not clear. What is important to recognize is that sharers' level of satisfaction in a traditional homesharing arrangement is at least in part a result of matching the sociability expectations of the homesharers. Clear-cut questions at time of application is one means of attempting to match expectations, but the questions need to be detailed concerning the sorts of interactions desired and not desired. Furthermore, matching agencies and sharers alike need to be sensitive to likely changes in sharer expectations as a match progresses; the dynamic between two (or more) sharers may very well produce a "change of heart" on the part of at least one participant. In such cases, if compromise doesn't work, it is likely that new sharers will have to be found for each.

*Access.* Two seemingly obvious places for conflict over access would appear to be the bathroom and kitchen. While adjusting to sharing the bathroom is a problem for some homesharers, in most cases it is not a major issue. Some typical problems include sharers' complaints that "One thing I didn't like was using the bath after a person had just used it," "It was hard in the beginning sharing the bathroom, because I'd never know when he'd come in," and "I can't run out to the bathroom unless I have my housecoat on." Because the bathroom is a very private space, it is probably the most difficult room in the house to share; and more homesharers probably would have cited it as a problem area were it not for the fact that many of the homes have more than one bathroom.

Interestingly, the kitchen is rarely mentioned as a problem area in terms of sharing space. However, the act of sharing a meal together as a social activity can be important. A person who expects the company of the homesharer will be disturbed if the sharer doesn't feel the same way or has a work schedule prohibiting this interaction. One provider, sharing with a younger couple, wishes they would spend more time with her. She particularly dislikes the fact that they eat their dinner at nine P.M. when she is used to eating at six P.M. She not only misses the company, but also believes the discrepancy in eating times disrupts a major part of her daily routine.

Some of the more problematic conflicts over access involve unresolved misunderstandings between sharers—a particular problem for lodgers. For example, a student lodger has become upset upon learning that he can't use the household washer or dryer or obtain a second phone at his own expense, even though the couple with whom he is living had not made these prohibitions explicit during their prematch discussions. Other conflicts concern access to the providers' refrigerator, and the lodger's stereo and friends visiting. In this case, neither sharer needs the social interaction, so the access problem is now driving the lodger to seek an apartment for himself.

In another case, a middle-aged lodger describes her living arrangement as somewhat dissatisfying, because she is not allowed to bring any of her own furniture, including a much needed desk, into her room. She also cannot use the house phone and is upset because it costs her so much more to use the pay phone. Another concern is that she is not allowed to keep her bicycle in the garage. Finally, she notes that she needs permission to take a bath. "I can't take one after she goes to bed which is early, and that's usually when I want to take one. Sometimes I can't take one earlier either."

In a final example, another female lodger complains that she isn't allowed to use the washer or dryer or iron and that her home provider "doesn't like me to be in the house alone when she isn't there." Presumably, the homeowner is afraid that her lodger will break these appliances and the way to avoid such potential damage is to deny her usage of them. Also, the lodger is an early riser while her partner sleeps late, creating concerns on the part of the lodger that she might inadvertently wake her sharer.

Despite these discomforts and inconveniences, the lodger describes her situation as "satisfying." Reflects the lodger, "I like the peace and beauty of the place and her open communication even if it is one of not always loving. Sometimes I feel she is checking up on me, but at least she openly expresses herself." Again it is important to note that specific discomforts and inconveniences do not automatically translate into overall general dissatisfaction with the relationship. Other positive attributes may offset the unpleasant aspects.

The homeowner in this relationship argues that she does not let her lodger have her own phone because, "I don't want to change anything." The provider asks her lodger to consult with her first about the best time to use the phone, because the provider is on a party line and doesn't want any trouble with the other phone party. "We got that pretty well adjusted," she adds. The provider also doesn't like her lodger to be alone in the house, because her present homesharer is forgetful. According to the provider, her lodger has forgotten to turn off the stove several times. Finally, the provider notes how hard it was at first because her lodger "stayed up nights studying the Bible. I'm a light sleeper and that disturbed me. We talked it over and got that settled." The provider's openness and directness, appreciated by her housemate, is illustrated in a concluding statement she made to us: "When you get to be my age you are pretty well set in your ways."

This particular sharing arrangement represents one of the few cases in which the homeowner comments at any length about her partner. In most cases, the lodger's need to make adjustments is unrecognized by a home provider who takes for granted the imposition of restrictions on the lodger's movement and access to household appliances. The homeowner may be unaware of the difficulty or hardship it causes the lodger, and so an evaluation by the provider about the relationship is meager in most interviews.

*Making Fair Exchanges in Traditional Matches.* Many of the problems that exist for traditional homesharers tend to center about different expectations regarding lifestyle, social interaction, and access to and the use of space and appliances. When evaluating their satisfaction with their sharers, homeowners tend to be most concerned about the responsiveness of their partner to their need for companionship and for fitting into their daily routine. The lodger usually has to make the greater number of adjustments in terms both of lifestyle and access to space and appliances.

In summary, the most satisfactory traditional sharing arrangements seem to be those in which the provider wants the lodger to feel at home and therefore, within reason, makes the home and its appliances available to the lodger. This has the joint effect of increasing interaction between sharers, which providers want, and maximizing freedom of movement within the home, which lodgers want. Finally, although their lifestyles may be quite different from one another, successful homesharers also develop a friendship based on fairly regular verbal interaction. Some of the most successful arrangements of this kind bridge age differences of seventy or more years.

## The Rule of Distributive Justice in Caregiving Matches

In caregiving arrangements, the frail elder appears to get more out of the relationship than does the caregiver, which appears to contradict the idea of a norm of reciprocity; but it is consistent with one aspect of Homans' (1961: ch. 12) notion of the rule of distributive justice: While exchanges between equals should produce equal rewards, when there is inequality in an exchange, the "better" individual should receive the greater reward. The remainder of this section attempts to define "better" operationally by considering two themes characterizing the caregiving relationship: gratitude and stress. The former is expressed by both the frail elders receiving care and their caregivers. The latter appears to be the sole province of caregivers.

*Two-Way Gratitude.* As is true in traditional homesharing relationships, the general level of satisfaction of the participants in the caregiving relationship tends to be very high. The employers, however, appear to be more satisfied than the caregivers. This is probably a function of the fact that the employers recognize they are able to remain in their own home only because of their caregiver. Furthermore, because they are in their own home and because their physical condition dictates the lifestyle of the home, employers can do little adjusting to their caregiver.

It is also possible that the employer's dependence on a caregiver makes them less willing to complain, but this does not appear to be the case. There was only one instance in which an employer says she does not want to verbalize her complaints because she is afraid she might lose her personal care companion. It is possible, however, that others may have been unwilling or unable to articulate this reason to outsiders.

Comments of homeowners typically tend to reflect gratitude for the services rendered:

I get taken care of well. I get three good meals a day and my health has improved. I am better than I was, because I have someone to talk to and to take care of the home.

She enables me to live in my home. She is a marvelous companion. She does things the way I do them. She's a good cook too and she's meticulous as far as the house is concerned. We think somewhat alike, we respect each other and she doesn't treat me like an old woman who occasionally loses her memory.

She's a good person, cook, homemaker and knows how to care for me. She helps get my housework done and helps me take care of myself. She's wonderful. I never have to tell her to do anything.

I feel comfortable at home. I don't worry about anything. She's right there to take care of everything.

One homeowner, very effusive in her praise of a live-in couple and their child, stresses how many changes they have made in the home to make life easier for both them and her. The couple has done some electric work, put shelves in the carport, put contact paper in the bath, fixed the hydraulic lift for her, and arranged the kitchen cupboards to suit their own purposes. She wants her personal care companions to make her home their home. "I always tell people when they come, to fix things and do things the way they want it done."

Caregivers' positive comments tend to center about the satisfactions that come from providing care to a needy person. One caregiver states that she "feels right at home" and that helping "[my sharer] is the major benefit I receive which in turn makes me feel good." Another caregiver remarks that she "could be lonesome in an apartment by herself without someone to care for." The benefits of her caring for a 97-year-old lady in her home are friendship, fellowship, and love. "I do love her, care about her, and watch her and give her the best service I can, because she is a special lady to me."

Another positive theme stressed by caregivers is the chance for personal growth. A young couple caring for a dying woman in her nineties note that they are "learning about death, compassion and about how a human being changes into a person no longer able to care for herself." A college student who provides live-in care only on weekends needs the income but also replies that "this situation is helping me know myself better. It's gratifying to help her." Another young person says that one gets to know oneself by virtue of having new experiences: "You get to know the process of aging of an older person."

The gratitude that stayers and movers articulate might appear to stem from somewhat different sources: For instance, employers are grateful for the opportunity to remain at home and, by extension, for the caregiver whose presence makes staying at home possible. Caregivers, on the other hand, are grateful for the opportunity to help someone in serious need and for the opportunity to see life from a different perspective. In both cases, however, the source of the gratitude is the frail employer's need for services. If the financial arrangements are not in dispute (and they rarely are), then the dependence of the frail employer on the caregiver is what directly produces the positive sentiments on each side. This is different from the traditional sharing situation in which the positive sentiments of providers and caregivers may or may not overlap very well.

*One-Way Stress.* Even when participants want to cooperate fully with one another, however, caregiver matches produce their own kinds of strains. For the frail employer, they are few and generally center around lifestyle issues. For example, one male employer is very satisfied with his female caregiver but observes that she does things differently from the way his (deceased) wife used to: "I don't like it, but I don't make an issue of it; so it's like a change of lifestyle. I got to a point where it didn't make any difference anymore. I just decided she was going to run the household and that she had to do it her way." Despite his reservations, the employer is very satisfied with the arrangement and very fond of his personal care companion.

Very rarely does one find the kind of dissatisfaction centering around aspects of lifestyle and access to space and appliances that is more typical of providers. In one case, however, an employer wishes her personal care companion would clean the house more thoroughly, not use the phone so much, and not do her own laundry every day. In the eyes of the employer, the caregiver also prays and goes to church too much and is too limited in the variety of ways she prepares meals. Despite this litany of complaints, the employer is reasonably satisfied with the arrangement and glad someone is in her home.

While complaints are rare among employers, caregivers—despite expressions of satisfaction with their arrangement—face continual stress in their caregiving role. At least half the personal care companions interviewed mention the demanding and confining nature of their job. Such comments do not necessarily indicate dissatisfaction with either the homeowner or the general living arrangement, but they are real nevertheless.

One woman who loves her caregiving role nevertheless remarks that she has to "give up a lot of her own life." She complains of having only one weekend off in six months—when her daughter stayed overnight. In another case, a personal care companion is willing to continue working as long as the agency will "find someone else to help me out and give me some time off. I would like to just take a walk."

A third caregiver laments that her time is not her own and she has to fit in free time between tasks, but even here "it's very difficult." Privacy is also very difficult to sustain in such a confining environment, because she has to provide continuous care: "I have no privacy. She [the employer] constantly questions me about everything I do. I never expected it to be so difficult." The caregiver in this case has arranged to terminate her present position within a few months and so notified her sharer's daughters.

The most confining situation occurs for a caregiver of a wheelchair-bound 82-year-old woman with Alzheimer's disease.

> If I went upstairs she would keep calling. She follows me from room to room. I have tried to emphasize the point that she would have to depend on someone else if I got sick. Sometimes I wish I was not quite so needed. I can't go in there and sew anytime. Your time has to be hers like a child. I used to leave the door open with the sewing machine in the bedroom but not anymore. She gets upset. She doesn't believe her mother and father are dead. When it gets to seeing things I tell her I'm going home and not coming back.

This caregiver eventually received help from other respite caregivers provided by Project HOME, a system discussed more thoroughly in the next chapter.

A final example perhaps best illustrates the strong contradictory feelings personal care companions have. A young caregiver in her twenties caring for a very frail older woman in her upper eighties now sees that she

> never realized how many responsibilities you had when you did a job like this. I had to learn that I can't come and go as I like and I had to learn to be confined. That was very hard to do and I had to get used to being a flexible person getting up at all hours of the night if needed to care for health problems. Also in the beginning I had to get used to not seeing my family anymore.

Fortunately, a college student was hired to provide respite care on weekends so the primary caregiver could take time off to visit her family.

Despite sometimes still regretting being a caregiver "when you don't get along real good and have arguments about silly things," the primary caregiver overall is very satisfied with her arrangement and very attached to her frail employer.

> I get the most satisfaction—now this sounds crazy—when I'm coming home and she's so glad to see me. Or if we've been separated for a little while, when she does see me she looks at me like she's seeing her best friend again. I don't know if that's stupid or not.

*Balancing Caregiving Arrangements.* The very deep relationship between employer and caregiver, while generally viewed in a positive light by both parties, nevertheless produces stresses in lifestyles. For employers, it seldom happens, but when it does it is a disruption of their routine, which they are willing to undergo in exchange for the help they receive. For caregivers, it is the too common problem of confinement necessitated by the tremendous demands evolving out of the employer's frail condition.

Of particular concern, therefore, are the stresses undergone by the caregivers. The above examples illustrate the two reasonable options open to caregivers. They either terminate the arrangement or ask the matching agency for help (e.g., a respite caregiver). Until they choose either option, however, caregivers are in an unbalanced exchange with their employers. The extent to which caregivers tolerate this "unfairness" is explained by the idea (borrowed from the rule of distributive justice) that the frail homeowner "deserves" the kind of continuous help the caregiver provides—even if it means great stress for the caregiver. Certainly, this belief is in the minds of the caregivers interviewed; but it also is shared by the agency, as will be shown in the next chapter.

# SHARING SATISFACTION ALONG THE CONTINUUM OF CARE

As described in chapter 1, in homesharing, an effort is made to match competencies with the "press" or demands of the environment. A range of types of support can be provided, at least theoretically, for people with different degrees of disability or be continually adjusted for people who physically deteriorate over time to prevent the press of the environment from exceeding their individual competencies.

The bonds of interdependence vary widely among homesharers along the continuum of care. In a simple homesharing match, the home provider may be relatively independent but need a slightly more secure environment at night should she fall and need help, or, perhaps, additional income from a sharer to maintain the home physically. At the other end of the continuum, a frail employer may need help in every phase of her daily living in order to remain in her own home. In between these two extremes is a large array of different combinations of physical environments and competencies necessitating different levels of personal support so that the press of the environment does not overwhelm the individual.

Key to understanding the process of homesharing is understanding the significance for the individual homesharer of what is exchanged between them and their partner and how they subjectively evaluate their partner and the exchange arrangement. The chemistry of a match that is satisfying to its participants depends on a great many personal and structural characteristics and expectations of each member in the homesharing arrangement. Needs, responsibilities, and expectations must be clearly defined ahead of time or dissatisfaction with the match can develop.

For home *providers*, the key to satisfaction in a match appears to be the fit between psychological needs and the degree to which a lodger is willing to share emotional space with the provider. In the previous chapter, the success of provider applicants in finding a lodger was dependent in large part on the expectation that the sharing arrangement would be a business relationship rather than a personal one. Here, it is clear that satisfaction in the sharing arrangement for providers stems largely from the quality of the interaction they have with their lodgers.

Environmental press appears to be primarily a psychological one for providers in traditional sharing relationships. Those providers who are "pressed" least psychologically (expecting a business relationship) have the least problem both in finding a sharer and getting along with a sharer. On the other hand, providers who say things like "I like company," "I don't like to be alone," and "I get too lonesome" need more than money and help with chores from lodgers; they need the companionship many lodgers are reluctant to provide.

It is not surprising that the *lodgers* most likely to find matches and to be satisfied in matches are those with a flexible attitude toward their potential relationship. Evidence from the follow-up sample of lodgers shows that they derive satisfaction in shared living not only from the lessening of financial burdens but also from the quality of interaction with their home provider, regardless of the differences in their lifestyles.

Perhaps even more important, however, is access to amenities around the house (space and appliances). In a paradoxical twist, lodgers' dissatisfaction often stems from the providers' restriction of access to the providers' most important possession—their home, while providers' dissatisfaction tends to come from the lodgers' restriction of access to their most important possession—their company.

These problems highlight the two areas in which the respective sharers have the most power to affect the arrangement in either a negative or positive way: Providers can limit access to their home severely, while lodgers can limit access to themselves as companions severely. On the flip side, it would appear that when providers and lodgers give a little regarding access to home and to themselves respectively, they strengthen the relationship greatly.

For personal care companion arrangements, the press of environment on the frail *employer* is mostly a physical one that restricts daily living. In terms of satisfaction with matches in process, the extent to which a caregiver looks after the employer's physical needs has the profoundest impact on employer satisfaction. Employers generally are quite satisfied with their arrangement when their physical needs are taken care of. This does not mean that social interaction is unimportant; indeed, in many of the arrangements studied, a deeply satisfying personal relationship had developed. What it means is that having one's physical needs taken care of and being able to remain at home cover a multitude of sins, in the eyes of employers. This is consistent with the evidence from the previous chapter showing that those employer applicants who anticipate an intensely personal relationship in the context of fee for service stand the best chance of getting matched.

For *caregivers*, the importance of expectations regarding fee for service and the necessarily personal nature of the relationship between employer and caregiver are reflected in both the reasons why caregivers get matched and the reasons they derive satisfaction from their matches. Dissatisfaction of the caregiver stems primarily from one source: the pressure associated with the continuous needs of the employer. Here it is important to distinguish the kinds of psychological baggage which sharers bring to a relationship. More than anything, this problem is inherent in any relationship between employer and caregiver and requires the understanding of the participants and the employer's family to provide respite care of some type to "spell" the caregiver.

When homesharing arrangements do not require clear roles for the participants, there is much room for negotiation covering access to room and appliances and for meeting social needs like companionship and friendship. Although both partners in such traditional homesharing matches are usually capable of leading quite separate lives within the arrangement, more often than not there tends to be an exchange of services and sharing of space. It is precisely this interdependence that is the source of the sharers' satisfactions and dissatisfactions with the arrangement. In the language of exchange theory, a "norm of reciprocity" needs to develop, so that both sharers give and take in a relatively equal way.

Indeed, evidence from the follow-up sample strongly suggests that willingness to compromise in the sharing of companionship and space in a traditional homesharing match goes a long way toward improving the quality of the shared arrangement. In this case, therefore, whether the instigator is one of the sharers or an outside agency, solutions to be found for improving a traditional sharing arrangement lie with altering expectations of the participants or, failing that, severing the relationship and finding new sharers for the participants.

In the personal care companion arrangement, however, the frailty and helplessness of the homeowner invoke aspects of the "rule of distributive justice" and thus dictate to a great extent the lifestyle of the household and the relationship of the homeowner to the personal care companion. Although close personal attachments often develop to the benefit of both participants, the arrangement is fundamentally a business one in which fees are paid the employer for the caregiver's services. Because of the relative physical powerlessness of the employer and her gratefulness for being able to remain at home, many areas of potential disagreement between sharers about lifestyle and access are simply not relevant for personal care companions and are avoided.

Personal care companion matches are likely to be very satisfying for most caregivers, or the match will dissolve, because the intensity of interaction is too great and persistent to survive a significant period of dissatisfaction. For the caregiver, her private living space is also her work space. The major drawback is that the responsibilities can become so demanding that they confine the caregiver too much.

As a result, the major source of improving personal care companion matches is a structural one, as opposed to the situation in traditional matches in which participant attitudes need changing. For caregivers, the matching agency needs to be available to work with the participants and the employer's family to organize a system of respite caregiving to give the primary caregiver some time off. Such a support network surrounding the primary caregiver is often necessary for the ongoing success of a match and will be the focus of the next chapter.

# 8

# Frail Elders and Their Caregiving Network

The evidence from Project HOME clients thus far presented strongly supports the idea that homesharing, while a deceptively simple concept, in practice actually a covers a wide range of sharing relationships. Furthermore, inherent in the variety of relationships considered thus far is the idea that homesharing is an important "stop" along the continuum of care. Indeed, the critical distinction between traditional and caregiving homesharing arrangements highlights the fact that there are at least *two* homesharing alternatives between so-called "independent living" on the one end and institutionalization on the other.

This chapter will examine one of these sharing alternatives—the caregiving arrangement—to develop a major empirical proposition, a conceptual point, and a policy statement. First, empirically, the existence of a support network is critical to the well-being of both homesharers in a caregiving arrangement. For the frail homeowner, family, friends, and neighbors provide secondary care to complement the work of the primary live-in caregiver. They also provide a kind of buffer for the homeowner when the primary caregiver leaves and the agency has not yet found another caregiver to live in. For the live-in caregiver, those providing secondary caregiving and coordination of services, whether they be family or friends or agency respite caregivers, are a welcome relief and tend to alleviate the primary caregiver's stresses described in the previous chapter.

Second, conceptually, live-in caregiving arrangements represent a relatively new home care model that can contribute important insights into the relationship between formal and informal home care services for elders. Especially useful is evidence suggesting the supplemental model described by Noelker and Bass (1989), but in a unique juxtaposition of roles regarding service provision. That is, rather than the usual situation in which an agency supplements the caregiving of family and friends, the caregiving homesharing arrangements observed entailed family and friends supplementing the work of the live-in caregiver.

Third, and having important policy implications, for the frail elder who is able to avoid institutionalization through homesharing, a continuum of care exists *within* homesharing. This will be documented with examples showing what happens within the homesharing arrangement when the frail homeowner's health deteriorates and what transition role homesharing can play when institutionalization is necessary.

# THE SUPPORT NETWORK OF THE FRAIL EMPLOYER

We begin by considering the human resources of the support network who directly provide help to the frail employer in whose home the homesharing usually takes place. The sample of personal care companion matches upon which the analysis in this chapter is based is part of the larger follow-up sample described in the previous chapter. It will be remembered that there are twenty-two employers and twenty caregivers, covering fifteen personal care companion matches.[1]

## Family Support

Although the personal care companion is usually crucial for the older person's ability to continue to live at home, a larger network of support consisting of neighbors, friends, and especially family, facilitates this arrangement in many significant ways. The first of these, the family, often tends to be considered irrelevant for the wellbeing of frail elders in this country, because an image has been developed over the last several decades of family life in the United States as becoming increasingly segmented—especially between middle-aged adults and their elderly parents.

This image is more myth than reality, as demonstrated by much research in the area. In the first place, elders and their children prefer to be close to one another—both emotionally and spatially—although not in the same household. Rosenmayr and Kockeis (1965) refer to this desire of elderly and their children to live close to relatives but not with them as "intimacy at a distance." Living apart yet nearby supports the feasibility of maintaining intergenerational family connectedness while preserving the autonomy of the family.

Is this concept of "intimacy at a distance" borne out by the facts? It would appear to be so for a large number of elders. About four-fifths of all elderly persons in a random sample conducted by Shanas (1979) had a surviving child and about three-quarters of those with a child lived within thirty minutes travel time of one another. Moreover, in the Shanas et al. (1968) large-scale study of elders in three industrial countries, 84 percent of the American respondents with living children had seen at least one of their children within the past week and 90 percent within the last month.

Furthermore, relatives tend to provide for the vast majority of the health care elders receive. A U.S. General Accounting Office (1977) study reports that families provide up to 80 percent of all home health care for elderly individuals in the U.S. Approximately 3 percent of noninstitutionalized elders are totally bedfast and an additional 7 percent are housebound (Shanas 1979). The majority of these sick and frail elderly are cared for by family members, particularly spouses and children. Elders without close family are more likely to be institutionalized. Thus, "the presence of immediate relatives makes it possible for bedfast persons to live outside institutions" (Shanas 1979:173).

The importance of family and kin for Project HOME lies in the various ways they provide emotional and material help to the homesharing couple. Rarely do a frail homeowner and her personal care companion live together without considerable external support. Organizationally, the staff of Project HOME is available to deal with small disputes and adjustments and make new homesharing arrangements should prevailing arrangements not work out or if the caregiver leaves after a predetermined commitment of time.

Often, these planned departures occur in the traditional homesharing matches. For example, sharers who are students leave when they graduate from college and move away, creating a request for a new homesharer. For reasons described in the previous chapter, caregivers, who generally are older and not in school, also may leave; but the leaving is often not planned.

In most cases, however, the role of the staff of Project HOME is small compared with the ongoing support provided by the families of the homesharers in a caregiving arrangement, particularly those of the frail employer. Not only do family members frequently play important active roles in supporting their elder relatives in their own homes, but they also may act as significant "fictive" supportive kin for the live-in caregivers as well. Even the families of the caregivers often play a supportive role for their caregiving children although the support may be less intense, direct, and continuous than is the case with the families of the homeowners. In general, families appear to help their elderly relatives in three ways related to homesharing.

One way family members frequently provide support for their elder relatives is as "connectors" with Project HOME. Sussman (1985:416) has argued that as societies become more complex, aged persons increasingly will have to deal with bureaucracies that provide human services. As a result, families of elders will be called on to "serve as a source of information and influence in making decisions and as a mediating link between the older individual and societal institutions and organizations." Several employers, when asked how they came to the decision to homeshare, would begin by saying that their daughter or son felt they should not be alone at home. The following explanations are typical:

> My daughter insisted I have someone here with me and not be alone. She felt I needed assistance with daily living like cooking and taking care of myself. Psychologically it would be better for me too.

> My child felt I should have someone here at night because of my age and all. I previously had only graduate students here at night.

Not surprisingly, therefore, initial contacts with Project HOME are frequently made by a relative rather than the elder herself. If at all possible, children do not want to put their relative in a nursing home. For most children, taking care of their elderly parent(s) is not practical or desirable either. One daughter, prior to matching her mother, cared for her five mornings a week in the mother's home. The effort was becoming too much for the daughter, so she contacted Project HOME who was able to find a caregiver for her mother to live in the mother's home. The daughter now converses with her mother several times a day on the telephone. Her granddaughter who previously helped with the housework sees her grandmother about twice a week. The daughter is very satisfied, remarking that her mother now "gets regular care all the time."[2]

Another kind of support provided by families can be described as "safety net" support. If a match breaks up before another personal care companion can be located, family members, usually children, will temporarily sustain the older relative in the relative's home. One 56-year-old paraplegic, who has had in-home care from many different personal care companions for the last fifteen years or so, has relied on her six children to fill in between caregivers both before and during her affiliation with Project HOME. In another situation, when a personal care companion left suddenly, a daughter came in during the day and a son stayed at night to provide temporary help until a new caregiver could be found.

In a third kind of supportive arrangement, the primary live-in personal care companion is given a respite by a family member who provides either a period of free time or a period of reduced obligations. The assistance may be relatively small and sporadic such as a child taking her mother on an occasional pleasure ride or to a bimonthly doctor's appointment. Or the assistance may be substantial and regular such as the case in which the niece of a 97-year-old woman assumes total responsibility for her aunt one full day a week to give the regular caregiver a respite. The daughter also transports the caregiver to the grocery store twice a week, since the caregiver does not drive. Most family assistance falls somewhere in between these two extremes. For example, in one case a daughter does all the grocery shopping and takes her mother to the doctor; they see each other about twice a week. In another case, a granddaughter visits her grandmother twice a week and the grandmother, in turn, talks to her daughter daily by phone.

Family, therefore, are often involved in the personal care companion sharing arrangement from the very beginning as facilitators who arrange the necessary contact with Project HOME, as support in crisis situations when caregivers leave, and, on a regular basis, as helpers or substitutes who attempt to alleviate the burdens of the caregiver.

## The Male as Family Resource

Although most research on caregivers asserts that daughters, or "women in the middle" as Elaine Brody (1981) refers to them, provide most care, there is evidence to suggest that sons are also important caregivers. For example, research conducted with a randomly selected sample of 900 noninstitutionalized elders living in eighteen different communities in six northeastern states has found sons to be as likely as daughters to help their elders (Rathbone-McCuan and Coward 1985). Elders interviewed name a daughter as a helper in 19 percent of cases, sons in 22 percent of cases, and both daughters and sons in 6 percent of the cases.

The Project HOME personal care companion arrangements include many instances in which caregiving for the frail employer is aided by the frail employer's son. Some of the more instructive cases are described in the following paragraphs.

In one example, a son arranged for his elderly mother and father to have a live-in personal care companion. The 90-year-old father is bedridden, and the 86-year-old mother is limited in mobility and suffers occasional bouts of confusion. The son calls the home every day, which is reassuring to the mother. Several times during the follow-up interview, the mother expresses gratitude for the concern of her son. She "thanked the Lord" her son is so near and she can call him any time. Her daughter lives in a neighboring state, so, not surprisingly, she says her son who lives close by is her major confidante and the one on whom she depends. This son is also the person to whom the male caregiver of the older couple looks for advice and support, an issue to be discussed later in this chapter.

In another case, the frail employer reports that her son takes her for rides or to appointments at least twice a week. He also buys groceries and "talks with me if I get depressed." Her son and his wife are jointly named as confidantes by the son's mother in response to the question in the follow-up interview that asks the client to name the individuals to whom they talk about important issues.

In another, very similar case, a son—described by his mother as a "mother hen"—visits her daily. He goes out to lunch with her twice a week, takes her to medical appointments and on other errands, and looks out for her financial well-being. His wife takes her mother-in-law out for lunch at least one other time a week. The mother also has a daughter who lives several hundred miles away and comes to visit whenever possible or when special care is needed (such as when she needed eye surgery).

In a case where the mother suffers from Alzheimer's Disease and could not be interviewed, the live-in caregiver remarks that the mother's son visits his mother frequently. Furthermore, the caregiver believes he is very appreciative and supportive of the caregiver's efforts on behalf of his mother. Several months after the follow-up interview, the mother moved into the home of a daughter who lives in another part of the state. The son was willing to provide considerable support when the mother was in her own home but, in this instance, it is the daughter who eventually takes the mother into her own home when "independent living" through homesharing is no longer feasible.

In another Project HOME caregiving arrangement, a wheelchair-bound father has a private nurse care for him every weekday from eight until six and an overnight caregiver every weekday night. His two sons alternate weekends away from their own families to care for their father. The sons change their father's urine bag, shower him, and help him get in and out of his bed. They also take him to the theater and out to dinner. The father perceives his condition as temporary, but if he ever becomes too much of a burden for them he will hire someone to come in on weekends.

In a final case in which a male support person is prominent, a son has come on weekends to cook for his paraplegic mother, when the couple acting as caregivers for his mother needed time off. At an earlier point in time, a previous caregiver walked out suddenly on the paraplegic mother. Support came from both her son and her daughter. The daughter helped the mother during the day, while the unmarried son stayed there overnight, living in the basement of his mother's home. Since the follow-up interview, the caregivers have gone, and the daughter has moved into the home—thus ending for a while at least a long period of homesharing. This case also illustrates how family can fill in during gaps in paid caregiving.

Although it may be true that daughters or female relatives provide more care for their parents than do sons, it is clear from the evidence cited earlier and from the Project HOME experiences described in the follow-up interview that sons frequently complement and assist their sisters in providing care for the frail parent(s). When there are no daughters in the family or when daughters do not live nearby, sons appear to be capable and willing to provide the needed support and coordination of services necessary to help their relatives remain in their own homes.

Regarding a related question, however, there is no evidence that sons would go so far as to take their parents into their own homes or move in with their parents as an alternative to homesharing. At the same time, despite the example given in this section, there is little evidence that choosing to live with a frail parent is preferred or utilized by many daughters either.

## Homeowners Without Children

In spite of the importance given to the role of children as facilitators and supporters of the homesharing arrangement, it is also true that about

40 percent of all homeowners have no children or children who live too far away to provide more than minimal support. Shanas (1979) found in her study of five industrial societies that one in five old people have no surviving children. Childless elders, without available family caregivers, are therefore an especially vulnerable population when the become frail. As a result, they are quite likely to need formal services; they also represent a disproportionate number of elders in nursing homes (Cantor and Little 1985).

There is evidence in this study that other relatives or even "fictive kin" can and do substitute for children. For example, in one case a niece arranges for caregiving help for her senile aunt because she feels an obligation to the woman who did a lot for her mother at an earlier time. In another case, a niece monitors the caregiving arrangement, provides time off for the caregiver, and takes the caregiver to the store as well as on an occasional pleasure outing. A nephew of this same aunt looks after his aunt's financial situation.

In yet a different situation, a male homeowner relies on a nephew as a confidante, although the nephew lives several hours away in Boston. The homeowner notes, "I call him on the telephone. We couldn't be any closer." For another employer, it is a brother who visits weekly, is named as a confidante and companion, provides services like help with bills, and rides in his car.

Finally, it is important to realize that the sort of dedication shown by a son, daughter, nephew, niece, brother, or sister to the well-being of an older relative also can be demonstrated by a nonrelated guardian. Technically, a guardian is recognized by the state as someone who looks after the social and financial interests of a handicapped or frail person. In one Project HOME match, an 82-year-old wheelchair-bound woman with a progressive case of Alzheimer's Disease is looked after by a dedicated 56-year-old neighbor who checks on the frail sharer's welfare almost daily. When the guardian does not make a daily visit, she talks with her frail neighbor by phone. The frail employer has four stepchildren whom she neither trusts nor believes to be helpful to her.

Because of the intense demand for personal care required by the frail employer, the guardian has had to make frequent matches and in the end patch together a group of several caregivers to provide services each week. One caregiver comes during the week and the other lives in during the weekend. In her legal role, the neighbor consults with the homesharers and is responsible for chores like bill paying, grocery shopping, and house maintenance; beyond being a guardian, the neighbor is also a warm trusted friend of the homeowner. Her case is unique in the comprehensiveness of the care and support she gives to the homesharing situation; aspects of this comprehensive care will be examined more thoroughly in the section on caregivers' support systems.

Overall, it is clear that kin other than immediate family and, in some few cases, guardians can play a critical role for the frail employer. As with immediate family support, the range of help of real and "fictive" kin includes arranging for and overseeing matches and providing direct services for the frail employer. Both emotionally and materially, guardians and relatives outside the immediate family are important sources of support in caregiver matches.

## Friends, Neighbors, and Formal Services

Friends and neighbors play a wide range of roles from no help to very helpful for the frail homeowner. In the many cases where frail homeowners are elderly, they tend to be quite isolated with regard to both friends and neighbors. In the first instance, death has taken away many long-standing friendships and new friendships have not necessarily replaced the old.

> I visit with friends now and then. All my friends passed away. I used to chum out with everyone of them. Three brothers died—two last year. I often think it is hell to see them all gone. I miss them. My closest friend died three months ago. Neighbors from across the street come over to chat about once every two weeks.

> I don't really know the neighbors. I don't have many close friends who are still alive. Many have died. I do talk to some friends once in awhile; maybe four times a week more or less. The fact that I speak with friends on the phone is an emotional support for me.

In each of the above two cases, neighbors are seen by the frail elder as providing some degree of solace.

Unfortunately, such frail elderly are limited in their own mobility and reluctant to initiate much contact with neighbors, although they do feel secure in the knowledge that neighbors are available in an emergency.[3] In the words of some of the employer respondents:

> Neighbors drop in to see how I am. They don't stay long. They would do things for me if I needed them.

> I don't see much of my neighbors. They're very kind. Mr. T. will do anything for me if I ask him. The pastor visits about once a month. People from church used to come over real often. Now not so much. A couple of weeks ago several ladies called. I wish they'd come over more often.

I know two or three neighbors real good and if I need them I know I can call on them. But I haven't had to. But if I really wanted anything the family across the street would help.

Neighbors mean an awful lot. They provide rides, bring food, flowers and company at least once a week, often times more often. Friends are here when I need them. They'll be here for anything I need.

Just as in the case of friendships, the transient quality of neighbor relationships can be a problem for very old homeowners who outlive their neighbors from earlier more active years and are unable to go outside enough to develop relationships with new neighbors. This difficulty is illustrated in the statement of an 87-year-old homeowner who notes, "I have great neighbors who drive—the old ones. I don't know the new ones." Because of mobility patterns and the mortality of their neighbors and old friends, current neighbors and friends do not provide a consistent support base. Neighbors tend to be younger, not have much in common and, in general might be called only in case of an emergency. As one 86-year-old homeowner reports, "One neighbor, we're sort of friends. They're much younger than I am and it's difficult to relate."

Because of their restricted interpersonal world, more indirect forms of communication become especially important for the elderly and disabled. Particularly important are mail and daily phone calls. One caregiver reports that the homeowner gets very grumpy and put out if she doesn't get a phone call or a visit every day. In another case, the son of a homeowner notified the post office to have his father's mail delivered to himself instead. The caregiver believes this to be wrong: "He doesn't receive any mail, which he misses. It's too bad it goes to his son; he used to look forward to it."

Another source of indirect support comes from services provided to frail home-bound individuals. For example, two of the homeowners cite the importance of having a "lifeline" that automatically connects the person with the hospital in case of medical emergency. This device seems especially reassuring to one woman, who reports having fallen and been rescued by police officers who had been notified by the hospital.

Pets constitute an additional source of support for the elderly. In some cases, the pet seems to be at least as important as kin in meeting the expressive needs of the homeowner. In the case of an 82-year-old widow, her cat, named Kitty, is a primary reason for wanting to homeshare. "Homesharing has been a major factor in my ability to stay here in my home. Probably I would not be able to move my kitty so I'd miss him terribly." Sadly, some family members and friends fail to acknowledge the significance of the emotional ties between the homeowners and their pets. For example, one 83-year-old homeowner, hospitalized for six weeks before starting to homeshare, reports that while hospitalized, "there was no one to care for the cat, B.J. My son put him to sleep. I really loved that cat." Although he wants another cat, he is reluctant to get one, since "if something happened to me, he would be left alone again."

Although many of the homeowners have been involved with community organizations, like church, most have limited contact at the present time, generally because of decreased mobility. Several report weekly visits by their ministers, or their wives, or church members, but few actually are able to attend church on a regular basis.

About two-thirds of the homeowners receive some formal public assistance which, in most cases, amounts to once-a-week visits from the Visiting Nurses Association. Generally, the duties of the Visiting Nurse involve giving the client a bath and helping with other aspects of personal care (e.g. cutting toenails). In only one case are visits made more than once a week. Even these brief visits can be helpful to personal care companions who are then free to run errands while the nurse is in the home.

In summary, the support network of the frail homeowners is comprised primarily of their families and individuals who are regarded as family. This network is supplemented by neighbors and friends, visiting nurses, and, in some cases, even the homeowner's pet. The functions of these resources are twofold: They perform tasks that directly help the frail homeowner; these range from being the tie between the homeowner and Project HOME and other service agencies to paying bills, grocery shopping, and respite care when the primary caregiver has time off. Invariably, when there is a gap in services (e.g., caregiver unexpectedly takes time off; caregiver quits), the family or fictive kin attempt to fill the breach.

Less easy to measure, the second kind of support provided by family and close friends stems from the security frail homeowners feel in having someone besides the caregiver be responsible for their needs. To the extent that family and others oversee the caregiving arrangement, as documented dramatically in the case of the guardian friend, the frail homeowner receives critical emotional support. The next section will show how this emotional support proves to be important also to the caregiver.

# THE SUPPORT NETWORK OF THE CAREGIVER

## Family Support

The social exchange involved in a caregiving homesharing arrangement is straightforward enough on the surface: The frail employer or her or his family pays a caregiver to provide important personal care services on a regular basis. As should be clear by now, however, the generally demanding nature of personal care and the deteriorating condition of many frail employers usually produce stresses on the caregiver that she or he is unable to handle alone. It is therefore important to examine the kind of supports caregivers themselves receive as they attempt to fulfill their responsibilities to their employers (see Clipp and George 1990 for a summary of the way caregiver needs and social support are related).

The caregivers often also receive support from family and relatives. Not only does support come from grateful relatives of the homeowner, but it also can be given by the care provider's own family. Some instances in which the family of the frail homeowner helps provide care for their relative and so indirectly aids the caregiver have already been described. Later in this section, more direct examples of support by the employer's family for the caregiver will be given, but, first, it is important to see how the caregivers' families provide support.

*The Caregiver's Family.* Usually the caregiver's own family is not directly involved in the homesharing matches but facilitates their child's participation in other, indirect ways. Some of these ways are illustrated by the following examples. In one case, a couple caring for a severely handicapped person visit both their sets of parents weekly. The husband and wife report that they don't need any particular assistance from their own parents but do find the time they spend with their parents helpful in getting away from their work. There are times when the parents also help out in a material way by agreeing to baby-sit at the last minute for their grandchild who is presently being raised in the home of the handicapped homeowner.

Another couple caring for a frail older person reports that their own families are proud of what they are doing and offer a lot of verbal support. In another case, the family of a young caregiver in her twenties provides a change of pace or a retreat from her caretaking job every weekend. Her family of orientation is where she goes to "enjoy life and be myself."

They make me laugh. They provide room and board for me and the transportation to get to and from St. Albans on the bus which I take from Burlington.

> It's a minivacation for me when I'm home and visit my family. I go out with my sister. I bowl, read books and see movies.

During the weekends, therefore, her family represents a refuge, a place to recharge and to enjoy the activities that are important for a young person who spends most of her weekdays caring for a frail 91-year-old woman.

Still another personal care companion with seven children sees at least two daughters each week and even cares for her grandchildren at times. Although not needing anything from her daughter, she feels secure in the knowledge that she can always ask her daughter for assistance should she need it.

While the evidence is sketchy, it is clear that their own friends can also play an important role for the caregivers. In many cases, however, those friends are seen only on days or weekends off. Furthermore, in the case of friends who live a distance away, the caregiver is often put in an uncomfortable position extending an invitation to visit the "shared home." As one caregiver has put it, "I have to be careful because it's Elsie's home. You tread on people's grounds and then you don't have a home."

As was seen in the discussion of how family supports the frail home-owner, caregivers themselves receive both emotional and material aid from their own families as they attempt to cope with the constant stress inherent in their work. Not surprisingly, while help with baby-sitting and other tangible examples of aid do exist, it appears to be the emotional release families can give their caregiver daughters or sons that is most important. As seen from the previous chapter, the single greatest source of dissatisfaction among caregivers is the constant stress of a demanding job that allows no time off if provisions are not made to give the caregiver some respite. Families of caregivers can and do provide such respite in the ways described above.

*The Frail Employer's Family.* The family of the frail employer can also be helpful to the caregiver. As already noted, family members often do chores or stand in during a period of time (e.g., weekends) for the caregiver so the latter can have a break from work. There are other ways the frail employer's family helps caregivers, however. Although it is possible to overdramatize the situation, many employer/caregiver relationships, because of the intimacy and intense contact involved, become like an extended family in which the caregiver is but another member. Here, too, the help received by the caregiver from her or his adopted family is both emotional and material.

One case in which both kinds of support are given involves a son and his wife who help both the son's mother and her personal care companion. The latter notes particularly the importance of the son's wife as a source of information and support. The caregiver speaks with the daughter-in-law several times a week on the phone. Since the daughter-in-law herself had cared for a sick mother at home for many years before placing her in a nursing home, she both empathizes with the live-in caregiver and provides her with useful information about the aging process and ways to cope with the needs of older frail persons.

An even more striking example of employer family support for the caregiver involves the one male caregiver in the follow-up sample. He was originally attracted to this particular homesharing assignment because of the support and concern expressed by the son of a frail elderly couple.

> I could tell that G. really cared about his mom and dad and it wasn't just going to be putting me here and forgetting about the situation. This was the main reason I took the job.

The family of the frail couple help the caregiver in material ways. For example,the son takes care of strenuous chores around the home like shoveling snow and basic repairs to the house, since the male personal care companion has asthma and finds these tasks difficult to complete.

The support is also emotional, as the caregiver reports that this homesharing arrangement and the support of the son and his wife are "the best things that ever happened to me."

> B. and G. are fantastic. I do get nervous sometimes. It's a job. But when I have a problem of any kind I call G. and it gets solved immediately. I love it. I even get use of the car. I was invited on their holiday and treated like family. I couldn't be happier if I was making $500 a week. B. and G. are closer to me than my own brother and sister.

In addition to having weekends off when the son and his wife look after the son's parents, the personal care companion was given time off and the use of the family car to visit a friend in Maine. The son's wife even baked a cake for him to take along on the visit. After being away for a few days, he longed to return to his "home." "I wanted to come back here. I like to have a home."

The most unusual personal care companion arrangement observed shows that the family of the frail individual cannot always help the caregiver; despite the best intentions and goodwill of family members, the caregiver may have problems that need professional help. In this case, a woman had been living with her mentally deteriorating and very demanding aunt. The niece felt a strong obligation to keep her aunt from entering a community care home. At the same time, the niece found living with her aunt so difficult that she applied to Project HOME and was matched with a young woman who was supposed to provide caregiver help for the niece to look after the aunt.

Initially, the arrangement appeared to be a godsend to the niece, who contrasts the period during which she was caring for her aunt on her own and the situation in which she has the caregiver:

> I love L. [the aunt] dearly but she's so demanding it's difficult for me to lead my own life as well. I had to provide 24-hour care. I had no privacy. She constantly questioned me about everything I did. I realized I couldn't handle it just the two of us, so that's when I decided I needed someone to help me out with L. and to share in the expenses. My aunt drives me bonkers. It's just so difficult to live with relatives. S. is wonderful. If she wasn't here I wouldn't have been able to stand it.

Unfortunately, the caregiver was herself in need of serious caregiving help. She had entered the arrangement without telling her sharers that she was pregnant. Furthermore, after a while it became apparent that she was also in need of psychiatric monitoring, so the niece, at the time of the follow-up interview, was planning to dissolve the arrangement because of the double stresses associated with her aunt and the caregiver.

After the interview, we learned that the aunt moved in with one of her daughters and the "caregiver" put up her baby for adoption and found another homesharing arrangement. In this particular case, the screening process had not uncovered the caregiver's situation, and so the arrangement proved to be far too stressful for any of the parties to overcome through family support, respite care, or any other intervention. Only dissolution of the match made any sense.

As a footnote, some rare instances in which the frail homeowner's neighbor plays the same kind of role as family members for the caregiver were uncovered. In one such case, a homeowner has a good 60-year-old friend of thirty years' standing who comes once a week to clean the apartment and take her for a ride. This is not only welcomed by the older homeowner but also by the young caregiver who remarks how this friend is a "cushion for her." "If I'm in a bind she'll help me out." Unfortunately this friend is planning to stop these visits in a few weeks because the weekly effort is tiring her too much.

Overall, therefore, their own families, the frail homeowner's family, and occasionally the frail homeowner's friends and neighbors can be welcome sources of emotional and more tangible kinds of support for caregivers. Unfortunately, as many of the cases illustrate, the relationship between employer and caregiver is often a changing one due to the deteriorating health of the frail homeowner (or, as in the last case, the homeowner's neighbor) and thus one that produces additional stress on the caregiver. The next section considers an increasingly important part of the network of supports for the caregiver: respite care.

## The Respite Caregiver

In addition to family and friends, a second, more formal source of support for the caregiver in a personal care companion homesharing arrangement is the respite caregiver who, as in the case of the primary caregiver, is found through Project HOME and whose specific duties are the care of the frail employer. As the demand for and supply of personal care companions grew during the second and third year of Project HOME's existence, so too did the need for caregivers who could provide short-term or occasional relief for the primary caregiver.

Unfortunately, the need for respite care frequently has exceeded the supply. Therefore, although family members have tried to fill in the gaps created by the primary caregiver's need for time off, such as caring for an elderly parent on weekends, the preference of family members continues to be having full-time live in personal care. As demands become more pressing on the primary caregiver, this means needing respite caregivers to supplement the work of the primary caregiver. This need for respite assistance generally increases over time as the condition of the homeowner deteriorates, as will be seen in some of the following examples.

In one case, the need for respite care and its provision were quite straightforward. The live-in caregiver at first was providing care seven days a week for her employer, but the demands of the job began to tire her until she reached the point where she was ready to quit the arrangement. Through Project HOME, a college student was hired to come in on weekends to give the primary caregiver time off. As she relates, the new arrangement meets her need for time away from her caregiver assignment perfectly:

> When I first began sharing I had to learn that I can't come and go as I like and I had to learn to be confined. That was very hard to do and I had to get used to being a flexible person. I had to get used to not seeing my family anymore.

> But that's no longer true because I see them on weekends now. With J. here it makes my homesharing much better for me. It gives me a break. With J. here, now I can go home on weekends.

As a footnote, it is interesting to observe that the son who coordinates this arrangement actually pays the primary caregiver less than the respite caregiver who comes on weekends. Just recently, however, he has offered to help make it financially possible for the primary caregiver to obtain a degree in nursing. It would appear, therefore, that all parties are now satisfied with the new arrangement involving coordination of care between the frail homeowner and primary and respite caregivers.

Another situation is somewhat more complex. This is the one involving the guardian who has been looking after her frail neighbor. In this case, the frail homeowner had a personal care companion only five days a week to begin with because she was able to get along on her own over the weekend when the live-in caregiver was away visiting family. However, as the homeowner's condition deteriorated, she began to need the caregiver for most of the weekend as well. Simultaneously, the live-in caregiver was realizing that she wanted even more free time for herself than just the weekends.

Again, the guardian went to Project HOME for help. In this case, a new primary caregiver was found to substitute for the previous one who herself eventually became a one-day-a-week respite caregiver. Therefore, the frail homeowner received the continuous care her deteriorating health was requiring and the original primary caregiver was allowed greater time freedom by becoming a respite caregiver in the same household.

Unfortunately, this satisfactory situation did not last long, because the homeowner's mental condition began to deteriorate along with her physical condition, creating additional stresses on the new primary caregiver. For instance, the primary caregiver reports that the only time she could leave the house was for a ten-minute walk to collect the mail once a day. Even for this brief interval, she would have to leave notes around the house reminding her homesharer where she had gone.

> The hardest part is not being able to come and go. She would keep calling me. I can't go into my bedroom and sew anymore. Your time has to be her time— like a child. I used to leave the door open with the sewing machine in the bedroom, but not anymore. She gets upset. I wonder if there is some volunteer organization where someone comes in and spends an hour when I go out for the mail so I will know she is not alone. I need to have someone I can call if I had a doctor's appointment so someone could come in.

This live-in caregiver eventually quit; and a third primary caregiver moved in to live with the frail homeowner during the working week, while a second respite caregiver came in during the weekend. As a result, the one-day-a-week caregiver was no longer needed. This situation worked for some time until still further physical and mental deterioration of the frail homeowner required her being placed in a nursing home.

In some cases the mix of primary care and respite care live-in companions is even more complex. In one case, a daughter working for her doctorate and living with her 90-year-old mother who had recently suffered a stroke, uses two different live-in companions. One person comes in eight hours a day during the week and a second person stays there during nights. The daughter has primary responsibility for her mother's care during the weekend; but the second caregiver also trades off every other weekend with the daughter, so the daughter can pursue her career and have a social life as well.

As a footnote, for those who want loose ends tied up, the personal care companion who only comes in during the day is now herself a home provider for the mentally disturbed pregnant woman who was helping the niece care for her ailing aunt. In this unusual sharing arrangement, it might be said that the homeowner is more likely to be giving than receiving services in what is certainly not a traditional homesharing relationship but rather more of a reverse caregiving arrangement in which the homeowner looks after the lodger.

# RETHINKING CURRENT MODELS OF CAREGIVING

The complicated relationship between the formal caregiving services provided by the live-in caregiver and the informal help given by family and friends suggests a need to reexamine contemporary perspectives on the ways in which informal and formal in-home care relate to one another.

## Formal and Informal Service Links

The nature of the ties between formal and informal support systems has a long history. Max Weber (1947) recognized the superiority of the formal organization with its specialization of skill, coordination through rules, and stress on informal relations over affectionate ties. The difficulty with Weber's position is that formal organizations work most efficiently through primary groups. For example, Litwak (1985) argues that the occurrence of unpredictable events, the presence of contingencies, and the fact that all tasks are not easily subdivided combine to enable primary groups to perform certain kinds of nonuniform tasks better than formal organizations: Neighbors watch homes, friends are companions, and kin assist in money management. Such evidence suggests that the dependency needs of the elderly are best met when there is a balance between formal services and informal supports with each performing the tasks it is best suited for.

Cantor has conceptualized the social support system as a series of concentric rings with the elder in the center. Each ring contains a different kind of support element with the innermost circles comprising the informal systems of kin, friends, and neighbors who provide the majority of care for elders. The assistance of such informal service providers tends to be nontechnical in nature and tailored to meet the idiosyncratic needs of the individual. It is more flexible in terms of time commitment and extends over the life cycle, and its provision of emotional support is as important as its instrumental assistance (Cantor and Little 1985).

Litwak's and Cantor's descriptions of the linkages between the formal and informal support systems are similar to the "dual specialization" model described by Noelker and Bass (1989), one of four models they propose to describe how formal and informal systems are linked together in providing service. The "dual specialization" model maintains that the informal system focuses on unpredictable and nonuniform tasks while the formal system specializes in predictable tasks in a *complementary* division of labor. The second model posits that the formal system *supplements* the efforts of the informal system. The third says that formal services *substitute* for or replace members of the informal system. Finally, the fourth model acknowledges *no relationship* between formal and informal services, emphasizing the overall lack of care provided by formal service systems.

There is considerable evidence that family members are the first group turned to by older people in need of assistance. A U.S. General Accounting Office (1977) study reports that families provide up to 80 percent of all home health care for elderly individuals in the United States. Elders without close families are more likely to be institutionalized.

Children, particularly middle-aged daughters, assume much of this care, which in turn can produce great strains for the caregiver (Brody 1981). As the numbers of these women who work outside the home increase, so too does the tendency for them to find time to caregive only by sacrificing their own personal lives (Brody 1981). Community services that share responsibility for elder care with families help to relieve some of the major demands of caregiving.

## A "Unique" Model of Formal and Informal Service Links

Homesharing, as a process mediated by paid staff, volunteers, or a combination of each in a formal agency (Shared Housing Resource Center 1988a), provides an especially fruitful way of studying the kinds of complex links that can arise between formal and informal service providers. In a general way it would seem that homesharing arrangements in which personal care is provided the homeowner are consistent with the "supplemental model" described by Noelker and Bass (1989) and with the research findings of Holmes et al. (1989) on Israeli kibbutzim and Edelman's (1986) research on homebound elderly. Their evidence suggests that community care more frequently supplements rather than substitutes for informal care, although the ratio of informal to formal care may vary with changes in the health status of the elder homeowner. Certainly in homesharing, the disabilities of the clients may require major service provision by the homesharer and a minor, albeit important, supportive role for family, friends, and neighbors.

Nevertheless, in its implementation homesharing is far more complicated. For one thing, family and friends have been unable to provide the elder with sufficient support to remain at home, so the agency is called in by either the elder or family members to find a homesharer who will reduce some of the elder's financial burdens, need for care, or social isolation. In this way, the homesharer substitutes for family and friends in some areas, while in other areas the complementary or supplementary models may be appropriate.

At the same time, in many sharing arrangements the health and well-being of the elder decline enough for the agency to seek help for the homesharer who has become the primary caregiver. In these situations, additional support comes not only from respite caregivers the agency finds but also from informal service sources such as family and friends. In this way, the family and friends supplement or complement the formal support provided by the homesharer. Thus, in a curious exchange of roles, it is not the agency that supplements the service provided by family and friends; rather, it is family and friends who supplement the services of the agency.

# THE LIMITS OF CAREGIVING IN THE HOME

The kinds of complex caregiving arrangements just described are becoming more and more frequent as the pool of people seeking rematches grows. Just as most divorces result in remarriage, so do dissolved matches frequently result in new matches, once again arranged by Project HOME. Indeed, the number of repeat matches is increasing faster than the overall rate of matches. This trend in part reflects the increased number of personal care companion matches where the population is fairly stable compared with the early populations of homesharers that included more transient college students. Both homeowners and personal care companions have continuous needs but require shifting casts of the same pool of characters to meet those needs.

How far can the patchwork of family, friends, community services, and primary and respite caregivers go to support the frail in their own homes? The limits of care in the home are tested in the follow-up sample with three clients who have Alzheimer's Disease. One homeowner was interviewed while still having periodic spells of lucidity. All information from the other two was collected from the personal care companion and the Project HOME director.

In the first of the three cases, two caregivers split the week; one cared for the homeowner four days and the other for three days. A devoted son was coordinating the care until the two caregivers had a disagreement with each other over jurisdiction and authority. No replacements were found to care for the son's mother, so she was then taken into the home of her daughter. In this instance, Project HOME was unable to continue the network of care through a caregiver or combination of caregivers.

In the second case, a young married couple has been very devoted to a 90-year-old mother who is dying of cancer and suffering from Alzheimer's Disease. They view their work as an educational experience in understanding the dying process. In contrast to almost every other situation in which younger relatives are involved in the care of older relatives, the family situation is not perceived by the personal care couple as a supportive environment.

> Before we arrived the family had stacked her refrigerator with frozen dinners. She was surviving on frozen food. Well, I cook all of us well balanced complete

meals. Mrs. W's family is constantly bickering about the food cost I give them saying "we don't need this or that." Also they have a habit of coming over and walking into the house at all hours of the day or night.

The family had been caring for the mother one weekend day a week but no longer wanted to do this and wished the live-in couple to assume this role at no additional pay.

The live-in caregivers are currently providing round-the-clock care seven days a week with a slight increase in salary. One of them must turn the mother in her bed several times each night. A neighbor does help out one evening every one to two weeks so the caretaking couple can enjoy a social outing. This couple remains with their frail homeowner basically out of fondness for the dying woman.

In this example, the conflict between family and the caregivers is an unfortunate, though rare, occurrence that has not yet caused the sharing arrangement to dissolve. Ironically, probably one of the more important reasons for the caregivers remaining with their dying charge is this conflict with the woman's family and their knowledge that she is dying.

The final case is the situation already referred to twice before—the elderly woman who has been deteriorating over time and had been looked after by a series of live-in personal caregivers under the overall monitoring by a devoted neighbor who is the woman's guardian. It will be remembered that, as the homeowner's condition deteriorated, even two alternating live-in caregivers couldn't manage her.

The homeowner would become irrational, screaming that "they" were banging the door down to get her and that her dead brother was still alive. Although she hallucinated a lot, the caregivers knew this would pass and were still able to manage. What tipped the scale toward institutionalization was her becoming a physical management problem. She became stubborn and refused to use the bathroom, take a bath, and go to bed, having temper tantrums when the caregivers would attempt to help her. Generally, it would take more than one person to get her to do things like go to the bathroom.

The nurse practitioner assured the guardian and the two caregivers that institutionalization was the appropriate decision. One of the caregivers now goes into the nursing home every day to provide the personal assistance the homeowner was used to in her own home and thus ease the transition to the new living environment. The guardian is paying for this service, an indication of her devotion to this woman. This is a good example of how every effort had been made to keep a person in her own home as long as possible. Had homesharing and a devoted guardian and caregivers not been available, this woman would have been institution-alized much earlier in her life.

This last example is also a good illustration of how a "continuum of care" may be provided in the home. As the woman deteriorated, increasing numbers and types of caregivers were employed so that she would not need to be institutionalized. The limits of home care are most likely to be reached when major mental deterioration has taken place and manifests itself in problematic physical ways, as was true in this case.

Although the primary personal care companion is crucial to the support of the frail homeowner, it is evident that the relationship itself is quite "frail." The homeowner's health, often quite poor to begin with, tends to deteriorate while the caregiver is present and often creates stresses on the caregiver that were unanticipated and, even if anticipated, too difficult for the caregiver to deal with alone. The problems are compounded when mental deterioration is acute.

At the same time, the caregiver has changing needs that will affect the relationship. Some couples serve as personal care companions in order to save money to purchase their own home. Some individuals provide care in order to save money to go to school. Others find their own health declining as they attempt to care for the frail homeowner. In all these and other cases, more often than not, the caregiver leaves when personal goals are realized or when circumstances make caregiving too difficult.

Fortunately, the frail homeowner and caregiver do not have to deal with these problems by themselves. Rarely a self-sufficient unit, they usually are dependent on an external support network of family, respite caregivers, friends, neighbors, and community services. Particularly important are the roles played by significant family members who oversee the caregiving of their mother or father and supplement caregiving themselves and the respite caregivers who provide critical relief to the primary caregiver.

As the clientele served by Project HOME continues to be the frail and dependent and as their health deteriorates, new and more complex supportive living arrangements will be necessary. Several caregivers may be needed for each case, in addition to the support provided by family, friends, and neighbors. In these situations, family and kin will play particularly critical roles as they are called on to coordinate and monitor the care as well as provide a safety net should the homesharing system temporarily falter.

For each homeowner, therefore, Project HOME represents not only a stop along the continuum of care but also an agency that potentially can provide for a continuum of care *within* the home. As relatively healthy homeowners experience physical (and even mental) deterioration, a traditional homesharing arrangement can be replaced by a caregiving one that, in turn, becomes more complex as the needs of the homeowner become greater. The last cases described suggest that, while extraordinary measures are needed to care for seriously incapacitated individuals, it *is* possible to maintain the very frail at home.

# 9

# Clients Speak About Project HOME's Service Delivery

In the previous seven chapters, the organization and clientele of Project HOME have been examined to show who the program's clients are, how homesharing services work in this program, how program services evolved in relation to changing client needs, what client characteristics facilitate their finding sharers, and what happens to clients once they have found sharers. In this chapter and the next, the answers to these questions will be used to help evaluate the service delivery of Project HOME. In the final chapter, this evaluation will be put in the context of homesharing programs throughout the country and of human service delivery programs in general.

The essential question in this chapter is: How well has Project HOME served its clients during the first five years of its existence? Specifically, three issues will be considered: How did clients remember their experiences with the application and introduction processes? How did they compare their current living arrangements with their situation when they first applied to Project HOME? How did they evaluate Project HOME's services? In the next chapter, attention will turn to a discussion of how the program has changed since the third director took over and to recommendations for improving homesharing services in Project HOME that also have relevance for other homesharing service delivery programs.

The analysis in this chapter will be based on follow-up interviews with 148 of the 616 who applied to the program during its first four years. About half of the clients contacted are those matched applicants whose living arrangements formed the bases for the analysis in the previous two chapters. In addition, we were able to contact and interview a number of unmatched clients as well as some additional clients whose matches had dissolved. (See appendix 4 for a detailed description of the follow-up sample which provided the information described in this chapter.)

## CLIENT VIEWS ON HOMESHARING APPLICATION AND INTRODUCTIONS

The evaluation in this chapter begins with an examination of how the clients remember their experiences with the application and introduction processes. Answers to the questions in table 9.1 tend to support the idea that most clients had good experiences: About half of all clients interviewed had been positive about the likelihood of finding a sharer, almost three-quarters had been introduced to one or more sharers, and most who met a prospective sharer rate their meetings with them as positive.

### Optimists and Pessimists

When asked to explain their answers, some clients provide illuminating insights regarding their prospects of getting matched at time of application: Among optimists, a few give structural reasons. These include, for example, homeowners who cite a low apartment vacancy rate and homeseekers who see the time of year as likely to produce less competition for housing among those who are willing to move. Others give personal reasons like the applicant who says, "I felt I had a lot to give somebody."

Even more mention the staff of Project HOME to justify their optimism in finding a sharer. For example, one unmatched applicant explains her great confidence is due to the fact that "the people at the program were so positive that someone could be found for me." Another adds, "That's what they're there for; they specialize in this," while a third points to the director, whom she believes to be "very competent."

Many pessimists cite their own situation. They include the woman who has two girls and doesn't think an older person would want to share

Table 9.1

*Client Views Toward Application and Introduction Process at Time of Follow-Up Interview by Sharing Status and Type of Applicant*

| Percent clients who | Total | Never Matched | Matched; No Longer Sharing | Still Matched |
|---|---|---|---|---|
| believed they were very likely to find a homesharer | 50.4 | 31.4 | 46.7 | 66.7 |
| (N) | (129) | (51) | (15) | (63) |
| were introduced to one or more applicants through HOME[a] | 71.4 | 39.7 | 100.0 | 90.3 |
| (N) | (147) | (58) | (17) | (72) |
| rate meeting(s) with prosp. sharer(s) as positive[b,c] | 60.0 | 22.7 | 82.4 | 87.5 |
| (N) | (55) | (22) | (17) | (16) |

| | Never Matched | | Currently Matched | | | |
|---|---|---|---|---|---|---|
| Percent clients who | Providers | Lodgers | Prov. | Lodge. | Employ. | Care. |
| believed they were very likely to find a homesharer | 28.6 | 42.9 | 54.5 | 72.2 | 81.3 | 52.9 |
| (N) | (28) | (14) | (11) | (18) | (16) | (17) |
| were introduced to one or more applicants through HOME[a] | 32.3 | 44.4 | 100.0 | 94.4 | 100.0 | 81.0 |
| (N) | (31) | (18) | (12) | (18) | (18) | (21) |
| rate meeting(s) with prosp. sharer(s) as positive[b,c] | 40.0 | 0.0 | 100.0 | 66.7 | 100.0 | 100.0 |
| (N) | (10) | (7) | (5) | (6) | (3) | (2) |

[a] In a small minority of cases there was no formal introduction before applicants agreed to share. They made their decisions on the basis of descriptions given by the director.

[b] Limited to those applicants who actually met prospective sharers.

[c] Question not asked of 60 applicants. See text for explanation.

with children, and the applicant who admits, "I'm not much at taking strangers in." A few others, however, cite the program's relative newness (at the time) or say the program wasn't explained very well.

## HOME Services at Application Time

When one considers how applicants feel retrospectively about the introduction process in general, it is clear that the great majority like how the director or volunteer allowed them to work out an arrangement themselves while still being available to offer support or suggestions if necessary. One homesharer, for example, notes how "every aspect of the homesharing arrangement was openly discussed." It is important for the agency to strike a balance between support and initiative on the one hand and a hands-off, nonintrusive role on the other so the couple can work out their own arrangement.

Several people wish they could have had more choices of partners or believe the agency was rushing them. One man complains that he was accused by the director of being too choosy by turning down five or six people when he really hadn't. Another homeowner complains that her perception of the introduction process was different from the director's. The latter brought a prospective sharer to meet the homeowner "expecting I'd accept her" when in fact the homeowner had unresolved questions about the prospective sharer.

The only other general comment concerning introductions between homeowner and mover has been the request that agency involvement extend beyond the introduction process and include more follow-up service. One woman notes that "they" [Project HOME] were "understaffed" and that "they should also have an official follow-up intermittently or every month or so." Another client hopes they will "keep track of me and my situation because I'm close to blind and I think its great to have you [the interviewer] here talking." Still a third person remarks that "they should periodically call or visit to keep lines of communication open between both parties." While the overall view of the introduction process has been positive, these last comments are important indicators of some critical gaps that existed in the early years of the program's service delivery: a somewhat unsystematic approach to keeping tabs on clients after the initial application interview. Even today, the gap in case management continues to some degree among all kinds of clients. As will be seen in the next chapter, the current director and her staff have recognized the problem and begun to institute measures to provide some case management follow-up of both matched and unmatched clients.

## Group Comparisons

When applicants who have never shared, those whose match has been dissolved, and those who are currently sharing are contrasted (table 9.1), expected differences are revealed: The never matched were least confident in believing they were very likely to find a sharer, were introduced to less than half as many sharers, and, when they did meet prospective sharers, were by far the least likely to rate their meetings positively. The lack of introductions among the never matched is largely time-bound, because many of the never matched applicants in the follow-up sample are from the program's first year.[1]

When never matched and currently matched applicants are further subdivided into type of applicant, two findings are noteworthy: First, unmatched lodgers were far less likely than unmatched providers to have had a positive experience during the introduction process. Part of the reason may be that many unsuccessful lodger applicants simply were not expecting the kind of sharing arrangement that many provider applicants wanted and were put off by the many strings attached to the prospective sharing arrangement. Living at home, providers are in a greater position of power when negotiating terms of a prospective living arrangement and thus likely to be very protective of their home. If, at the same time, homeowners are also confident that the agency is likely to find an appropriate sharer, then their position on various issues in the negotiations may well border on intransigence.

The second finding, the importance of money, is indirectly indicated by the evidence that lodgers and employers were more confident of being matched than were providers and caregivers, among all those currently matched. It is likely that the relatively greater confidence of the first pair is based, in part at least, on their having money to pay their sharer and the clients in the second pair being dependent on sharers with money.

Overall, therefore, the numerical data and comments together combine to show that most clients are satisfied with their experience in the application and introduction processes; differences among subgroups, furthermore, are in the expected direction with matched clients perceiving their situation most positively. Finally, while generally pleased with program service, several clients are concerned with lack of follow-up contact by the program.

## PAST, PRESENT, AND FUTURE LIVING ARRANGEMENTS

The second issue concerns clients' views of their living situations. Over three-quarters of the clients view their current living arrangement as satisfactory or better. Even more telling, three times as many (43.0% to 14.0%) view their current situation as better rather than worse than the arrangement in which they lived when they first contacted HOME (43.0% see no difference) (table 9.2). Thus, the expected positive tie to home would seem to emanate not only from the generally good feelings one always tends to have about home but also from something connected with the Project HOME experience.

TABLE 9.2
Client Views Toward Living Situations at Time of Follow-Up Interview by Sharing
Status and Type of Applicant

| Percent clients who | Total | Never Matched | Matched; No Longer Sharing | Still Matched |
|---|---|---|---|---|
| rate present living arrangement as satisfactory[a] | 77.4 | 75.9 | 76.5 | 83.3 |
| (N) | (93) | (58) | (17) | (18) |
| rate present living arrangement as *better* than when first contacted HOME | 43.0 | 34.5 | 35.3 | 77.8 |
| *worse* than when first contacted HOME[a] | 14.0 | 15.5 | 23.5 | 0.0 |
| (N) | (93) | (58) | (17) | (18) |
| want present living arrangement to last at least two more years | 56.1 | 61.8 | 46.7 | 53.2 |
| (N) | (132) | (55) | (15) | (62) |
| are interested in meeting prospective sharers either now or in the future | 72.0 | 68.4 | 64.7 | 76.8 |
| (N) | (143) | (57) | (17) | (69) |

| Percent clients who | Never Matched | | Currently Matched | | | |
|---|---|---|---|---|---|---|
| | Providers | Lodgers | Prov. | Lodge. | Employ. | Care. |
| rate present living arrangement as satisfactory[a] | 77.4 | 72.2 | 80.0 | 100.0 | 66.7 | 66.7 |
| (N) | (31) | (18) | (5) | (7) | (3) | (3) |
| rate present living arrangement as *better* than when first contacted HOME | 22.6 | 55.6 | 60.0 | 71.4 | 100.0 | 100.0 |
| *worse* than when first contacted HOME[a] | 16.1 | 16.7 | 0.0 | 0.0 | 0.0 | 0.0 |
| (N) | (31) | (18) | (5) | (7) | (3) | (3) |
| want present living arrangement to last at least two more years | 66.7 | 56.3 | 41.7 | 57.1 | 70.6 | 41.2 |
| (N) | (30) | (16) | (12) | (14) | (17) | (17) |
| are interested in meeting prospective sharers either now or in the future | 77.4 | 58.8 | 91.7 | 75.0 | 84.2 | 68.4 |
| (N) | (31) | (17) | (12) | (16) | (19) | (19) |

[a] Question not asked of 60 applicants. See text for explanation.

Despite positive feelings about their current situation, a little over half of the clients neither want nor expect their current arrangements to last two years or more. Part of the reason is that about 40 percent of the clients interviewed still want to meet prospective sharers now, and, altogether, almost three-quarters want to meet prospective sharers either now or in the future.

## Never Matched Clients Speak

Among unmatched applicants, the reasons for rating current living conditions, wanting living arrangements to last a certain time, and interest in looking for new sharers vary considerably. For many never matched homeowners who feel better about their current living arrangements than those they were in when they first contacted the program, for example, either objective circumstances or their perceptions have changed. Some have finally moved into community care or nursing homes where their needs appear to be met. Several have found substitutes for homesharers, like the woman who now has a walker, a three-wheel cart, and someone who comes in regularly to help her with housework. Another homeowner says she now finally has come to grips with the death of her spouse, while yet another is "getting more used to living alone."

Most negative comments concerning current situation indicate the homeowner's health has deteriorated since their application, including one who has recently had a hip operation and therefore needs even more care now. Another former homeowner has moved to a community care home that she "hates."

The majority of never matched homeowners want to remain in their own homes but are still looking for someone to share, in the words of one homeowner, "because I don't want to move again; I feel comfortable here." A large number who are willing to keep looking for a sharer add a qualifier: "If I become more ill," "If I get lonely and need someone," "If I can find someone compatible." Negative comments are few but revealing. One homeowner, for example, doesn't want to seek a homesharer any more, because he is afraid the sharer would sponge off him. Another is living with a daughter and not interested in leaving that situation.

Many unmatched homeseekers have found better living accommodations either by themselves or with friends. When there are complaints, it is usually about money; one mover, for example, laments that the rent has increased. Unmatched homeseekers generally want their situation to remain stable but would entertain the idea of a sharer now or in the future. Those who don't often cite the problems of adjustment involved: "[Sharing] would take my liberty away." "I don't wish to be bothered with other people's problems."

When the never matched are subdivided into providers and lodgers in table 9.2, two comparisons are striking: First, the lodgers are much more likely to view their current situation as better than it was when they first contacted HOME. Second, not surprisingly, providers are more likely to want to meet prospective sharers than are lodgers. Both findings underscore the importance of the program to providers, many of whom are elderly or frail and who have far fewer options to improve their living situations than do those in the younger, more mobile lodger group.

## Previously Matched Clients Speak

Among those whose matches have dissolved, one former homeowner puts the most positive light one can apply to a homesharing experience that has terminated: "I was satisfied with homesharing but am also now satisfied to be alone." The majority of homeowners, however, rate their current position as about the same as it was when they first contacted HOME and are still hoping for a rematch. Others have experienced deteriorating health and rate their current position as better or worse, depending on whether they have found someone from outside of HOME to help them; a few have, while others have not.

The vast majority of previously matched homeowners, when asked about their future plans, indicate that they want to share again, some for the help they would get around the house and others for the companionship. Among those who say they don't want to homeshare in the future, the reasons generally have nothing to do with their previous sharer. One is too ill to share, another likes being alone, and so forth.

Among the very few movers whose matches had dissolved, there is a generally upbeat outlook, because they have found (short-term) housing superior to that which they had when they first applied to the program. Only one indicates a dissatisfaction with the homesharing experience: "I felt I was expected to pay more as time went by. The elderly are hard to deal with."

## Currently Matched Clients Speak

Among those currently matched, the numerical data in table 9.2 has shown quite positive views concerning current living arrangements, and the comments by sharers reflect this. Homeowners are happy to have someone stay with them and provide companionship (in some cases), help with chores around the house (in other cases), or at the least a presence (in almost all instances). Most homeowners want their sharing to last at least two years but recognize that their sharer is the one who will determine how long the relationship will last. One points to her sharer's student status, while another says simply that the arrangement will last until the sharer "gets pregnant."

Homeseekers, on the other hand, speak almost exclusively about the independence they now have and the better financial situation they are in. One currently matched mover, for example, exclaims, "I wanted to be independent from my friends and have more control over my own finances, and this situation makes that possible. One negative comment by a mover indicates that some arrangements are meant to last as short a period of time as possible: "We can't get along. [The homeowner] is very demanding and nasty. Old people are set in their ways and they're not going to give."

As seen in chapter 7, the fit between the desire for companionship by home providers and the need for cheap housing and maximum personal space by lodgers is always a complicated matter, and the above statements reflect these different reference points for each of these groups. Among those involved in personal care companion matches, the in-depth interviews detailed in chapter 8 show that the interpersonal fit is better—but certainly no less intense. Here, the satisfaction of employers in having their health needs attended to is balanced by the caregivers' satisfaction in having a job and in helping another person. Stress to the caregivers is the major negative aspect to this relationship.

Among the currently matched, two group differences in table 9.2 are worth noting: First, not unexpectedly, employers are most likely to want their match to last at least two years; after all, they are the individuals with the need for continuing care. Second, providers and employers are most likely to be interested in meeting a prospective sharer now or in the future, again suggesting the importance of homesharing to these two groups of stayers who are the primary target groups of the program.

## Group Comparisons

Somewhat unexpectedly, a comparison among never matched, previously matched, and currently matched does not put the never matched at a disadvantage to the other two groups. For example, table 9.2 shows that about three-quarters of each group is satisfied with their present living arrangement, and the never matched and previously matched groups both compare their current arrangements favorably to arrangements at the time they first contacted HOME and in about the same proportions; currently matched clients are even more positive, as three-quarters say their current arrangement is better and none say it is worse than before—a definite selling point for Project HOME.

At the same time these positive feelings are being expressed, about half of those currently matched want their living arrangements to last no more than two years, the never matched wanting more permanence and the previously matched desiring more change. As another indication of their continuing commitment to the program, about two-thirds to three-quarters of each group are willing to meet with prospective sharers now or in the future.

Overall, the evidence from table 9.2 and from client comments show that, whether they were ever matched or not and regardless of the type of applicant, clients appear to be satisfied with their current living arrangements and view them as better than or about the same as their situations before contacting Project HOME. Superficially, this might appear to show that homesharing doesn't matter, since most clients, unmatched as well as matched, feel good about their living situation during the follow-up interviews.

Two points are relevant here. First, it is likely that just participating in the process has a salutary effect on all applicants, with the unmatched clients learning to cope with their situation, as some of their comments suggest. Second, most clients are willing to continue to meet new sharers, if not at present, then in the future. These results clearly suggest a positive effect from having applied to the program. In general terms and through group comparisons, therefore, the results show perceived benefits from sharing and a continued willingness to be served by the program.

## CLIENT ASSESSMENT OF PROJECT "HOME"

As important as the above information has been, the previous questions do not ask clients directly how they actually feel about the program itself and how they have been handled by the director and the staff. To get at these issues, it is necessary to turn to questions that more directly deal with client perception of Project HOME. If one looks only at the first column in table 9.3, it will be clear that the clients sampled generally feel positive about homesharing, are satisfied with Project HOME's services, and don't believe HOME could have done much more for them

Client Views Toward Project HOME at Time of Follow-Up Interview by Sharing Status
and Type of Applicant

| Percent clients who | Total | Never Matched | Matched; No Longer Sharing | Still Matched |
|---|---|---|---|---|
| feel positive about homesharing[a] | 62.6 | 57.1 | 64.7 | 77.8 |
| (N) | (91) | (56) | (17) | (18) |
| are satisfied with Project HOME services | 77.6 | 57.4 | 70.6 | 94.4 |
| (N) | (143) | (54) | (17) | (72) |
| believe Project HOME could do more for them | 25.2 | 36.4 | 25.0 | 16.7 |
| (N) | (143) | (55) | (16) | (72) |
| have recommended Project HOME to other(s) | 45.3 | 32.8 | 47.1 | 54.8 |
| (N) | (148) | (58) | (17) | (73) |

| | Never Matched | | Currently Matched | | | |
|---|---|---|---|---|---|---|
| Percent clients who | Providers | Lodgers | Prov. | Lodge. | Employ. | Care. |
| feel positive about homesharing[a] | 56.7 | 52.9 | 80.0 | 100.0 | 66.7 | 33.3 |
| (N) | (30) | (17) | (5) | (7) | (3) | (3) |
| are satisfied with Project HOME services | 53.3 | 75.0 | 91.7 | 100.0 | 89.5 | 95.0 |
| (N) | (30) | (16) | (12) | (19) | (19) | (20) |
| believe Project HOME could do more for them | 48.3 | 23.5 | 16.7 | 5.3 | 0.0 | 38.1 |
| (N) | (29) | (17) | (12) | (19) | (18) | (21) |
| have recommended Project HOME to other(s) | 16.1 | 61.1 | 66.7 | 52.6 | 47.4 | 52.4 |
| (N) | (31) | (18) | (12) | (19) | (19) | (21) |

[a] Question not asked of 60 applicants. See text for explanation.

—to the extent that nearly half of the sample have actually recommended the program to others.

## Clients' Views on Homesharing

The reasons for positive attitudes toward homesharing across all groups boil down to two kinds of explanations: philosophical and practical. The philosophical range from the large number of never matched applicants who say merely that homesharing is "a good idea" to the currently matched client who stated, "As humans, we need to live together—not build walls between [people of different] ages."

The practical reasons for viewing homesharing positively tend focus on companionship, money, and health. The major reason among these appears to be money, according to several currently matched clients. Two currently matched clients echo this notion:

> It's a good opportunity to live comfortably on limited income.

> It helps people survive financially.

A client whose match dissolved, argues that homesharing is positive because of "company sharing"—adding that it's "good for morale."

On the other hand are the minority who believe homesharing is not a positive alternative. These include a large number of applicants who view the process in a neutral light; they maintain that homesharing *would be* a good thing *if* certain conditions could be obtained. When asked to elaborate, these clients, many of whom have never been matched, mention that the key is finding the right kind of person with whom to share.

A few clearly negative responses from matched clients, while part of a minority view, illustrate the problems of homesharing that their speakers have experienced or anticipate. One currently matched lodger complains, "Old people are set in their ways, and they're not going to give." Echoing this view is the dissatisfied lodger whose match dissolved; she complains about having to deal with intransigent elders.

Generally, the homeowners who are still matched or whose matches have dissolved are positive about sharing, but one woman had a bad experience with her sharer and therefore feels very negative about homesharing. While she could only reiterate that she "didn't have a good experience" in response to the question "Why do you feel that way?" about homesharing, during another part of the interview she complains that her sharer hardly ever cleaned the snow off the steps, even though she said she would keep them clean. Furthermore, when the homeowner told her sharer she would have to look for other arrangements because the homeowner was planning to enter senior housing the sharer "began screaming and got hysterical" at which point the homeowner called the police.

Applicants who were never matched yet say they feel negative about homesharing are a small minority but perceptive in their vision of homesharing:

> It would be OK if it was a "50–50" arrangement.
>
> I feel homesharing is where you live 50–50, and I wouldn't like that.
>
> I'd rather be alone.

It's not clear why these individuals applied to homeshare in the first place, although each of the above three individuals is an older person who, since first applying to HOME, has made arrangements to meet health and other needs through living in a community care home, having someone come in to clean, or having family look after them and their home.

## Unmatched Clients' Views on Project HOME

Table 9.3 shows that a majority of unmatched clients are satisfied with Project HOME services. For the minority who find fault with the organization, the obvious dominant complaint is that the agency has not found a partner for them. Of even greater concern, is that applicants feel they had not been provided with updated information about the status of their application once the application interview was administered. There is considerable anxiety from those applicants who have been screened but never called back about the status of their application.

> I wish they would explain to me more what they are doing.
>
> They should have contacted me to see if I still needed someone else. They should have followed up.
>
> In two years they could show me more people than they have.
>
> They never contacted me. It would have been nice to have heard from them every so often to update the situation.

Better case management could have reduced this as a problem. It is also possible that the difficulty of making a match was not realistically presented to the client at the time of application. The client may have been left with unrealistic expectations about a quick match. However, again, it should be noted that the majority of unmatched clients are not critical of Project HOME.

## Matched Clients' Views on Project HOME

Among those who had been matched at one time or another, the data in table 9.3 show even more positive sentiments toward the program. The criticisms, understandably, are also even fewer. They center about lack of information of either the other homesharer or about the living situation they would encounter when they lived together. A married couple with an infant caring for a quadriplegic believe they had not been adequately informed by Project HOME about their future personal care responsibilities.

> They should have explained more about quadriplegics. When we first met [the director], the understanding was that we'd give [the homeowner] her tea, clean the house and make dinner. That's all. We thought the V.N.A. would come each morning, but she only comes on Monday, Wednesday and Friday. It takes two people to get [the homeowner] out of bed.

They have had to do more personal care tasks than they had originally been led to believe and are understandably upset about their situation.

In a similar situation, a caregiver wishes she had been given more thorough background information on her employer who needed more care than she was told would be necessary. "[The program director and her staff] didn't tell me the seriousness of her situation." Critical responses generally center about lack of information or the unmet expectations of either the homeowner or the mover.

> I don't think Project HOME goes into people's backgrounds enough before matching them up.

> I think they should have told me more about [my sharer's] character. I should have been given the phone numbers of her previous live-ins.

> One woman said she could cook so well she could cook with her eyes shut but I wish she would open them. She was from——and cooked weird stuff which I couldn't eat. If [Project HOME] had called her mother-in-law she would have told them the daughter wasn't right for me. They didn't follow a reference; they should have.

Another person, a lodger, wishes he had known ahead of time he would not have access to the homeowner's phone and laundry facilities.

The great majority of comments are laudatory and supportive of Project Home, its director and her volunteers. The most frequent themes of praise center about the program's promptness in obtaining a match for them and the empathic personal style of the director.

> [The director] has helped me when I needed it. She gave me a boost when I needed it. She called my daughter-in-law to talk to her about my feelings and being really dragged out and in need of some help.

> They were very kind to me and they are really quick about matching people into living arrangements.

> She [the director] was terrific. She explained the whole process so clearly.

Both times she had someone ready to move in on the dates she needed someone.

They were very helpful and understanding to me and my situation. They found a place for me quickly.

They made me feel comfortable by coming with me to the people's homes.

[The director] is a very giving person. She shines. She's wonderful—a great interpersonal agency.

Clearly, many Project HOME clients believe the program has served them well.

## Group Comparisons

When the never matched, previously matched, and currently matched clients are compared, three clear-cut patterns are revealed (table 9.3). First, as already seen, a majority of each group feels positive about homesharing in general and Project HOME in particular, and only a minority of each group believes Project HOME could have done more for them. Second, for each of the four questions, not surprisingly, the never matched are either less positive (questions one, two, and four) or more negative (question three) than the currently matched clients. Third, just as important, those clients whose matches have dissolved are not, overall, bitter about their experiences but rather fall somewhere between the other two groups—not as positive as the currently matched but not as negative as the never matched.

When the never matched are subdivided into providers and lodgers, one interesting contrast is apparent: Provider applicants expected more from Project HOME and therefore perhaps have told fewer people about the program when they found no sharer than did the less expectant (and therefore less disappointed) lodger applicants. Given their relative youth and the larger number of housing options at their disposal, it is not surprising that lodger applicants feel less grievously hurt by the program.

When currently matched are subdivided, an interesting contrast of results appears. On the one hand, almost every one of the four groups of currently matched applicants is satisfied with Project HOME's services, and this is good. At the same time, caregivers believe the program could have done more for them. This finding again underlines the kinds of special stress caregivers experience and suggests an area in which the program may be able to help sharing arrangements. This issue will be discussed more in the next chapter, which explores case management and the respite program.

When one considers the overall pattern of information in the tables (especially table 9.3) and the comments by the clients themselves, two things are clear: First, the vast majority of clients believe the program satisfies their needs or is trying to satisfy their needs, whether one is currently matched, previously matched, or has never been matched. Second, and of greater interest here, is the fact that those complaints that do surface speak to a weakness in the program's follow-up of clients —not only clients for whom no matches have been found but also clients who are in matches that are causing problems.

Two specific groups of clients who are especially thus affected are the unmatched home provider applicants in relatively frail health but without sufficient finances to pay for a caregiver and caregivers who are in matches that are causing them great stress. Previous chapters have already addressed the problems facing both groups, but the criticisms raised by clients in the follow-up interviews indicate that these two groups of clients are especially vulnerable to a program that does not follow its clients through on a case management basis.

In general, the client data demonstrate that the first five years' clients have been satisfied overall with the program's service delivery. Still, clients' comments have indicated concerns about the lack of follow-up by the staff. The next chapter will describe how the current director and her staff have made a conscious effort to follow clients more closely after their applications, utilizing a case management approach that appears to have met with some degree of success.

# 10

# An Entrepreneurial Program Begins to Manage

After hearing what the clients say about how well Project HOME has served them during the first five years of its existence, it is appropriate to turn to organizational responses to the concerns raised by clients and the implications of such "dialogues" between client and agency for service programs in general. This chapter will use the summary results from the analysis in the previous chapter, in-depth interviews with the second and third directors and three of their staff (two volunteers and the Respite Coordinator), program documents, and our own observations to describe programmatic response to concerns raised by both clients and the evaluators. At the end will be recommendations for improving homesharing services in Project HOME that also have relevance for other homesharing service delivery programs.

## CURRENT AGENCY PRACTICES

*Responses to Client Concerns*

*The Evolution of Case Management.* The themes of discontent that surfaced among clients during the follow-up interviews presented in the last chapter have centered on the need for more introductions, the lack of contact from the agency, mismatching of some clients, and a need for the director and her staff to explain the program better. While these complaints clearly represent a minority point of view, they are nevertheless serious. In order for a service agency to continue to attract clients, it must have credibility; and these criticisms tend to undermine that credibility.

The major intent in this chapter is to show how problems brought to the attention of the program have been addressed to the degree that limitations of field and administrative staff allow. This includes consideration of how the program changed after the second director took over and how two important mechanisms have contributed to the addressing of these problems. One is the very open relationship that existed between the director who oversaw the major growth and expansion of Project HOME during its second, third, and fourth years and the evaluators of the program.

This relationship has been reported in detail in chapter 4, showing how it operated on the principle of social exchange: At the same time the director gave the evaluators complete access to all applicant files and other agency data, she received both formal and informal feedback concerning how the program was doing. Chief among the concerns clients raised early and often to the evaluators (and, in some cases, to the director and her staff) was the problem of following the status of both matched and unmatched clients. Indeed, the evaluators' follow-up interviews often were the only contact many clients had with the program.

The second major mechanism by which the program began to address client concerns has greater importance in the sense that it represents a more formalized response than the relatively informal exchange between director and evaluators. It will be remembered that during the fifth year of the program the second director resigned to pursue academic studies in preparation for the ministry; her replacement brought to the program a similar proprietary concern over clients but also some experience in administration. As a result, her tenure became one in which the dramatic initiatives made by her predecessor became institutionalized through the rationalization of service delivery. Foremost among the new formalized procedures was the use of a case management model to keep track of clients.

Key to this rationalization was the granting of agency status to the program by United Way (one of several important legacies left by the second director) and, later, the program's becoming a "line item" in the state's budget. These financial changes allowed the program to hire administrative staff to take the day-to-day clerical burdens off the hands of the director and her volunteer staff, thus freeing them up to do the kinds of follow-up many clients were clamoring for.

*Current Case Management Practices.* The central importance of the volunteer in the staffing of Project HOME has been a constant from the program's inception to the present. At the same time, as was described in chapter 3, the particular form of volunteer participation has evolved in three analytically distinct stages: interviewer, executive, and, most recently, case manager. Especially important for the latter role has been the support of an expanded paid staff. The hiring of an administrative assistant has permitted a more efficient coordination and utilization of the volunteers' time and skills, because the assistant now assumes many of the routine filing and telephone duties centered in the office that formerly were handled by the volunteers.

Originally, the volunteers had done interviews as a team but with little responsibility for the actual matching of clients and subsequent monitoring of matches. Today, the director and her volunteer staff attempt to be case managers for each Project HOME applicant. As described by the current director, the change in duties for the volunteers has been particularly important:

> When I started, [the volunteers] were doing the interviews and bits and pieces of other things. But what they are doing now is following a case management model and following through on the people in all aspects of the match. Their role has expanded. They actually are working with people's live-in agreements and helping people with introductions.

This live-in agreement (appendix 1) is processed by the volunteer and signed by both partners in the homesharing arrangement. Responsibilities and duties of each member in the match are specified and accessibility to appliances and living spaces is spelled out.

In caregiver situations, the salary and job expectations are made very explicit. The process is described by one volunteer who has been with the program since its inception.

> When I go out for the introduction I take [the live-in agreement] with me and I listen to their expectations and I will go over it with them. Afterwards I say this is what was said and you should try it for a couple of weeks and then we'll come back and finalize it.

Whenever possible, family is brought directly into the process in the role of intermediary to represent the homeowner, particularly in caregiver matches. Usually a daughter or daughter-in-law is the intermediary, but some sons play this role too, as seen in chapters 7 and 8.

Despite the desire of program staff to emphasize the importance of family members as resources to whom sharers can turn, program volunteers are still quite central to the needs of homesharers. Volunteers help arrange the introduction, the caregiver's hours, payments to the caregiver, and establish a caregiver agreement. Volunteers also act as mediators when there are conflicts between the employer and caregiver.

One particularly important change has been the emphasis on specificity in the live-in agreement. The volunteer now encourages the members in the match to be as specific as possible in this agreement. "Companionship," for example, says one volunteer, "is a loose word and I get them to talk about it and if they expect the other to play cribbage three nights a week we get them to talk about it." A trial period for a week or two is recommended and then the agreement is signed. This allows for some adjustments that surface only when a couple actually is living together.

This procedure has reduced some of the major problems of adjustment. The expectations of the matched couple regarding interaction, personal habits, and accessibility to shared spaces and appliances can now be discussed beforehand and agreed upon in a relatively systematic way. The more clients are clear about their sharer's (and their own) expectations, the more likely they both will be satisfied with their living arrangement.

In addition to interviewing potential applicants, checking their references, arranging the introductions, and mediating the live-in agreements, the volunteers also contact their matches after two weeks and occasionally act as arbitrator should difficulties between the homesharers develop. For example, a 79-year-old bachelor having increasing problems with dementia was facing likely institutionalization until Project HOME became involved. The director describes the problem:

> He gets in his truck and drives down the driveway and can't remember how to turn to go to places. He had been very intensely independent but ended up in a hospital very recently. His nephew, who is his closest relative, was looking for nursing homes for him. [Meanwhile a] clerk in a local hardware store talked to the nephew about a place to live.

At this point Project Home was called by the nephew, and a volunteer was assigned to interview the old man and the clerk and to screen the references of the clerk. After the match was made, it became clear that the young clerk enjoyed doing things around the house like cleaning and cooking. At the same time, the older man had difficulty accepting help from the younger person, a conflict discovered by the volunteer after a routine two-week follow-up call. According to the director,

> [The homeowner] doesn't like having the dishes done. He just prefers clutter and dirt and doesn't want anyone around helping with things. [The volunteer] has been talking with the two of them to get that worked out.

Where there is a great deal of conflict or where the volunteer is uncomfortable in the problem situation, the director accompanies the volunteer.

The follow-up phone call after two weeks usually results in a very positive assessment if the volunteer asks general questions. However, the staff and volunteers of Project Home have developed a precisely worded questionnaire that now asks specific questions like: "How is communication done?" "How are things managed?" These questions tend to turn up more problems than "How are things?" In addition, the director also checks resumés and files to be sure no one is missed in the follow-up calls.

The initial contract signed by the sharers also benefits them when the volunteer checks after two weeks. According to one volunteer, having a contract probably has "saved" some matches, because it provides a starting point for discussion when two sharers are in conflict. The volunteer and the sharers then can sit down and reexamine the contract and look for the places where it has been misinterpreted.

As described above, one of the major early complaints of unmatched applicants had been that they were not informed of developments in their case after completing their application. The present case management procedure has been designed to correct that problem. Says one volunteer:

> We are responsible for keeping our people "alive" and in the group. We are supposed to keep in touch with them and let them know we are still trying and see if their situation has changed. Unfortunately they don't always tell us when they have solved their situation. I also call some of my matches if I haven't heard from them in some time.

Overall the volunteers now assume much more responsibility for their clients than they did earlier. Although they do less in office administrative service, they have greatly expanded their role in client service delivery. The result is a program that serves its clients better, because it is now tailored to anticipate problems before they occur and to deal with them in a systematic and fair manner when they do occur.

Still, both the director and the volunteers feel the need for more follow-up assistance. As the director states: "After the match it is difficult for us. We have a live-in agreement but we don't have a policy on how often people are to be followed up after the match." When asked about follow-up interviews, one volunteer has noted: "We should do it more often, which we don't do because we think things are going well." Awareness that more follow-up work would be useful often surfaces when a person in a match is contacted for other purposes such as for publicity. One woman who felt "left out" by her homesharer complained to the volunteer only after she had been contacted when the agency was seeking her participation in an advertising spot.

Just how much responsibility the agency should assume after the match has been initiated is an ongoing concern. The general feeling among staff is that after the two-week follow-up the client should be responsible for contacting the agency, particularly the volunteer who acted as case manager. Considering current practices among clients, however, the director and her staff agree that making the client responsible for contacting the program is inadequate.

## Current Project HOME Concerns

Despite uninterrupted service to homesharing applicants for nearly seven years and despite rearranging the director's and volunteers' roles to provide case management support to the program's clients as financing would allow, Project HOME continues to face new challenges. Each in itself is the kind of ongoing issue that tends to confront all homesharing programs at one time or another, so while we will describe the particular case of Project HOME, the applications to other programs should be evident.

The issues discussed briefly in the following sections are: the central problem of finding matches for clients, new initiatives in respite care matches and rural outreach, how volunteers best fit into the program, and the never-ending problem of fund-raising.

*Finding Matches for Clients.* There always will be challenges to the staff as they try to match people with special interests, requests, and needs: A frail employer with pets, a caregiver who must have regular "time off," students who must be within walking distance of campus, and homeowners who, in the words of the current director, are "looking for that ideal woman of sixty in good health who is going to be a friend and companion" all need to be accommodated.

In addition, however, there are basic structural limitations that also limit options in forming matches. For instance, finding caregivers and lodgers for homeowners in rural areas is difficult since many movers do not have cars. One other group is particularly important in this context, because their problems stem from structural limitations as well. These are homeowners who are frail enough to require caregivers but who lack the finances to afford them.

The current director notes that Project HOME now attempts to put together a patchwork of services that will enable these frail homeowners to remain in their own homes. One part of this patchwork is a new program called "medicaid waiver," which will pay a live-in respite person $5.50 per hour for up to seventeen hours a week. In situations in which the homeowner qualifies for the medicaid waiver, Project HOME tries to place a respite caregiver in the home.

When considering the costs of maintaining elders in their own home, it is necessary to look at the direct costs of live-in and respite care and the food and utilities consumption of the caregivers. The director estimates the current average cost of a live-in caregiver to be about $200 per week. Estimating another fifty dollars a day for two days of respite care, she projects the total direct cost for care to be around $300. Adding another $50 for food and utilities usage brings the total cost of keeping a frail elder at home to about $350 a week. When one compares this with area nursing home charges, which run from $600 to over $800 per week, homesharing as a source of caregiving makes economic sense.

The director is now also looking into the use of reverse mortgages to help frail homeowners with financial problems raise sufficient money to pay for caregiving. The reverse mortgage is a process by which the bank provides payments to the homeowner during the homeowner's lifetime and then assumes ownership of the home at the time of the homeowner's death. The homeowner is guaranteed the right to live in the home as long as he or she lives.

Two obstacles have prevented the reverse mortgage initiative from becoming a reality, however. First, all but one local bank have thus far been reluctant to get involved particularly since Congress mandated that counseling had to be included but did not provide funding for it. HUD is now supporting counseling but, as yet, none of the homesharers have utilized this provision. As the director reports, "people are reluctant to give up the ownership of their home and the assets of the home. I have confidence this will change, although it will be slow." Many may also want to have ownership of the home to pass on to their children. The director sympathizes with such homeowners: "It is sad that people are forced to give up the equity in their home that has been built up over many years."

A final structural problem facing Project HOME and all other home-sharing services is having a sufficiently balanced pool of owners and movers, and of recipients and providers of services. The director and her staff face a continuing challenge to maintain a balance in the program's pool of clients in the face of changes, often external to the agency, that are constantly causing imbalances in the types of clients who seek assistance to Project HOME.

For example, recently homesharing matches have leveled out, but there has been a decline in the numbers of caregivers available to share with homeowners willing to pay for their services. Fortunately, at the same time there has been an increase in the number of respite caregivers. It is likely that the cause of the live-in caregiver decline has been the robust economy and low unemployment in the area. As the director observes, "People can find jobs with benefits and much better pay than they can get through homesharing." To deal with this problem, the program is trying to recruit more caregivers by running advertisements in less financially prosperous communities outside the area served by Project HOME. The assistant director is also talking with people in the state department of education about building in a nonmedical caregiving component in some rural high school job training programs for students who might be attracted to this form of employment.

This last instance clearly illustrates how the larger community has an important, often direct impact on the ability of a homesharing program to deliver its promised services. As long as program leaders understand this relationship between their local program and the larger societal context in which it exists, they will have a chance to alleviate the negative effects when they occur. Of course, program leaders also need to realize that certain kinds of applicants—those in rural areas and those with caregiving needs but no ability to pay for care, for example—will have constant problems in getting matched and so require the kinds of new and unusual initiatives described above to help them.

*The Rural Outreach Programs.* Since the current director took over, two new programs have been developed under the umbrella of Project HOME in response to client needs. The less successful of these is the rural outreach program. A local foundation had provided funding for release time for one of the regular Project HOME staff members to coordinate. Volunteers attempted to get the word out to recruit people from the area for potential rural matches, and posters were distributed in prominent places around rural towns.

The director has become pessimistic about being able to support a rural outreach program. She notes that there *is* a "rural need," but early on it became clear that "the majority of seekers were looking for an urban situation." She believes that other counties in Vermont now trying to develop homesharing programs will have difficulties "without a good population base" (see Maatta et al. 1989 for description of a rural home-sharing program that is working).

*The Respite Program.* Nevertheless, the director is a strong advocate of diversification within Project HOME to complement the basic homesharing service function of the program. Recently as the number of clients served through the homesharing portion of HOME has leveled off, the program has begun to emphasize relief help for caregivers, or respite care. Currently, in fact, there are often as many respite as homesharing matches made during any given period of time. The respite component of Project HOME is an outgrowth not only of the need for relief help for caregivers within the program but also the considerable encouragement from other agencies in the community who are themselves involved in long-term care. Although still a part of Project HOME, the respite program is designated as a separate program when it is time to approach funding sources like United Way.

As the current director describes it:

> The respite program arose when we found ourselves entering into agree-ments with caregivers who wanted time off, and there was no one to cover for them and come in. Two days is often not enough time off. You also may need a few hours in the middle of the week to go to church, visit a friend, or just get out. It was hit or miss whether we could find anyone.

The respite worker is distinguished from the primary caregiver only by the amount of services provided. A respite worker offers short-term care either as a live-in worker for a few days, as on weekends, or as "day help" for a few hours during one or more weekdays. Therefore, the distinction between primary caregiver and respite caregiver has nothing to do with whether one lives in or not: Some primary caregivers, for example, work eight hours a day for five days a week but do not live in. In some such cases, a family member provides care on nights and weekends, while in others a combination of family and respite caregivers living in share the work. Rarely does a respite situation involve more than three days of live-in care.

According to the administrator of the respite portion of HOME, the general rule concerning which respite workers live in and which do not is based on how many days a week they put in. Respite caregivers who work three days or less a week do not live in and are paid by the hour. Those who work more than three days a week do live in and receive a flat fee for service. The amount of respite care provided, therefore, ranges from a one- or two- to forty-hour week.

There really are no "typical" respite situations, because each is tailored to client needs, which vary tremendously. For example, in one case a respite caregiver's duties are confined to going into a home two hours a day to fix dinner for the homeowner who has no one living in. In another, more complex arrangement, one respite caregiver lives in during the weekend while another comes in for an hour or two a day to provide relief for the primary caregiver who lives in and provides care the rest of the time.

Thus respite arrangements vary along several criteria: Some are long term, while others are for a short duration. For example, there have been temporary situations in which respite workers have filled in during the family or primary caregiver's vacations. As seen above, some arrangements involve only one respite caregiver, while others are based on multiple caregivers. The status of the respite workers differs also: Some are married, others single. Some are in the work force, some are keeping house, while others are students.

As far as money goes, however, most respite caregivers are paid. The fees range between five and eight dollars an hour, the average fee being from six to seven dollars an hour. Respite care is arranged through Project HOME's respite coordinator, who functions like the director and her volunteers when they arrange homesharing matches. At the same time, neither the respite coordinator nor the agency sets rates since that is part of the negotiations between the frail elder and the respite caregiver.

A recent modification to the respite program has been the use of volunteer as well as paid respite caregivers. Volunteers normally put in no more than four hours a week; respite workers providing more hours of care usually are paid. The coordinator of the respite program plans to expand the number of volunteers in the future, especially in cases where respite care is needed for short periods of time. Paid caregivers are hard to find for such short-term needs, because it is not worth the paid caregiver's time and effort if the period of service is minimal. As the respite coordinator observes, volunteers can fill in for paid workers in a variety of situations:

> One person wanted someone to come two days a week for one to two hours to make lunch for her mother. I found her someone eventually, but it would have been easier to find a volunteer to do this kind of short-term service. Volunteers would be useful if the clients had fairly limited needs or were difficult people to manage or needed help while living in the country. A volunteer could work with a difficult person because there is never enough money if the person is difficult. If you are a volunteer you can feel like a rescuer. It is a different motivation.

The respite coordinator's plan is to recruit as many as thirty volunteers to supplement the present number of thirty paid caregivers. She already has begun eight-week training sessions for the volunteers. Adding volunteers means that the program is likely to expand because "we are going to have people seeking services who couldn't afford it." She would also like to develop a support group for paid caregivers and for family members who provide caregiving services, because intervention and support in the initial stages of an elder's deterioration can prove more effective than waiting for the deterioration to reach an advanced stage. Recently, a student intern has been helping the respite coordinator with telephone inquiries, interviewing applicants, and reference checks, so that the coordinator would have time to work on recruiting volunteers and developing a volunteer training manual.

> I am putting an interpersonal component into the training aspect of the volunteer program, such as the reality of dealing with Parkinson's or Alzheimer's or a hearing defect. People assume that Parkinson's is just a muscle disorder. They don't know about the depressions and moodiness that often accompanies it. They need to know that ahead of time and be effective in helping that person. That helps them stay.

With respect to staffing, the coordinator is also planning to recruit an older volunteer who will be assigned specifically to the respite portion of Project HOME, because directing the volunteer component of respite care will be a full-time job. Just as the second HOME director oversaw a significant increase of client demand and consequent division of labor within the agency, the respite coordinator stands at the beginning of a potentially significant growth period that would require additional staff or volunteer resources. If she gets the help she wants, the respite coordinator plans to devote more time to public speaking, recruiting, and advertising.

Despite some clear-cut parallels between the early years of HOME and the current situation of the respite part of HOME (e.g., early success, rapid growth, the use of volunteers) and despite the fact that the respite program has its own funding from United Way, neither the HOME director nor the coordinator foresee the respite part of HOME becoming an independent agency in its own right in the way HOME split off from RSVP. The coordinator of the respite program appreciates having "a support system around me" as she deals with the stresses of managing the new program.

The respite component obviously has been a successful addition to the services offered by Project HOME, once again illustrating the advantages of being flexible in the face of changing community needs. By growing and diversifying its service delivery, the agency is able to balance the demands of several different client groups. At a time when homesharing has leveled off, the respite component of the program is expanding its services both to more clients and also to the trained volunteers who will serve those clients.

*Wither the Staff Volunteers?* The number of staff volunteers has declined to three, although the director hopes to recruit one or two more in the future. Each volunteer puts in about six to eight hours a week of service and is clearly dedicated and loyal to Project HOME. They look forward to their volunteer days and talk about the cases they have matched with exuberance. As one volunteer put it, "I love the interaction with the people. Monday never seems long enough." The volunteers believe they are busier now with more cases than they were when the program was young. A large part of the reason probably is increased case management.

After each interview, the volunteer writes up a resumé and places it in one of six large notebooks representing all the various combinations of respite and homesharing caregivers. All staff then have access to these notebooks when looking to match one of their clients. The only disappointment expressed by volunteers interviewed stems not from the program but from the weeks that it may take to arrange a match. A volunteer reports that "I do four interviews a month, but I may go months without making a match."

A continuing problem with using volunteers, of course, is that they can reduce their service and commitment at almost any time, as described in chapter 3. Unfortunately, such withdrawal may come at a time when more, not less, service is needed. The director laments that "our newest volunteer is going to take a leave of absence because her husband just had a heart attack and they will do the cardiac rehabilitation program at the hospital together. So we are missing a person coming out of a very busy summer." While it does take service time to coordinate the volunteers, the director continues to believe the effort is worth it.

Fortunately HOME almost always is able to recruit very capable student interns from the colleges in the community. The intern provides an additional resource when there is a sudden surge of applicants or reduction in staff. According to the director, the intern "is part of the team and does most of the things elder volunteers do. She fills in gaps of the older volunteers."

The director further notes that making the volunteer component effective and efficient takes considerable staff support. In addition to the weekly group meetings, she believes it is important for the volunteers to have "one-on-one meetings with paid staff persons to review people interviewed in the past to talk about potential matches and to help with the logistics of setting up introductions." Not forgetting hard-to-place people requires constant vigilance. She continues, "[It is] a struggle to follow up" and "when times are busiest it is easier to take new people in to do the interviews and let the folks in the system fall behind unless there is an obvious match."

Since so much paid staff effort goes into coordinating, monitoring, and supporting the efforts of the volunteers, the question obviously arises as to whether such efforts could be more efficiently spent in direct service to clients. When asked whether an all paid staff might have some advantages over a large volunteer staff the director responds,

> I think so. When you are in the office for such a short time every week you miss the connections that a paid staff person does. For a volunteer model to continue working while the staff becomes more professionalized you need one-on-one staff support.

Still, the program continues to use volunteers in important ways. Their coordination and support is now largely the responsibility of the administrative assistant. One of her key roles is to schedule client application interviews, some of which require as much as a month's lead time. The assistant also types, files, orders supplies, and recently has become involved in data management as she enters client information into a newly purchased computer. Eventually the director hopes all clients will be on the computer.

Originally much of the work the administrative assistant now does had to be done by the volunteers, which decreased the time they could work directly with clients. The administrative assistant also does more "sifting out" calls than was done in the past. For example, according to the current director, "If a student calls us in August and says he needs a room within two weeks and within walking distance of campus and we don't have anyone, we will discourage them from coming in. If we have someone we will act quickly."

Although the administrative assistant does several other tasks, as shown above, her primary function is to assist the volunteers in the interview process. For her part, the director does *not* believe the assistant's time would be better utilized in direct service delivery. This is consistent with her belief that service delivery by volunteers, while perhaps not as efficient as the work of paid staff, nevertheless brings the intangible qualities of motivation and empathy essential for working with the program's clients.

> Purely from an organizational point of view it would be more efficient to have paid staff people, but I think you miss a lot given [the volunteers'] life experience and concern for elders. So, at this point, it is worth it for the program to give them the support so they can do their job. It is less efficient, but qualitatively it is worth it.

Obviously the volunteers were essential at the inception of the program when no financial support was available and innovation, flexibility, and high motivation were essential ingredients for success. As the program and paid staff expands and as it becomes a more professional program with a need for greater standardization and coordination, it is possible that the utility of a volunteer staff will diminish and eventually result in greater costs than rewards to the success of the program. At this point, however, the director and her staff appear to be satisfied with the arrangement of administrative staff support for the volunteers as they provide services to Project HOME's myriad clients.

*Fund Raising.* If there is anything a homesharing program needs to pay attention to as much as matching clients, it is making sure the program can operate on a day-to-day basis. For a program like Project HOME, which has paid staff, this means worrying about money. In Project HOME, not surprisingly, this responsibility has generally been the director's. From the hectic early grant-application days to its present United Way agency status, Project HOME's directors have always had to grapple with funding questions.

The program also is currently a "line item" in the state budget with funding channeled through the State Office on Aging. Coupled with the ongoing funding from United Way, this has given the program a much more sound ongoing financial base—quite different from the annual scramble for financial support during the program's early years. The budget has also grown dramatically, from $35,000 to over $100,000 during the nearly four years the current director has been in place.

When money concerns in the program are mentioned, it is in two contexts: Obviously, the director has to continue to be concerned about money for Project HOME, the agency, but she also is concerned about money for clients of the program. These include homeowners who cannot afford to pay a caregiver for services or lodgers who cannot afford to pay rent to a provider.

With respect to fund-raising for the agency, the program's advisory council is supposed to take on a large part of the burden of raising additional needed monies. In fact, council members have generated worthwhile fund-raising ideas and provided direct service in raising money, including the use of their ties with state officials and legislators to help the program become a line item on the state budget.

Unfortunately, fund-raising initiatives from the council recently have involved staff personnel in ways that detract from service delivery. For example, during the last two summers the council has raised money through a home tour in which several private homes having particular qualities, like being especially equipped for a handicapped person, were opened to the public for a ten-dollar donation. According to the director, "It was the paid staff that put hours and hours of work into what was supposed to be a volunteer and council and community friends effort." Although the tour was a successful fund-raiser, the director hopes to restructure it differently in coming years so that it does not absorb so much staff time. Likely candidates to take the place of staff volunteers are members of the advisory council or the assistant director, who is directly responsible for fund-raising.

Concerning financial support for clients, the director hopes more can be done with Section Eight money to make homesharing more affordable to renters. "Section Eight" is a federal housing subsidy program that was developed in the 1960s to allow people to pay only a portion of their income for rent. Congress has extended the program to include home-seekers in programs like Project HOME, although regulations do not yet exist that would allow the subsidy to be put into effect. Its application to Project HOME clients will be limited even if it is implemented, since these federal monies apply only to persons who are over sixty or disabled.

Although few in number, some seekers are over sixty years old and thus eligible. In addition, there are a small number of homeseekers under sixty who are disabled but still can provide a protective presence and help with services for some homeowners. According to the current director, however, more will need to be done for those "people who cannot afford the rent and end up committing themselves to an exchange of services they are unwilling or unable to provide." A final limitation to the subsidy, of course, is that it does not help homeowners who cannot afford to pay caregivers what they are asking for. Some hope exists in the "medicaid waiver" and reverse mortgage initiatives described earlier, but these solutions are not without their own set of problems.

## Summary of Current Practices

Clearly important in the evolution of Project HOME has been the stabilization of its financial base. With the director and her volunteer staff able to concentrate more on service delivery, important case management initiatives have been developed that lessen the chances that clients will be unintentionally ignored, as happened to some during the program's early years.

At the same time, current concerns over the factors from outside the program adversely affecting the staff's ability to match, new programs in respite care and rural outreach, attempts to maintain the delicate balance of administrative support for the volunteers doing service delivery, and continuing problems of fund-raising for the program and its clients all together ensure that the current "stable" regime of Project HOME still faces many critical challenges. The next section briefly highlights some additional concerns we have as evaluators with respect to the program's development and its current practices.

## An Evaluation of Project HOME

In one sense, both this and the previous chapter have already presented the major critiques of the first five years of the program through the description of clients' concerns and the ways in which the current director and her staff have dealt with them. In brief summary, we have come to two conclusions concerning homesharing service delivery and client satisfaction in the program. The first is that Project HOME, one of the earliest homesharing programs in the country, has had a good track record of serving clients—as measured by client perception of their living arrangements during follow-up interviews and as assessed by questions directed toward client experiences with the program.

Second, those client dissatisfactions that occurred during the program's hectic earlier growth period have been addressed through reallocation of staff resources made possible by an increased and consistent source of funding. The transformation from an entrepreneurial to managerial service agency model has been completed, and the program's clients are better off for it.

*Tactics.* At the same time, the discussion of current practices in the previous section suggests some additional comments concerning tactical and strategic considerations in the evaluation of Project HOME. At the tactical level, we suggest an expansion of the case management role of the staff volunteers.

At present, two gaps appear to exist in the program's follow-up of clients. In the first place, there is no systematic follow-up of those who are unmatched. Volunteers do care about "their" clients and do attempt to keep them updated, but they are not always successful at doing so. We recommend two things: Telephone contact should be made at regular intervals if no possible sharer has been found. Further, it would be useful if the program were to employ a brief telephone questionnaire of perhaps a couple of questions to be asked of each unmatched client when the volunteer calls. Through these questions the program would find out whether there have been any major changes in the applicant's situation and, if so, what they are.

A second problem area we see has to do with the lack of any systematic follow-up after the volunteer checkup on clients when they have been matched for two weeks. The director points out that currently any sort of follow-up beyond the initial one is likely to be "hit or miss," depending on the volunteer. The homesharers are encouraged to get in touch with the program if problems arise, but there is no systematic provision for agency-initiated follow-up.

Obviously, needs of participants change, particularly in the case of frail homeowners whose deteriorating health may be producing strains in the arrangement. Also, past experience has shown that not all sharers will contact the program on their own to complain about problems; yet, when a staff member contacts them, evolving problems are mentioned. We recommend follow-up telephone calls at regular intervals after the two-week trial period in order to spot changes in the sharers' needs and expectations before major intervention is required. The number of follow-ups and the length of time between them will depend, of course, on staff resources; but, at a minimum, one call a month for half a year seems reasonable (see Howe and Jaffe 1989 and Underwood and Wulf 1989 for examples of how follow-ups are done in other programs).

One area in which the program has made inroads, in addition to the two-week follow-up of matched clients, is in employing an exit survey to be administered when sharers dissolve their matches. At this time, clients are asked how the match went and whether they have thoughts about a rematch. The director explains:

> This [exit survey] helps us know whether or not to rematch either party and what to look out for if we rematch again. This is done with everyone matched.

The reality, of course, is more complicated, because the director and her staff are dependent on at least one member of the match alerting them about the match's dissolution. Therefore, only those who themselves choose to contact the program are picked up through the exit interview.

If follow-ups beyond the initial trial period are instituted, as suggested above, then the program should have higher visibility to its clients and be more likely to be contacted when matches dissolve. Based on the information she does have, the director tells us that the major reasons for the breakup of matches is that the elders want more services and companionship and the seekers, particularly lodgers, want more freedom.

*Strategy.* While the suggestions concerning tactical approaches to improving follow-up of clients are dependent on the availability of staff time to perform the various required duties (e.g., making the calls, noting the information, saving the information in a systematic way so it can be utilized properly), we have one final recommendation that we believe is easily manageable within the current structure of Project HOME. This has to do with the broad issue of program evaluation. It has already been shown in chapter 4 how program evaluation was part of the exchange that existed between the program and its evaluators during the first five years. As we have come closer to full disengagement from the program, no mechanism to replace us has been introduced.

The director admits that she "does not know where to start in program evaluation," and at the moment says she has none. Referring to us, she states that "for several years I have put in your research findings to help us obtain grants. But now that your role is ending we need to look elsewhere." She acknowledges it is "important for people who manage programs to step back and see what is done."

Despite the lack of a formal mechanism for evaluation, the program must "claim we do it," states the director. In fact, evaluation of a sort does go on in the program. For one thing, the director, the paid staff, and the volunteers discuss service matters with one another routinely, especially at the weekly meetings. In addition, information about numbers of people served and goals of the organization are regularly generated for reports. Finally, since hearing our concerns about the lack of current evaluation, the director has indicated that the Planning and Evaluation Committee on the Advisory Council intends to address the need for evaluation through a variety of mechanisms, including the contact of clients for their views of the program in much the same way that we did in preparing the material for the previous chapter.

Nevertheless, at the moment, evaluation, which was such a significant process for the current director's predecessor when she was trying to define the program's goals and establish its legitimacy, has been in a subordinate role to that of fund-raising and publicity. Except for general information about seasonal trends in applications, numbers of clients served, and duration of matches, and limited data on dissolutions of matches, no ongoing formal mechanism for evaluation is now in place.

Although the director is sympathetic to the importance of evaluation in fostering improvement in service delivery, the ongoing daily demands of servicing clients and seeking financial support have an immediacy that has taken precedence over long-range planning. It is possible that the recently announced intentions of the Planning and Evaluation Committee will come to fruition and redress this imbalance to produce a comprehensive internal evaluation of the program, but for now their thinking is still in its early stages and much remains to be done.

Systematic evaluation of the program is both necessary and desirable, not so much from the viewpoint of the two research-oriented sociologists who are finally coming to the end of their formal ties to Project HOME but from the point of view of the program itself. The final section of this chapter addresses in some detail the variety of ways in which Project HOME, as it currently is constituted, can provide for its own systematic evaluation.

# THE HOMESHARING AGENCY AND
# ITS EVALUATION

## The Continuing Need for Program Evaluation

The very special, and one could argue "unique," relationship that characterized the social exchange between the second director and the evaluators has highlighted the great potential that exists between evaluators and evaluated if the two parties have mutual goals in mind, if the evaluated does not feel threatened by evaluation, and if the evaluators are not afraid to become emotionally involved in the program they are evaluating. In chapter 4, we argued that such a relationship not only *can work* but actually produces optimal results for both the evaluated and the evaluators. It is not necessary, however, that all service agencies and would-be evaluators emulate our experience. The time and emotion spent in developing the kind of social exchange that existed in the Project HOME case are unlikely to be duplicated in any but the most unusual instances.

Nevertheless, some form of evaluation is necessary for any homesharing program to succeed, including the current Project HOME. There are two simple reasons for supporting systematic, ongoing evaluation: First, the agency needs to know how well it is serving its clients. Certainly, staff will have anecdotal evidence and an intuitive feel for how well things are going, but without systematic evaluation the chances for errors in this method are far too great. Second, the agency's funders will demand evaluational information, as they consider whether to fund the agency or not, and, if they do fund, how much. Sadly, evaluational information has the potential for being used as a weapon by the funding agency to rationalize a negative decision, but without evaluational information homesharing programs are quite likely to be "dead in the water."

Therefore, while there might be rare exceptions, *both* the funding agency and service agency decisions are served by pretty much the same kind of information. In the case of homesharing programs, some of the most important questions concern the number of inquiries received and by whom, the number of referrals made and to whom, the numbers and types of applicants, and the numbers and types of applicants who are matched. Also vital to know are the characteristics of applicants, characteristics of applicants matched, satisfaction of matched clients with their sharing arrangements, reasons for dissolving matches and for requesting rematches, and attitudes of all applicants toward the program and its services by type of applicant among matched and unmatched individuals.

While some of these questions can be answered easily enough merely by noting the relevant information during inquiries and on application forms and then organizing the information on a regular basis (e.g., monthly, quarterly), other questions require a larger expenditure of effort (and, in some way, cost). In particular, follow-up interviews are resource draining. For one thing, locating applicants after a period of time often requires a great deal of persistence, especially in the cases in which applicants have changed residences and not kept the program informed. For another, even without the problem of locating what has proven to be a geographically very mobile population in the case of lodgers and caregivers, staff time often has to be diverted from what is perceived as direct service delivery functions to what is often perceived as the "It would be nice to know but we don't have the resources" type of indirect service delivery/evaluation function.

## Three Models of Evaluation

If the kind of social exchange relationship that evolved between evaluators and evaluated during the early years of Project HOME is not likely to apply to many homesharing arrangements, then what sorts of evaluation models are possible? There are at least three functional equivalents, that is, evaluation arrangements that can substitute reasonably well for the type detailed here. (These models are also applicable to service delivery agencies that are not engaged in homesharing, because the major ingredients—service delivery, outside funding, evaluation—are present in most such agencies.) Evaluation in this context means the data gathering, data management, data analysis, and data presentation concerning client needs and service upon which funding agencies base their decisions to allocate or not allocate support for homesharing programs and upon which homesharing programs make internal decisions concerning expansion and curtailment of services regarding particular target clients. The three models are different from each other primarily in terms of who does the evaluating: the funding agency, a third party, or the homesharing program itself.

The first is the *funding agency evaluation model,* which places evaluation of a program exclusively in the hands of the organization funding the homesharing program. Homesharing agencies *could* ask funding agencies to gather, organize, analyze, and interpret their own data about the homesharing service, but there are too many practical arguments against this strategy. In the case of Project HOME, the initial problem is deciding which funding agency should do the evaluation, since both United Way and the State of Vermont provide important monies to the program.

A further problem, from the agency's perspective, is even more loss of autonomy. Homesharing programs today usually exist at the pleasure of one kind of funding source or another, so they clearly are not fully autonomous units. Nevertheless, with the funding agencies taking on the role of evaluation as well as funding, the homesharing program becomes more like a subunit of the funding agency, rather than an independent body.

Finally, despite limited record-keeping concerning numbers of clients served, it is simply unlikely that the funding agencies themselves would even want to consider the additional burden of integrating an evaluation team into their organizations. Those who fund homesharing programs, such as United Way and the State of Vermont, are involved with too many programs to make this suggestion practical.

Altogether, incorporating the evaluation process into the money giving process appears to raise many practical barriers to its implementation. While there is something philosophically satisfying about the money providers doing their own legwork to get sufficient data to make a reasoned financial decision regarding a beneficiary homesharing program, the objections that would be voiced by funding agency and beneficiary program alike would probably be far too strenuous to give the suggestion much chance of making it.

We label the second model the *third-party evaluation model*. Within this approach one can distinguish two subtypes: the disinterested or "hired gun" and the interested evaluations. In the case of the *disinterested* evaluator, an outsider with expertise in research and/or evaluation is hired by the homesharing agency to gather, analyze, and present data on the program's goals and its success in meeting those goals. For Project HOME, researchers from the university or another local school or professional consultants or research firms not affiliated with any school could be hired.

There are two major benefits to receiving a paid evaluation of the program: First, the third party doing the evaluating is likely to be accepted by the granting agency as a truly disinterested, objective evaluator of the program. Second, the agency can look for experienced, qualified

evaluators, not "settling" for just anyone who is interested in homesharing programs, as might be the case in an exchange agreement with a
university researcher. The homesharing program can check the references of its evaluators beforehand in the same way that it checks the
references of its clients before attempting to match them.

On the debit side there are several problems to hiring an outside
evaluation team or individual. First, of course, is cost. As indicated
throughout this book, raising money to operate has been a dominant goal
of Project HOME almost since its inception as an RSVP experiment.

A second, equally strong argument against hiring an outside evaluation
is the likely intransigence of homesharing staff. While we have had a
relatively good relationship with Project HOME, it is clear that the
current director is not nearly as comfortable with us as her predecessor
was. We believe a large part of the reason stems from the fact that our
role currently is closer to that of outside evaluator than it was during the
program's early years. The disengagement which we initiated some two
years ago has reached the point where we clearly are more outside than
inside the program.

Indeed, homesharing directors often refuse cooperation with outside
evaluators (Mantell 1988). The reasons vary, but one important one is
that they fear such evaluation will somehow compromise their program.
Many are simply concerned that the evaluation will find fault with the
program and their management of it, and they don't want that kind of
criticism. In some cases, it simply may be that the director does not have
a strong enough ego to tolerate constructive criticism that could actually
lead to improvements in the program. In other cases, however, it is most
likely that directors honestly believe that (1) the evaluators don't really
have the program's best interests at heart (and this is probably true of
paid evaluators) and (2) the evaluators could seriously jeopardize the
service delivery of the program through unwarranted, unfair criticisms.

One solution to these kinds of concerns is the second type of third-
party evaluation, that done by an *interested* third party. This category
includes the kind of exchange that existed for several years between
ourselves and Project HOME, described in chapter 4; but it also includes
a special kind of third-party evaluation: the Shared Housing Resource
Center survey of homesharing programs.

While not an evaluation in the strictest sense, the Center's survey
does perform an important service to both homesharing programs and
their granting agencies by describing both median tendencies and ranges

for a variety of important organizational and client-related indicators. Even with the avowed purpose of disseminating important information on homesharing to its newsletter subscribers, the Center is still an outsider and thus subject to the same kinds of responses from wary directors as are paid evaluators.

The third model, *evaluation by the homesharing program itself* is, we believe, the most desirable practical alternative to the first two models, because it can work within the organization of the homesharing program as it currently exists or with minor modifications, it maximizes organization autonomy, and it minimizes the kinds of financial strains usually associated with evaluation.

Consider the case of Project HOME. According to the current director, the only kind of evaluation now being done is the record keeping of numbers of inquiries, applications, matches, duration of matches by type of client and time of year, and staff time use. As indicated earlier in this section, this information is quite important, but in itself not enough to paint an adequate picture of the program's service delivery. Additional information needs to be extracted from the application form to show the kinds of breakdowns on both applicants and matched clients as were done in chapters 5 and 6 to determine whether there are any discrepancies between target populations at which the program is aimed and those clients who are actually being helped. For example, it is important to know if clients with hearing problems are not being matched because of a difficulty in communicating with potential sharers through telephone introductions. This was a problem, incidentally, for the program during its first two years and was corrected after we shared our findings with the director and her staff.

While such information exists in the program records and needs only to be extracted, there is an additional need to contact clients systematically who have not been matched by follow-up interviews, so that follow-ups of both unmatched and matched clients can be compared to see how well the program is serving them and to locate areas that can be strengthened, such as was done in chapters 7, 8, and 9. This strategy will require the development of a (probably brief) follow-up questionnaire for clients who have not been matched that can be administered over the telephone in the same way that follow-ups are now done for clients whose matches have dissolved.

How can this be done? There are essentially two answers. First, the work can be done by the staff. The paid administrative assistant could collate the additional information needed by putting application data on the computer, as is now being done. The director and her volunteers could put together the follow-up questionnaire for unmatched clients in the same way that they did for clients whose matches have dissolved, and this information too could be computerized. The result would be an ongoing database to which the director, her staff, and the advisory council could refer both to keep track of the program's success in meeting stated program objectives and to update information when funding time comes around.

The second way by which the program could do its own evaluation is through its advisory council. As previously described, a central focus of the council when it was set up was planning and evaluation, in addition to volunteer support, publicity, and fund-raising. There is even a Planning and Evaluation Committee on the council. Unfortunately, as we have disengaged from the program, the program's commitment to planning and evaluation began to disengage as well. When the two researchers did not choose to serve second terms on the council, their places were taken by individuals with fund-raising experience rather than with either research or evaluation experience. Thus, unless the director and her staff explicitly acknowledge the need for an evaluation perspective on the council, natural attrition will have removed the last vestige of a research/evaluation focus from the advisory council and, given the interests and abilities of the current staff, from the program entirely.

If, on the other hand, one or two of the positions to open up next on the council are filled with "research types," then the council could take the lead in gathering, managing, analyzing, and presenting evaluational data for the program. This strategy, of course, has the dual benefits of keeping all staff time free for service delivery while a committee of the council takes charge of evaluation as an insider who nevertheless has some distance from the actual delivery of services in the program.

Given a choice, we would opt for the council-organized evaluation of Project HOME, but only if the council contains at least one interested individual who is qualified to oversee evaluation. Funding agency evaluation is impractical because of the multitude of funding agencies and poses a serious threat to Project HOME's autonomy. Third-party evaluation, aside from the sorts of perceived threats it represents, costs money the program doesn't have and likely wouldn't want to raise. Between the two kinds of in-house strategies, giving the council responsibility for evaluation is both consistent with one of the four main charges of the council and potentially makes use of appropriate professionals. They are appropriate in the sense that they have an interest in and experience with evaluation, and because they also have a commitment not only to homesharing but to the program on whose council they sit.

While the best strategy for evaluation may differ from program to program, the in-house council committee model has much to recommend it. Whatever choice a homesharing program makes, if it chooses to incorporate a systematic evaluational component alongside its service delivery then it will be demonstrating the kind of concern for its clients that is needed.

As funding allowed, the current director and her staff have made a conscious effort to follow clients more closely after their applications, utilizing a case management approach that appears to have met with some degree of success. Currently, while one follow-up does occur regularly with matched clients, a need is perceived to widen the case management net to follow up all clients, matched or not, in more systematic ways. Clearly staffing limitations are a key determinant as to how much follow-up can occur.

Finally, we have proposed a set of functional equivalents to the kind of evaluation process that the first five years of Project HOME saw and for which the current program must find a substitute. While one should not expect Project HOME, or indeed any homesharing agency, to duplicate the sort of evaluation we were able to provide the program during its early years, adequate functional alternatives exist; and, in the case of one of them, the mechanism is already in place to make that alternative work.

In the final chapter, the idea of homesharing will be reconsidered as an alternative to institutionalization and as a living arrangement itself providing for a continuum of care within the home. Also, the important findings concerning Project HOME clients will be summarized and shown to represent important groups of potential homesharers throughout the country. Finally, the original organizational analysis of the program will be reconsidered through a review of the importance of social exchange in service delivery programs like Project HOME.

# 11

# Homesharing:
# Beyond the 1980s

The grassroots phenomenon analyzed through the in-depth case study of Project HOME appears to be much more than a ten-year fad. From its humble beginnings in a few scattered sites just a few years ago, homesharing has expanded into well over two hundred communities throughout the country and promises to grow even more in the years ahead. Of primary interest to social service program directors and social scientists alike are questions dealing with the ways this relatively new housing alternative will affect and itself be affected by family structure, medical care delivery, government and private funding sources for service delivery programs, local housing conditions, and local attitudes about homesharing.

While a detailed examination of these issues is beyond the intent of this book, the analyses contained here should provide a solid foundation for such further inquiry (see Jaffe 1989a; Mantell and Gildea 1989; and Robins and Howe 1989 for good overviews on important homesharing issues). This chapter will return to the major themes discussed in the previous ten chapters. We will place the Project HOME experience in the context of homesharing as a general phenomenon with certain common elements shared by almost all programs—no matter how large or how small, how new or how old.

Not surprisingly, the emphasis will be on the two major concepts that have been developed in this book: a continuum of care and social exchange. Consideration of these two ideas has produced four major themes to be underscored in the next few pages. Together these themes provide important insights into both the practical and conceptual meaning of homesharing. Furthermore, as we have attempted to do throughout the book, they focus on both the individual and organizational aspects of homesharing. The first two themes relate to the idea of a continuum of care.

## THE CONTINUUM OF CARE

Chapter 1 argued that homesharing is an important innovation along the continuum of care for elders and frail individuals who find themselves faced with undesirable alternatives. Between the extremes of living alone without help for necessary daily tasks and institutionalization, homesharing provides yet another choice for those individuals who want to retain as much independence as circumstances will allow. Responding to the environmental press of which Lawton speaks, these people no longer need consider perhaps unwanted intrusions on family or expensive medical care delivery to stay home.

Chapter 8 showed that homesharing fits into the continuum of care in yet another way. Several of the clients whose sharing arrangements were analyzed showed that the deterioration of health of the homeowner produced a "naturally occurring" continuum of care within the individual's home. As the homeowner's health required more care, some individuals went from traditional homesharing arrangements with a lodger to more complex arrangements often involving family members, one or more caregivers, and homesharing program staff. In this way, homesharing has been continued, but in arrangements requiring greater caregiving to keep environmental press at an acceptable level.

This section explores these two continua of care, showing how Project HOME's experience demonstrates the importance of homesharing as an alternative housing arrangement that can reduce environmental press for elders and frail individuals who desire to remain at home.

### Homesharing is a Choice along the Continuum of Care

Chapter 1 described the variety of housing options theoretically available to elders in this country and in other countries. Between the traditional options of living alone at home and living in a nursing home are a wide range of alternative housing schemes like congregate housing, retirement and life care communities, domiciliary and personal care homes, and, of course, homesharing.

Nationally, there is only indirect information about the desirability of homesharing as an alternative housing form. The Andrus Foundation funded a study of attitudes toward homesharing nearly ten years ago that shows that, among homeowners fifty-five years of age and older, 34 percent express positive attitudes toward homesharing, while 51 percent are negative toward homesharing. Favorable views come particularly from those living in large houses, those who perceive they live in a high-crime area, and those who rate their health as poor and income as less than adequate. Not surprisingly, loss of privacy is the most frequently mentioned disadvantage of homesharing, while having someone around in case of illness or emergency is the most frequently mentioned advantage (McConnell and Usher 1980).

Much more recently, the state of Vermont commissioned a statewide needs assessment survey of elders, including in its telephone interview schedule a series of questions about current living situation and about alternative housing options (Vermont Office on Aging 1988). Two points are important to note here. One is that the state of Vermont, while clearly more rural than the rest of the country, is nevertheless quite representative of the nation in terms of the proportion of the population sixty years old and over (about 12 percent for Vermont and the nation). Second, Project HOME is the only homesharing program in the state, covering less than one fifth of the state's population; so direct, or even indirect, knowledge about homesharing because of Project HOME is likely to be limited.

The 1986 study reports that four out of five respondents own their own homes. Almost nine out of ten of them are very satisfied with their present housing. Of the remaining tenth, the concerns and problems tend to be ones addressed by Project Home as well as other alternative kinds of housing. These include problems associated with the cost of upkeep and physical maintenance of their home; furthermore, many of those dissatisfied complain that their house is too big and that they have no one to call for help. This latter concern is especially frightening for an older person living alone who fears having an accident at home and being unable to contact anyone for help. A smaller, but nevertheless important, minority of elders also express concern about having no one to talk with. All of these major problems of homeowners can be alle-viated by homesharing.

Elders in the survey were also asked whether they would like to share a home with someone else; 26 percent express at least some interest. Significantly, interest in this form of alternative housing grows when information about the benefits of house sharing are added to the question. For example, 27 percent are attracted to the idea of sharing their house and sharing costs, 29 percent to the idea of sharing their house and having company, 35 percent to sharing their house and having someone to do the chores, and 39 percent to sharing their house and having someone to help in an emergency.

While homesharing is a relatively new concept for many people throughout the state compared with the more traditional congregate or cooperative housing options existing in several communities, it is signifi-cant that from one-quarter to over one-third of the elder respondents are receptive to the idea of homesharing under certain conditions of assis-tance. Many of the features desired in congregate and cooperative hous-ing are also incorporated into homesharing, and it is likely that many respondents became more positive toward homesharing when these simi-larities were pointed out. For example, homesharing allows elders to remain in their own home and in control of the decision-making that takes place in it. Further, they can control the amount of rent and the length of the lease in their sharing agreement.

The Andrus and Vermont studies together indicate several things about elders' receptivity toward homesharing. First, when given home-sharing as an alternative to their current living situation, only a minority of elders seize on it as an option. This is not surprising, considering that homesharing is still a relatively new phenomenon about which people surveyed know very little. As the Vermont study shows, the more kinds of potential benefits that can be highlighted for respondents, the more positive their attitudes become.

More important than the numbers, however, is the fact that respon-dents even would be willing to consider a housing option sight unseen. The kinds of housing problems elders currently face, as indicated by the Vermont study, obviously have much to do with people's willingness to consider having a stranger come live with them.

This brings us to the last observation about homesharing as an alter-native housing form along the continuum of care. Homesharing is an *alternative* to people's current housing situation and to other potentially practical living situations they might choose. We are not promoting it as the option of choice for all people. Homesharing is not meant to replace other choices. Indeed, the Vermont study has discovered considerable interest among its respondents in congregate housing and in smaller cooperative housing apartments.[1]

Nevertheless, the popularity of homesharing likely will grow as its presence becomes better known by potential clients, their families, and service providers. Project HOME is a good example of how increased awareness of a homesharing program in a community can result in rapidly expanding requests for its services. Agencies contemplating supporting homesharing services should be aware, however, that there is also likely to be a period of at least a year or so before the publicity for such a program has any serious impact and produces the kind of increased demand Project HOME experienced.

The Shared Housing Resource Center's (1988a) recent survey of homesharing programs shows that nationally almost 100,000 people request information on shared housing over the course of a year, almost 40,000 actually apply to homesharing programs, and over 15,000 actually end up homesharing.

Clearly homesharing is an alternative that fits the needs of many individuals, particularly the old and the frail. Hopefully, our analysis of Project HOME has shown the variety of shared housing options within the context of this alternative living arrangement. At one end of the spectrum are home providers and lodgers who tend to share a relatively minimum amount of space and time together. At the other end, caregivers provide aid to homeowning employers in an intensive, around-the-clock arrangement. In between are home providers and lodgers who spend much time together in a satisfying exchange of space for services and companionship for companionship. We have also witnessed the evolution of complex sharing arrangements in which the homeowner shares with one or more individuals and receives respite care from yet other sources.

As an alternative living option, homesharing has much to recommend it for those elders who are dissatisfied with or unable to cope with their current housing. When such elders contact homesharing agencies, they at least expand their living options, even if they choose to pursue another one such as congregate housing. Once elders do choose to homeshare, their living arrangements become a dynamic. The changing conditions of homesharing arrangements are summarized next.

## Homesharing Provides a Continuum of Care within the Home

> [I]t can be argued that the agency-assisted homesharing arrangement occupies a unique status within this continuum of care.
>
> The uniqueness of this option lies in the opportunity to respond to a wide range and changing set of needs within the private residence. In other words, it is possible to receive an increasingly rich mixture of assistance over time within an individual's home (Jaffe and Howe 1988:318).

The above observation has been demonstrated empirically quite well in our analysis of Project HOME, especially through the information gleaned from the in-depth follow-up interviews with homesharers described in chapters 7 and 8. Importantly, caregiving was never an explicitly stated goal of Project HOME when it first began to function, nor did its early staff and volunteers themselves really understand the full ramifications of the match-making they were undertaking on behalf of the program's clients.

What started Project HOME to think explicitly about helping to arrange for a continuum of care within the home for its clients were the changing circumstances in which its clients found themselves. As described in chapters 2 and 4, the second director's strong commitment to serve needy clients who could somehow benefit from homesharing was equaled only by her entrepreneurial drive and willingness to try new things in the program. Because of the program's early flexible structure, such initiatives as she developed became informal, then later formal, policy.

In the meantime, there are three key points to remember. First, it was client needs that initially created the sense in Project HOME staff that they were part of an ongoing process to help those clients who wished to remain at home do so through a variety of homesharing arrangements that would change as the clients' needs changed. Project HOME, as did numerous programs like it, started out with the idea of matching up applicants who wanted to homeshare in the traditional sense of home provider and lodger. Once caregiving needs for home providers were recognized, staff energies were focused to help those whose matches had fallen through find another sharer, and to help those whose current match did not provide enough care to get additional care from respite caregiver(s). Ongoing client needs, in fact, helped promote an active respite care component to the program that now has its own staff coordinator and is operating as almost an independent entity.

Second, for homesharing service providers in other communities and for those who might be planning to develop a homesharing service, the Project HOME experience demonstrates a clear need existing in all communities: Elders and frail individuals who live in their own homes (1) usually want to remain there rather than enter a nursing home or some other congregate facility, (2) usually continue to experience declining health, and (3) often have family who are willing to help them remain at home but who are unwilling or unable to provide full-time caregiving services.

While homesharing certainly won't work for those individuals who prefer some form of congregate housing or other alternative arrangement to homesharing, and while homesharing is only now beginning to deal with the limitations involved for those who want caregiving services through homesharing but can't pay for them, for many others homesharing arrangements can provide a continuum of care within the home. As evident from some of the matches involving clients with Alzheimer's Disease, the limits of homesharing care are only now being approached.

Finally, while, organizationally, the Project HOME experience serves as a model for how programs evolve to deal with changing client needs, it also should prepare those who currently are starting up homesharing programs or plan to do so in the near future. Forewarned is forearmed, in a sense. Those who do *not* wish to get involved in arranging caregiving services need to rethink their motives in arranging homesharing matches. On the one hand, they may decide that expanded services are a necessary part of homesharing and thus be prepared to deal with the added drain on staff time involved with the kinds of case management procedures Project HOME has developed. If so, then program directors can go to their funding agencies with a clear-cut idea and demonstrable evidence (from Project HOME, for example) that homesharing staff time will involve more than simple match-making.

On the other hand, agencies may choose, for a variety of defensible reasons, to limit their services to the more traditional sharing arrangements involving a home provider who requires a presence around the house and perhaps help with some chores and a lodger who requires a reduced or no rent arrangement. If this be the case, however, we submit that such agencies should be morally obligated to give some minimal referral service to those agencies or individuals in their community who *can* provide the caregiving that may be required for a homeowner whose health is deteriorating. Therefore, at the very least, as stated in the previous section, homesharing agencies should accustom themselves to the role of referral agency within the network of services available to the elderly and disabled within their community.

In summary, the idea of a continuum of care within the home is certainly not a new one. Families historically have taken care of their old and their ill within the home, until recent technological advances and changed values concerning care have handed over the job to outside agents like hospitals and nursing homes. Today, however, modern medical science has helped create circumstances substantially more complicated than they were in early rural America or during the flowering of technology just a few score years ago.

As we approach the end of the twentieth century, we encounter circumstances produced by life expectancy rates for men and women that are significantly higher than those at the beginning of the twentieth century. Living longer means meeting a larger number of challenges to make that longer life meaningful.

Among those challenges is the ability to keep up one's own home. Is it reasonable to put one's widowed mother in a nursing home when she is in reasonably good health and needs help only in doing some heavy chores around the house and in paying for the upkeep of her large house? Probably not, and among the choices she now has in many communities is homesharing—an arrangement that not only can alleviate the environmental press she currently experiences but that also conceivably could help keep her independent even in the face of further deterioration of health.

## SOCIAL EXCHANGE

Social exchange represents an important concept in homesharing service delivery in at least two ways. The following sections will reexamine the role that exchange, or bartering, plays in the homesharing arrangements between clients and between the program and those who volunteer on its behalf. The underlying theme in the following pages is that understanding the dynamics of exchange will benefit clients, staff, and researchers alike in their efforts to understand why homesharing has become such an important alternative in the continuum of care and to appreciate how the homesharing process can be maximized. While the following arguments stem from our experiences with Project HOME, they are easily generalizable to other homesharing programs because of the basic exchanges that all programs include in one way or another.

## Homesharers and Social Exchange

While seeming to be too simple a truism to contemplate spending time discussing, the idea that homesharers must barter with one another, giving and taking in ways they had not originally anticipated, is in fact too important to ignore. Chapters 5 through 8 described typical home-sharing applicants and then the typical kinds of applicants who got matched, and finally examined in detail what the homesharing matches of such clients were like during Project HOME's first five years. From the general patterns revealed by the application interviews to the in-depth insights of the follow-up interviews, the consistent message seems to have been: Applicants who succeed in getting matched are the ones who appear to understand the importance of bartering.

*Prelude to Bartering: A Complementarity of Applicants.* Chapter 5 showed that Project HOME was originally set up to accommodate two kinds of clients—stayers and movers—but found itself with divisions within each of those groups that clarified the complementarity of client needs even better. Among traditional homesharing applicants, when compared to lodgers, home providers are more likely to be: older, financially better off but less educated, in good but not as good health, living alone, and, of course, homeowners.

This background "fit" of characteristics, however, is only the beginning of a basis for exchange between the two groups. Key to any sharing arrangement is the *perception* of what homesharing involves. In this respect, the fit between provider and lodger applicants is not bad either, as represented by traditional sharer attitudes toward household and nursing service. Over half of the provider applicants want to share or have each partner do his or her own services, while almost all lodger applicants are willing either to share/do their own or provide services. In addition, lodger applicants generally have no objection to sharing with a disabled home provider.

The only warning sign is the length of time each type of applicant wants to share: Providers are much more likely than lodgers to desire an indefinite homesharing arrangement. This should not be too surprising when one considers where each type of applicant is in the life cycle.

Jaffe, finding similar patterns in his study of homesharers in Madison, Wisconsin's Project SHARE, puts these differences in the context of "status passages." He argues, "For the homesharing participants interviewed in this study, status passage involves a movement along the continuum of independence-dependence (Jaffe 1989b:40).

What makes the status passages of homesharing applicants so important, he adds, is that home providers and lodgers are proceeding in different directions. The older homeowner is moving "from independent living as widows to complete dependency or death," while the very much younger lodger is moving in the opposite direction, "from dependency to autonomy" (Jaffe 1989b:41–42). Concomitant with these changes, of course, are perceptions as to their desirability; thus, it should be no surprise that the older homeowner wants to resist any further deterioration of position by living in a homesharing arrangement that will last indefinitely, while the younger lodger really wants to move on with her or his life once their particular crisis is resolved and they are on their feet financially.

Among applicants classified as personal care companion sharing clients, the fit between stayers and movers appears to be even stronger. Employers are like providers but are better off financially and have more health problems. Caregiver applicants are likewise similar to lodgers but much more willing to provide household and nursing services.

These distinctions create the apparently perfect fit between employers and caregivers. The former are in poor health but not concerned about finances, and are therefore willing to pay for caregiving services, while the latter need a job and are willing to provide caregiving services. What could be simpler? As seen in chapter 8, when employers and caregivers do begin to share, concerns do arise to complicate the arrangement. These concerns are discussed below.

Together, then, the four kinds of homesharing applicants who represent typical stayers and movers appear to have fit together well. One important exception has been mentioned in previous chapters and needs to be mentioned again. Homeowners who are in failing health but who do not have the financial resources to pay for a caregiving sharer face a dilemma when they apply to homesharing programs. Given the nature of social exchange, they are quite unlikely to find someone willing to do the kinds of chores and services they require unless rent is waved and some fee paid to the caregiver; but the homeowner wants the rent and certainly cannot afford to pay for services.

The previous chapter showed that Project HOME has begun to address this particular problem. Nevertheless, until Project HOME and her sister programs can find practical creative solutions to this dilemma, homeowners will continue to have difficult choices to make in the context of homesharing. Many in Project HOME have attempted to manage with a traditional lodger and hope the lodger will be able to perform enough household chores to help the homeowner (and her or his family, if they are nearby) to cope. Many other homeowners are not even matched by the program, because appropriate lodgers cannot be found for them.

*Understanding Social Exchange Facilitates Match-Making.* Chapter 6 described the kinds of client characteristics that helped each of the four types of applicants get matched. Here social exchange shows itself to be the foundation of homesharing matches. Among traditional homesharing applicants, providers and lodgers benefit most from possessing two qualities: flexibility and a realistic expectation concerning homesharing and what it involves.

In terms of flexibility and realistic outlook, traditional homesharing is not unlike marriage. In both arrangements, the participants must be willing to accept their mate as she or he already is and to gave as well as take. In both situations, therefore, the rewards one is gaining from the relationship must be tempered by an understanding of the rewards the other person is gaining from the relationship. For homesharing applicants, this means that one should approach both prospective sharers and an anticipated sharing arrangement with an appreciation of the give and take involved in sharing.

For personal care companion applicants, flexibility was also found to facilitate one's chances of getting matched. Among employers, it is a willingness to share with a caregiver who has children or who is a student; among caregivers, flexibility is indicated by a lack of concern over sharer's lifestyle and a willingness to share with someone who is disabled.

Of particular interest, the desire for an indefinite sharing arrangement actually seems to *help* both employers' and caregivers' chances of getting matched. Both types of applicants seem to expect to be in the arrangement for "the long haul"; in this sense, the outlook of successful employer and caregiver applicants is "realistic." This differs dramatically from the attitudes of successful providers and lodgers who want an arrangement of finite duration.

*Social Exchange Facilitates Shared Living.* Once clients actually begin to share, the ideas of social exchange, flexibility, and realistic expectations become paramount. As was discovered in the in-depth follow-up interviews described in chapters 7 and 8, the characteristics that help applicants find a sharer also help applicants once they have begun to share.

In traditional sharing arrangements in which the respective roles of provider and lodger have some degree of flexibility, there is a great deal of room for negotiation as to what each will give and take in their exchange. Further, despite the possibility of sharing very little in the way of time and space, many providers and lodgers in fact do exchange services and share space. Central to the satisfaction of the partners in these arrangements is the amount of social interaction they have.

For the majority of the homeowners, having someone present and willing to spend time with them is even more important than the useful tasks their sharers perform. Not surprisingly, the amount of interaction was found to be an area in which the sharers must bring their flexible and realistic approach to homesharing to bear. For many lodgers, access to space and lifestyle conflicts represent problem areas. To the extent that sharers compromise in seeking solutions, they succeed in improving the quality of their relationship, whether the initiative to sit down and discuss mutual problems comes from one or the other of them or from the homesharing agency.

Sharing arrangements involving employers and caregivers involve what we call "two-way gratitude." Most employers genuinely appreciate the efforts their caregivers are making on their behalf, while the caregivers for their part receive not only money but also intense satisfaction from the help they are providing the homeowner. Originally unanticipated by employer or caregiver applicants or by Project HOME staff, the stresses caregivers undergo in their work looms as a major obstacle to satisfaction in many personal care companion shared living arrangements.

In this case, the idea of social exchange has its limitations, except to indicate that as caregiver stress increases, it reduces the salience of the rewards the caregiver receives from the sharing arrangement and one of two things inevitably happens. Either the caregiver quits and looks for another employer or some other accommodation, *or* the agency finds respite help, like that described in chapters 8 and 9. In any event, despite needing the money and gaining much satisfaction from the help they are giving their sharer, caregivers face tremendous problems in attempting to manage alone; they need the help of the employer's family and the homesharing agency to ensure that their frail employer receives the necessary care.

In summary, actual matches exemplify a variety of social exchanges. In traditional sharing arrangements, a provider's home in exchange for rent, reduced rent and services, or only services is merely the starting point. More important to the arrangement are the attitudes of the parties toward companionship and time and space use. Those who bring flexibility and realistic understanding of the arrangement are most likely to gain satisfaction from the match.

In personal care companion matches, the starting point really is the exchange of the employer's money for the caregiver's services. The fact that the service takes place inside the employer's home, however, adds a critical dimension to the relationship, because it draws the sharers close together in ways that often produce an overdose of stress for the caregiver. In those cases, the imbalance of exchanges is not rectified by a willingness to compromise. Rather, it is accomplished by the intervention of family and/or homesharing agency so that respite help can be provided to alleviate the caregiver's burden.

## Homesharing Service Delivery through Social Exchange

As described in chapters 2 through 4, social exchange has played a critical organizational role in the evolution of Project HOME. Of particular importance have been the exchanges between the second program director and the volunteers and between the director and us, the university researchers. While we do not necessarily suggest that all homesharing programs must follow the organizational structure and dynamics of Project HOME to succeed, it is nevertheless important to understand *why* these exchanges have been so important to the program's success and *how* they may be borrowed by other agencies. We shall review briefly the whys and offer some suggestions regarding the hows for each type of exchange in the next few pages.

*The Importance of Volunteers to Homesharing.* At the very outset of Project HOME, of course, volunteers were deemed to be critical to the program in two ways: as *providers* of homesharing service delivery but also, because of their role as service providers, as *receivers* of meaningful RSVP experiences. Both roles were equally important. Chapters 3 and 4 described how the program, especially under the second director, did indeed use volunteers extensively during the program's first five years, as a small number of volunteers came to perform critical executive tasks. Chapter 10 showed how the third director, as a result, is now able to use volunteers as case managers to improve the program's matching and follow-up services.

Throughout this book, we have argued that the work of the volunteers has been very important to the survival and later growth of Project HOME. While functional equivalents to the volunteers might have been found along the way, they weren't. The volunteers filled in where they have been needed. In fact, it is no exaggeration to say that, throughout Project HOME's existence, volunteers have performed every type of job in the program except for grant application writing, which has been the sole province of the director.

Furthermore, whether or not substitutes for the volunteers could have been found (a very unlikely event), there are three instances in which the volunteers contributed significantly to Project HOME's development. In the beginning, volunteers provided the needed "bodies" to do the necessary interviewing. A few did their work quite well, many were at least adequate, and a very small number really were doing a task they were ill-equipped to do; but the fact that the volunteers could supplement the director's interviewing efforts meant that more applications could be processed and more matches likely made. This became especially important after the first year when the number of applications began to grow dramatically.

During the third year especially, the volunteers made another important contribution. While their numbers were dwindling, the few who remained with the program began to take on many more tasks besides interviewing, so that the second director could devote more of her energies to the necessary fund-raising to keep the program going. This escalation of volunteer duties gave rise to the executive volunteer role discussed in chapter 3. From clerical office work to media campaigning to match-making, the volunteers became the critical "right hand" of the director.

Today, volunteer work is being supplemented by the paid staff made possible by increased funding for the program. Again new challenges have been found for the volunteers in the current director's efforts to provide case managers for each applicant. Today, applicants are less likely to be lost among the myriad cases being daily considered by the program, because each client has a volunteer whose responsibility is the client's well-being.

Not surprisingly, the Project HOME model is quite consistent with what is happening to homesharing programs across the country. As stated in the first chapter, the Shared Housing Resource Center has found that most homesharing programs use at least one volunteer. In the most recent issue of their quarterly, the Center reports findings from in-depth interviews they did with the twenty-five programs who use the greatest number of volunteers:

> All match-up programs surveyed use volunteers in the intake and screening process. Most programs use volunteers to interview and match clients, check references, visit homes and perform clerical work. Volunteers do counseling, follow-up and marketing/publicity for 60 percent of the programs. In some 40 percent of the programs volunteers provide information and case management referrals. (Shared Housing Resource Center 1988b:1)

Clearly, some seven years after Project HOME began using volunteers as one of only a handful of homesharing programs in the country, incorporating unpaid staff into homesharing service delivery has now become the norm.

Indeed, the Shared Housing Resource Center argues, "In many instances, the contributions of dedicated volunteers are crucial to the success of the program" (Shared Housing Resource Center 1988b:1). As a result of this belief, they devote much of their fall 1988 issue to discussing how homesharing programs can maximize their use of volunteers. Topics covered include: recruitment, interviewing, training, and retaining volunteers.

Of special relevance to the Project HOME experience is the argument that volunteers need to be treated like coworkers and shown that their efforts are being appreciated. Both of these retention "strategies" have been a part of the Project HOME experience from the beginning, but they may not be enough. As pointed out in chapter 4, after a while, the program had to start making matches so that the volunteers could feel that they were accomplishing something. Without that sense of success, they would have been less willing to stay with the program.

We *do* agree with the Shared Housing Resource Center's conclusion regarding volunteers:

> While shared housing programs may vary according to focus, location and resources, almost all could benefit significantly from the increased use of volunteers. The time and effort invested in volunteer development is likely to pay lasting dividends in terms of organizational growth, expansion of services and increased community awareness and involvement. (Shared Housing Resource Center 1988b:3)

Volunteers represent a marvelously deep well of resources for homesharing programs. The evidence is there for all to see in terms of the general tendencies from across the country that have just been described and through the case study we have offered in this book.

Furthermore, if the Project HOME experience is any indication, using volunteers also represents an important application of the notion of social exchange. On the one hand, volunteers receive meaningful life experiences and a sense of well-being from the good they do. On the other hand, the homesharing agency receives "free" work, which is often unavailable from traditional sources (i.e., paid staff for whom little or no money exists).

This is particularly important in the early stages of development of innovative programs such as those offering homesharing services for two reasons. First, community acceptance is just evolving and means are necessary to "get the word out" about the program; volunteers are a good grapevine. Second, traditional sources of funding may not yet be forthcoming to support a program with a relatively unproven service record, so the work of volunteers substitutes for paid staff until the program gets enough financial support (and perhaps even beyond that time, as in the case of Project HOME).

There is another consideration as well. By using volunteers, homesharing programs *underline* the importance of social exchange. Exchanging becomes not just a goal to be accomplished for pairs of clients; it also comes to represent an ambience within the program. At least, this has been our experience with Project HOME. "Giving and getting" in nonmonetary ways is what volunteers do in a homesharing program, and, after a while, it becomes an important value in the program and emphasized in staff relations, hopefully spilling over into staff-client relations and finally into client-client relations.

*Other Exchanges Involving Homesharing Programs.* Chapter 4 spent some time describing our own role in Project HOME, and chapter 9 suggested ways the evaluation role could be substituted for. Whether outside evaluators like us or internal evaluators such as a committee on an advisory council are going to provide important feedback to a program's director, we maintain that the critical thing is to have some sort of ongoing evaluation. When this occurs, social exchange again becomes manifest.

If evaluation gets done without money changing hands, there is, of course, the danger that the arrangement will deteriorate. A paid consultant or evaluator will have a financial incentive to provide the information the agency needs. As seen in the case of Project HOME, however, exchanges between evaluators and the agencies they evaluate is somewhat more delicate when no money is involved.

While we were getting useful information from the director, her staff, and the program's files on clients, writing papers for professional presentations, and preparing material for this book, it was in our interest to keep helping Project HOME. The conclusion of these tasks, however, meant that we either continue providing feedback to the program for altruistic reasons or we terminate those ties involving the exchanges discussed in this book. Given our interests in other research projects and a sincere desire to put some emotional distance between ourselves and the program before we attempted to write up some of this book's chapters, the decision to disengage was a relatively easy one.

From the point of view of the program's staff, our decision to disengage was not difficult to accept for two reasons. First, as indicated in chapter 4, additional funds for clerical work, paper and the like and using volunteers in an increasing diversity of roles meant that many of the in-kind services we were giving the program in its infancy were being provided without our help. Second, during the last couple of years, the program's emphasis on evaluation has become overshadowed by its concern over fund-raising. To be sure, finding money to run the program has been with Project HOME from the beginning; but, as described in the previous chapter, the current director believes advisory council energies need to be oriented toward raising additional financial support for the program.

Therefore, volunteers and staff have taken over what small direct service role we had in the beginning of the program, and the advisory council's increasing concern with publicity and fund-raising has reduced its commitment to ongoing evaluation. We have no quarrel with the substitution of volunteer and paid staff for our early direct services; it was inevitable. As explained in the previous chapter, however, Project HOME should continue to provide for program evaluation in some way, such as through the advisory council.

There are other kinds of exchanges that can augment volunteer and evaluation contributions to homesharing programs, and we take a bit of space to mention two of them. All homesharing programs are near one or more hospitals. It seems reasonable to suggest that, if a program is going to attempt to match employers and caregivers, as Project HOME has done, then hospitals might be interested in supporting such endeavors in a variety of ways. Two questions naturally arise. First, why should hospitals get involved? According to Hare and Haske (1984), homesharing programs, by providing someone to live with frail elders in their own homes, allow earlier discharge of these elders when and if they become hospitalized, because they have someone (more likely a combination of someones, as described earlier) to look out for them. To the extent that hospital space is at a premium, it is in the hospital's, as well as society's, best interests to discharge patients as soon as is medically feasible.

The second question has to do with the kinds of things hospitals could do to cooperate with homesharing programs. Here the answers are not as clear cut, depending really on the ingenuity of the participants involved. A partial listing of possible hospital involvement might include direct funding for any homesharing program in the community that matches caregivers and frail elders, because support of such a program is in society's best interests and because such a program will ultimately benefit the hospital, however indirectly.

While such altruism might be slow in coming forth (and, strictly speaking, it is not the kind of exchange emphasized in this book), there are other ways hospitals might come to the aid of homesharing programs. Hare and Haske (1984:33–34) argue, for example, that hospitals "could provide emergency backup services. They could train potential caregivers in necessary skills and in brokering services. They could assist with liability questions." In addition, hospitals might list and advertise the homesharing program's services for their patients; such help could range from posting information on bulletin boards to providing patients with handouts on the program to having either hospital or homesharing program representatives speak with patients about the program's services.

Many homesharing programs are also located near universities. If our own community is any indication, the university students contribute to a shortage of decent affordable rental units, because there is not enough university housing for them and because they are often able to afford the kinds of rent that local citizens cannot. This opens up several opportunities for joint ventures between the school and the community. Indeed, some homesharing programs like Independent Living, Inc. in Madison, Wisconsin actually specialize in matching university student homeseekers with elders living in the community.

At this level of cooperation, the university or college actually becomes a partner in the program. Homesharing agencies not currently connected to any such schools but that are located near them, however, might profit from contacting them in an effort to augment the pool of home-seekers. The extent of university involvement could parallel that of the hospitals discussed earlier.

In both of these suggested exchanges, the institution, be it a hospital or university, has a stake in supporting local homesharing agency efforts. In the former case, it means earlier discharges and more available hospital beds; in the later case, it means finding both housing and worthwhile life experiences for some of its students. For the homesharing agency, of course, these are two more kinds of social exchange opportunities.

By all objective indicators, Project HOME is a success story. More than that, however, the story of Project HOME is a case study of how a service agency can begin with a good idea—bartering services for a place to live—and expand on that idea to make barter not only the essence of its clients' matches but also the essence of its own operation. In addition, Project HOME is a case study showing not only how the continuum of care works within the community but also how it can work within one's own home.

In our analysis, we have attempted to show, through a detailed examination of Project HOME, that homesharing is a grass roots phenomenon that reaffirms old values and gives new meaning to others. In emphasizing the value of remaining relatively independent in one's own home, homesharing tells elders and young people alike that there are alternatives to staying home alone or succumbing to an institutionalized setting. In providing for a variety of services for elders, homesharing tells all of us that the continuum of care that exists institutionally also can be made to exist within the home. Finally, in the context of its delicately constructed service delivery programs such as Project HOME, homesharing tells us that the exchanges between homesharers is but a mirror of the exchanges that exist within these programs themselves.

Indeed, Dorothy is correct. There really is no place like home. Yet, for those elders and other individuals who desire to live at home but face a press of environment in their daily lives, the solution need not require a wizard. Indeed, along the continuum of care there are a number of alternatives available to these individuals. It should be clear from this book that, on the basis of its flexibility within the continuum of care and its exemplification of social exchange principles, homesharing is an important one of those alternatives.

*Appendix 1*

# Application Form, Interview Schedule, and Live-In and Nonliability Agreements

The application form and interview schedule represent the most detailed ones used during Project HOME's first five years. Both earlier and later ones were much smaller, as described in chapters 2 and 4. The live-in and nonliability agreements are the ones in current use.

## APPLICATION FORM

The first set of questions numbered 1 through 77 is taken from the provider/ employer form. The lodger/caregiver form is identical except with respect to Neighborhood Considerations (questions 44 through 49) and Home Considerations (questions 50 through 59). This form was filled out by each applicant before staff conducted a personal interview with the applicant.

Project HOME    Application Form    Applicant No. ☐☐☐☐

Name _____

Present Address _____
                     Number        Street      Apt. #        City

        Telephone _____   _____   _____
                    Home          Work        Best time to be
                    reached

Immediate need? _____

Reason _____

Please circle appropriate response or fill in blank for each question

*Personal Information*

1. Sex: _____ male      _____ female

2. Birthdate _____
              Month     Day     Year

3. Birthplace _____
                        Town     State

4. Length of time in Vermont _____

5. Length of time in this home/apartment _____

6. Present place of residence: _____ own home        _____ live in trailer

   _____ rent home        _____ other (specify) _____

   _____ rent apartment    _____

7. Number of rooms in present residence (including kitchen, bath) _____

8. Marital status: _____ married      _____ divorced      _____ never married

   _____ widowed      _____ separated      _____ other (specify)

   If married, widowed, divorced, or separated, how long have you been? _____

9. Highest grade in school that you finished and got credit for _____

10. Are you presently under legal guardianship or permanent supervision?

    _____ yes    _____ no

    If yes, name of person _____

    address of person _____ phone _____

11. Employment status:

    _____ full-time worker      _____ unemployed, looking for work

    _____ part-time worker      _____ student

    _____ retired              _____ other (specify)

    _____ homemaker

12. Your occupation when working (please be specific) _____

13. Present/most recent employer_____

                                       name/company

                         _____

                          address                   telephone

14. Length of employment at most recent job_____

    If student, name of school_____

    What year?_____   _____

                                 Address                   Telephone

    What major?_____   _____

                                      Contact Person

15. Your total monthly income:

    _____less than $100     _____$400–$599     _____$1000–$1249

    _____$100–$249       _____$500–$749     _____$1250 & over

    _____$250–$399       _____$750–$999

16. Please check income sources:

    _____Soc. security     _____Food stamps

    _____S.S.I.             _____Fuel Assistance

    _____Pension           _____Other (Specify_____)

## *Support Networks*

17. How many people are presently living here with you?_____

    If there are people living here with you, please give the following information about each:

| First name or initials | Relationship to you | Age | How long living with him/her |
|---|---|---|---|
| _____ | _____ | \_\_\_\_\_ | _____ |
| _____ | _____ | \_\_\_\_\_ | _____ |
| _____ | _____ | \_\_\_\_\_ | _____ |
| _____ | _____ | \_\_\_\_\_ | _____ |
| _____ | _____ | \_\_\_\_\_ | _____ |

18. How many living children do you have?_____

19. How many of your children are living within a day's drive of you? _____

If you have children within a day's drive of you, please give the following information about each son/daughter:

| First name or initials | Sex | Marital status (single, married, widowed, or divorced/ sep.) | How frequently do you see him/her? (daily, weekly, monthly, a few times a year, hardly ever) | Does he/ she have any children? |
|---|---|---|---|---|
| _____ | ___ | ___ | _____ | ___ |
| _____ | ___ | ___ | _____ | ___ |
| _____ | ___ | ___ | _____ | ___ |
| _____ | ___ | ___ | _____ | ___ |
| _____ | ___ | ___ | _____ | ___ |

20. Do you have any other living relatives (excluding your spouse and children) living within a day's drive of you? _____

If you have any other relatives living within a day's drive of you please give the following information about each relative:

| First name or initials | Sex | Marital status (single, married, widowed, or divorced/ sep.) | How frequently do you see him/her? (daily, weekly, monthly, a few times a year, hardly ever) | Relationship to you (e.g., cousin, sister, etc.) |
|---|---|---|---|---|
| _____ | ___ | ___ | _____ | _____ |
| _____ | ___ | ___ | _____ | _____ |
| _____ | ___ | ___ | _____ | _____ |
| _____ | ___ | ___ | _____ | _____ |

*Services and Health*

21. Are you presently participating in any of the following services?

Visiting Nurses Association (VNA)        Area Agency on Aging (AAA)

_____ yes    _____ no              _____ yes    _____ no

Home Delivered Meals          Retired Senior Vol. Program (RSVP)

_____yes  _____no          _____yes  _____no

Transportation Assistance      Senior Companion

_____yes  _____no          _____yes  _____no

Home nursing                   Other

_____yes  _____no          _____yes  _____no

                               (please specify)_____

22. In general, would you say your

| vision is | hearing is | mobility is |
|-----------|-----------|-------------|
| _____excellent? | _____excellent? | _____excellent? |
| _____good? | _____good? | _____good? |
| _____poor? | _____poor? | _____poor? |

23. Here is a list of things that people usually have to do during the day. After each, check the answer which best describes how well you can do the activity.

|  | Can do without help | Can do, but need help | Can't do |
|---|---|---|---|
| dressing and putting on shoes | _____ | _____ | _____ |
| bathing | _____ | _____ | _____ |
| cutting toenails | _____ | _____ | _____ |
| readings | _____ | _____ | _____ |
| preparing meals | _____ | _____ | _____ |
| going on walks outside | _____ | _____ | _____ |
| climbing stairs | _____ | _____ | _____ |
| cleaning house | _____ | _____ | _____ |
| hearing over the telephone | _____ | _____ | _____ |
| going grocery shopping | _____ | _____ | _____ |
| riding a bus | _____ | _____ | _____ |
| driving a car? | _____ | _____ | _____ |

24. Are you on a special diet?     _____yes  _____no

    If yes, what diet are you on?_____

25. Are you taking any medications regularly?     _____yes  _____no

    If yes, what medications?_____

26. Have you ever suffered from the disease of alcoholism? ＿＿＿yes ＿＿＿no

    Comments＿＿＿＿＿＿＿＿＿＿＿＿＿＿＿＿＿＿＿＿＿＿＿＿＿＿＿＿＿

27. Has drinking ever caused a problem for you or your family?

    ＿＿＿yes ＿＿＿no    Comments＿＿＿＿＿＿＿＿＿＿＿＿＿

28. Who is your physician?

    Name＿＿＿＿＿＿＿＿＿＿＿＿＿＿＿＿  Telephone＿＿＿＿＿＿＿

29. How often do you see your physician?＿＿＿＿＿＿＿＿＿＿＿＿＿＿＿

30. Whom would you contact in an emergency?  Name＿＿＿＿＿＿＿＿＿

    Address＿＿＿＿＿＿＿＿＿＿＿＿＿＿＿  Telephone＿＿＿＿＿＿＿

31. What is this person's relationship to you?＿＿＿＿＿＿＿＿＿＿＿＿＿

32. Have you been hospitalized within the last six months?  ＿＿＿yes  ＿＿＿no

33. Do you have a health condition a home sharer should know about?

    ＿＿＿yes ＿＿＿no

    If yes, what is it?＿＿＿＿＿＿＿＿＿＿＿＿＿＿＿＿＿＿＿＿＿＿＿＿

34. Do you have any recurring health problems that affect your activities?

    ＿＿＿yes ＿＿＿no

    If yes, what are they?＿＿＿＿＿＿＿＿＿＿＿＿＿＿＿＿＿＿＿＿＿＿

    If yes, how do you cope with them?＿＿＿＿＿＿＿＿＿＿＿＿＿＿＿

35. Have you ever been arrested or convicted of a crime?  ＿＿＿yes  ＿＿＿no

    If yes, please explain＿＿＿＿＿＿＿＿＿＿＿＿＿＿＿＿＿＿＿＿＿

*Interests*

36. What activities are important to you? (hobbies, church and other activities, social engagements, sports, volunteer assignments, etc.)

    ＿＿＿＿＿＿＿＿＿＿＿＿＿＿＿＿＿＿＿＿＿＿＿＿＿＿＿＿＿＿＿＿

    ＿＿＿＿＿＿＿＿＿＿＿＿＿＿＿＿＿＿＿＿＿＿＿＿＿＿＿＿＿＿＿＿

37. How would you describe your lifestyle? For example:

    Do you follow a daily routine?＿＿＿＿＿＿＿＿＿＿＿＿＿＿＿＿＿＿

    Are you neat or sloppy?＿＿＿＿＿＿＿＿＿＿＿＿＿＿＿＿＿＿＿＿

    Are you easygoing?＿＿＿＿＿＿＿＿＿＿＿＿＿＿＿＿＿＿＿＿＿＿

    Are you out of your home frequently?＿＿＿＿＿＿＿＿＿＿＿＿＿＿

    Are you a private person?＿＿＿＿＿＿＿＿＿＿＿＿＿＿＿＿＿＿＿

What kind of music do you like?_____

Anything else?_____

_____

38. Do you want your homesharer's lifestyle to be similar to yours?

_____yes _____don't care _____no

39. How much time do you expect your homesharer to spend with you?

_____

_____

40. How would you feel if the first thing someone did was clean up your kitchen?

_____

41. What irritates you about people?_____

_____

42. What would someone like about you?_____

_____

43. What wouldn't someone like about you?_____

_____

*Neighborhood Considerations*

44. Are you a walker _____yes _____no

45. Do you drive a car _____yes _____no

46. Do you use the bus? _____yes _____no

47. Do you own a car? _____yes _____no

48. What type of transportation do you usually use?

_____walk _____car _____bus _____other (specify)_____

49. Are the following near your home?

grocery store                    hospital

_____yes _____no          _____yes _____no

shopping areas                   laundromat

_____yes _____no          _____yes _____no

church                           school

_____yes _____no          _____yes _____no

senior center                     other

_____yes  _____no            _____yes  _____no

                                  If other, specify_____

## Home Considerations

50. Do you have off-street parking for your homesharer?

    _____yes  _____no

51. Is there public transportation within a few blocks of your home?

    _____yes  _____no

52. Is there a private bedroom for your homesharer?

    _____yes  _____no

53. Will your homesharer need to use stairs?

    _____yes  _____no

54. How many rooms do you have for a homesharer's belongings?_____

55. How much of this space would be for the homesharer's private use?

    Remarks_____

56. What is the minimum rent per month you are willing to receive?_____

57. Are you willing to

    receive reduced rent for services?

        _____yes  _____no

    provide free rent for services?

        _____yes  _____no

    provide free room and board for services?

        _____yes  _____no

    provide free room and board plus compensation for services?

        _____yes  _____no

58. If Project HOME has difficulty in matching you with a homesharer who is willing to move, but finds a good prospective homesharer who has a home to share, would *you* be willing to move?    _____yes  _____no

    Remarks: _____

59. Will you need or can you provide the following services?

cooking                              nursing

_____ need              _____ need

_____ can provide    _____ can provide

_____ neither           _____ neither

housework                         maintenance

_____ need              _____ need

_____ can provide    _____ can provide

_____ neither           _____ neither

laundry                             errands

_____ need              _____ need

_____ can provide    _____ can provide

_____ neither           _____ neither

gardening                          driving

_____ need              _____ need

_____ can provide    _____ can provide

_____ neither           _____ neither

observing health problems     other (specify what it is and

\_\_\_\_\_need                   whether you need or can provide it)

_____ can provide    _____

_____ neither           _____

Remarks     _____

## Homesharing Preferences

60. *Do you*                                              *Remarks*

smoke?     \_\_\_\_\_yes   \_\_\_\_\_no        _____

drink?     \_\_\_\_\_yes   \_\_\_\_\_no        _____

have pets?     \_\_\_\_\_yes   \_\_\_\_\_no    _____

have overnight guests?     \_\_\_\_\_yes   \_\_\_\_\_ no    _____

use a walker?     \_\_\_\_\_yes   \_\_\_\_\_ no    _____

use a cane or crutch?     \_\_\_\_\_yes   \_\_\_\_\_ no    _____

use a wheelchair?     \_\_\_\_\_yes   \_\_\_\_\_ no    _____

*Can your homesharer*

smoke?  _____ yes  _____ no

drink?  _____ yes  _____ no

have pets?  _____ yes  _____ no

have overnight guests?  _____ yes  _____ no

use a walker?  _____ yes  _____ no

use a cane or crutch?  _____ yes  _____ no

use a wheelchair?  _____ yes  _____ no

61. What is your religion? _____

62. Does your homesharer's religion matter?  _____ yes  _____ no

    Remarks _____

63. What temperature range in the home do you prefer in the winter?  _____

    in the summer?  _____

    Remarks  _____

64. Would you consider sharing with a

    _____ male  _____ female  _____ doesn't matter?

65. Would you consider sharing with a college student?  _____ yes  _____ no

66. Would you consider sharing with children?  _____ yes  _____ no

    Remarks on sharing preferences  _____

    _____

*General Issues*

67. Have you shared before (other than with family)?  _____ yes  _____ no

    Situations  _____  Length  _____

    _____  _____

68. If you shared before, what was successful in these arrangements?

    _____

    _____

69. If you shared before, what problems did you have?

    _____

    _____

70. What is your reason for wanting to homeshare now? (economic, companionship, influence of other people, safety, etc.)

_____

_____

71. What concerns do you have about homesharing?    _____

_____

72. How did you hear about Project HOME?    _____

73. Are you seeking a homesharer through any other means? (commercial service, advertising, etc.)

_____ yes  _____ no    remarks  _____

74. If you find a homesharer through other means, will you notify us of this?

_____ yes  _____ no

75. Are you investigating other housing possibilities like selling, moving, etc.?

_____ yes  _____ no

76. How long do you want this homesharing arrangement to last?

_____ 3 months or less  _____ about a year  _____ permanently

_____ about 6 months  _____ 2 years or more

77. Who are two people we can contact as references?

| Name | Address | Telephone | Relationship |
|------|---------|-----------|--------------|
| Name | Address | Telephone | Relationship |

Thank you for your cooperation in filling out and returning this application. We will be in touch with you as soon as we can.

## INTERVIEW SCHEDULE

The following set of questions numbered 1 through 36 are taken from the provider/employer schedule. The lodger/caregiver form is identical except with respect to question 36. This interview schedule was administered by one of the staff volunteers or the director after the application form was filled out and brought in by each applicant.

PROJECT HOME          Applicant No.

Date _____

Name _____

Address _____

_____

Telephone (home) _____    (work) _____

Referral Agency _____

Assisting Friend's or Relative's Telephone _____

Interviewer Assigned _____

START INTERVIEW HERE

(Introduce yourself if you haven't already done so. Ask follow-up questions on confusing or missing answers from application form. Introduce interview you are about to administer by saying:)

Now I would like to ask you a few more questions concerning your feelings about homesharing and about your life generally that will help us in our efforts to find a good match for you and that will help researchers at the University of Vermont to evaluate our homesharing program properly. Only limited information from the application and this interview will be shared with prospective homesharers. All the rest of the information will be used in the matching and evaluation process without your name being attached to it.

(Give applicant release form, let her/him read it over, answer any questions, and make sure it is signed and returned.)

1. How do you now feel about homesharing—positive, neutral, or negative?

_____ positive      _____ neutral      _____ negative

2. Let me read you the most mentioned possible benefits of homesharing. Would you please tell me how important they are to *you*. Are they very important, somewhat important, or not at all important? (HAND RESPONDENT CARD #1).

|  | Very Important | Somewhat Important | Not Important |
|---|---|---|---|
| Sharing expenses | _____ | _____ | _____ |
| Companionship | _____ | _____ | _____ |
| Sharing driving | _____ | _____ | _____ |

Having someone to help you if
  there are things you cannot do    _____  _____  _____

Sharing household tasks            _____  _____  _____

Having someone around in the
  event of illness or emergency     _____  _____  _____

Safety—criminals are less likely
  to bother people living together  _____  _____  _____

3. Now let me read the most often mentioned possible problems of homesharing. Would you please tell me how important these are to *you*. Are they very important, somewhat important, or not at all important?

| | Very Important | Somewhat Important | Not Important |
|---|---|---|---|
| Not having enough privacy | _____ | _____ | _____ |
| Having difficulty adjusting to other person's routines | _____ | _____ | _____ |
| Having someone who might meddle in your business | _____ | _____ | _____ |
| Not being able to share expenses | _____ | _____ | _____ |
| Being set in your ways | _____ | _____ | _____ |
| Not being able to keep all your own furniture and other possessions | _____ | _____ | _____ |
| Being likely to do more than your share | _____ | _____ | _____ |
| Worrying that you will get close to the person you share with, who may then decide not to live with you anymore | _____ | _____ | _____ |
| Worrying that once you start homesharing you are stuck with a person | _____ | _____ | _____ |

4. What would you say are the three most important things you could offer to the person sharing a home with you.

  first _____

  second _____

  third _____

5. Considering everything—amount of room, structure, condition, and so forth, how satisfied are you with your present home? (PROBE: If they just say "Satisfied" or "Dissatisfied" ask how much)

_____ very satisfied                          _____ somewhat dissatisfied

_____ somewhat satisfied                      _____ very dissatisfied

_____ neither satisfied nor dissatisfied

6. Here are some reasons for people's concerns with their present living arrangements; tell me which of them is a major concern for you with your present arrangements.

inability to keep up house          dislike neighborhood

_____ yes   _____ no            _____ yes   _____ no

expenses too great                  fear of crime (specify crime)

_____ yes   _____ no            _____

                                    _____ yes   _____ no

loneliness                          other

_____ yes   _____ no            _____ yes   _____ no

inconvenient location               specify _____

_____ yes   _____ no

7. What type of transportation do you usually use?

_____ car   _____ bus   _____ other (specify) _____

8. In general, how frequently do you have trouble getting around; that is, how frequently does lack of transportation keep you from doing the things you want to do?

_____ always   _____ often   _____ sometimes   _____ never

9. Compared with others your age, would you say your health is:

_____ better than average?   _____ about average?

_____ worse than average?

10. How do you feel about your present financial situation?

_____ pretty well satisfied

_____ more or less satisfied

_____ not satisfied at all

11. During the last few weeks, did you ever feel:

proud because someone complimented you
on something you had done?                        _____ yes   _____ no

| depressed or very unhappy? | _____ yes | _____ no |
|---|---|---|
| bored? | _____ yes | _____ no |
| pleased about having accomplished something? | _____ yes | _____ no |
| on top of the world? | _____ yes | _____ no |
| very lonely or remote from other people? | _____ yes | _____ no |
| so restless that you couldn't sit long in a chair? | _____ yes | _____ no |
| that things were going your way? | _____ yes | _____ no |
| particularly excited or interested in something? | _____ yes | _____ no |
| upset because someone criticized you? | _____ yes | _____ no |

12. Taking all things together, how would you say things are these days? Would you say that you are:

    _____ very happy?    _____ pretty happy?    _____ not too happy?

13. What organizations in this community do you belong to? (List the first five organizations mentioned.)

    _____

    _____

    _____

    _____

    _____

14. (Note: Did applicant list more than five organizations?)

    _____ yes    _____ no

(For each of the above organizations ask:)

15. How often do you attend or participate in (name organization) activities—at least once a week, a few times a month, once a month, or less than once a month? (Circle appropriate number below.)

| | At least once a week | A few times a month | Once a month | Less than once a month |
|---|---|---|---|---|
| Org. mentioned first | _____ | _____ | _____ | _____ |
| Org. mentioned second | _____ | _____ | _____ | _____ |
| Org. mentioned third | _____ | _____ | _____ | _____ |
| Org. mentioned fourth | _____ | _____ | _____ | _____ |
| Org. mentioned fifth | _____ | _____ | _____ | _____ |

16. How many of your friends live in this area or neighborhood?

    _____all    _____most    _____a few    _____none

In the next few minutes I would like to get an idea of the people who are important to you in a number of different ways. I will be reading descriptions of ways that people are often important to us. After I read each description, I will be asking you to give me the first names, initials, or nicknames of the people who fit the description. These people might be friends, family members, teachers, ministers, doctors, or other people you might know.

I will want you to give me only the names of people you actually know and that you have actually talked to during the last month. It's possible, then, that you won't get a chance to name some important people if for one reason or another you haven't had any contact with them in the last month.

If you have any questions about the descriptions after I read each one, please ask me to try to make it clearer.

*Private Feelings*

17. If you want to talk to someone about things that are very personal and private, who would you talk to? Give me the first names, initials, or nicknames of the people that you would talk to about things that are very personal and private.

    _____    _____

    _____    _____

    (PROBE) Is there anyone else that you can think of?

18. During the last month, which of these people did you actually talk to about things that were personal and private?

    _____    _____

    _____    _____

    (PROBE: Ask specifically about those who were listed in response to question 17, but not listed in response to question 18)

19. During the last month, would you have liked:

    _____a lot more opportunities to talk to people about your personal and private feelings?

    _____a few more opportunities?

    _____or was this about right?

20. During the past month, how much do you think you needed people to talk about things that were very personal and private?

    _____not at all

    _____a little bit

    _____quite a bit

*Material Aid*

21. Who are the people you know that would lend or give you $25 or more if you needed it, or would lend or give you something (a physical object) that was valuable? You can name some of the same people that you named before if they fit this description, too, or you can name some other people.

———————————————     ———————————————

———————————————     ———————————————

(PROBE) Is there anyone else that you can think of?

22. During the past month, which of these people actually loaned or gave you some money over $25 or gave or loaned you some valuable object that you needed?

———————————————     ———————————————

———————————————     ———————————————

(PROBE: Ask about people named in response to question 21 that were not named in response to question 22)

23. During the past month, would you have liked people to have loaned you or to have given you:

———a lot more?

———a little more?

———or was it about right?

24. During the past month, how much do you think you needed people who could give or lend you things that you needed?

———not at all

———a little bit

———quite a bit

*Physical Assistance*

25. Who are the people that you could call on to give up some of their time and energy to help you take care of something that you needed to do—things like driving you someplace you needed to go, helping you do some work around the house, going to the store for you, and things like that? Remember, you might have listed these people before or they could be new names.

———————————————     ———————————————

———————————————     ———————————————

(PROBE) Is there anyone else you can think of?

26. During the past month, which of these people actually pitched in to help you do things that you needed some help with?

_____    _____

_____    _____

(PROBE: Ask about people who were named in response to question 25, but who were not named in response to question 26)

27. During the past month, would you have liked:

    _____a lot more help with things that you needed to do?

    _____a little more help?

    _____or was this about right?

28. During the past month, how much do you feel you needed people who would pitch in to help you do things?

    _____not at all

    _____a little bit

    _____quite a bit

*Social Participation*

29. Who are the people that you get together with to have fun or to relax? These could be new names or ones you listed before.

_____    _____

_____    _____

(PROBE) Anyone else?

30. During the past month, which of these people did you actually get together with to have fun or to relax?

_____    _____

_____    _____

(PROBE: Ask about people who were named in question 29, but not in question 30)

31. During the past month, would you have liked:

    _____a lot more opportunities to get together with people for fun and relaxation?

    _____a few more?

    _____or was it about right?

32. How much do you think that you needed to get together with other people for fun and relaxation during the past month?

_____not at all

_____a little bit

_____quite a bit

## Negative Interactions

33. Who are the people that you can expect to have some unpleasant disagreements with or people that you can expect to make you angry and upset? These could be new names or names you listed before.

_____     _____

_____     _____

(PROBE) Anyone else?

34. During the past month, which of these people have you actually had some unpleasant disagreements with or have actually made you angry and upset?

_____     _____

_____     _____

(PROBE: Ask about people listed for question 33, but not for question 34)

## Personal Characteristics of Network Members

35. Now I would like to get some information about the people you have just listed. For each name on the list, could you tell me this person's:

| Name | Relationship to you* | Age (in years) | Sex | How many years have you known this person? |
|------|------|------|------|------|
| _____ | _____ | ____ | ___ | _____ |
| _____ | _____ | ____ | ___ | _____ |
| _____ | _____ | ____ | ___ | _____ |
| _____ | _____ | ____ | ___ | _____ |
| _____ | _____ | ____ | ___ | _____ |

(*For family members get exact relationship, e.g., husband, wife, son, daughter, etc.; for professional people, get exact profession, e.g., minister, M.D., etc.)

36. Finally, I'd like to ask you about the specific kinds of things you would be willing to receive in exchange from someone moving into you home.

Would you want to receive money? \_\_\_\_\_yes \_\_\_\_\_no

(If yes) How much per month?_____

Would you want to have someone
who prepares any meals? \_\_\_\_\_yes \_\_\_\_\_no

(If yes) How many meals per day?_____

Would you want to have someone who
does any household tasks? \_\_\_\_\_yes \_\_\_\_\_no

(If yes) What kinds of tasks?_____

Would you want to have someone who
provides transportation? \_\_\_\_\_yes \_\_\_\_\_no

(If yes) How often: every day, a few times
a week or what?_____

Would you want to have someone who keeps an eye on any health
problems you might have? \_\_\_\_\_yes \_\_\_\_\_no

(If yes) How much responsibility would you want your housemate to have?

_____

_____

Would you want to have someone who does any household maintenance, such
as fixing things up that need repair, and so forth?

\_\_\_\_\_yes \_\_\_\_\_no

(If yes) What kinds of things?_____

_____

_____

Is there anything else you would want your housemate to do in exchange for
their living in your home? \_\_\_\_\_yes \_\_\_\_\_no

(If yes) What kinds of things?_____

_____

_____

Those are all the questions I need to ask. Thank you very much for your cooperation!

# PROJECT "HOME" HOMESHARING
## LIVE-IN AGREEMENT

The persons_____and_____
              home provider                    homesharer

have agreed to participate in the following arrangements to begin on_____, 19 .

I, _____, agree to provide the following:
              home provider

*Yes/No*                      *Specifications*

_____private room_____

_____common living area_____

_____kitchen privileges_____

_____door key_____

_____transportation reimbursement_____

_____parking_____

_____linen_____

_____laundry facilities_____

_____storage space_____

I, _____, agree to provide the following:
              homesharer

*Yes/No*                      *Specifications*

_____financial contribution in the amount of $_____due on_____

_____exchange of services for_____hours per week

_____share of utilities_____

_____housekeeping_____

_____simple household maintenance_____

_____meal preparation_____

_____grocery shopping/errands_____

_____transportation_____

_____companionship_____

_____yardwork or shoveling snow_____

_____laundry_____

We also agree to the following items:

   *Yes/No*                                 *Specifications*

_____meal planning_____

_____eat together_____

_____smoking areas_____

_____phone sharing_____

_____visitors: daytime/night-time_____

_____pets_____

_____schedule: home_____

           away_____

_____emergency contact list_____

In the event of a health-related emergency we agree to notify the appropriate persons including relatives, doctors, or hospitals and to initiate emergency services to the fullest extent possible.

We also agree that in the event of a hospitalization of the home provider, the homesharer will be able to reside in the home for a period of_____

We also agree to the following: _____

_____

_____

_____

In the event that an alteration of this agreement is required, or termination of the homesharing match is desired by either party, Project HOME must be notified and a period of_____will be given as notice in advance.

| Staff Contact | Phone # | Signature of Home Provider | Date |
|---|---|---|---|

| Signature of Witness | Date | Signature of Homesharer | Date |
|---|---|---|---|

# PROJECT "HOME" LIVE-IN COMPANION/ CAREGIVING AGREEMENT

The persons_____and_____
    home provider                              caregiver

have agreed to participate in the following arrangements to begin on_____, 19 .

I, _____, agree to provide the following:
    home provider

*Yes/No*                          *Specifications*

_____salary, in the amount of $_____to be paid on_____

_____private room_____

_____common living area_____

_____food_____

_____door key_____

_____transportation reimbursement_____

_____employer payments_____

_____linen_____

_____laundry facilities_____

_____storage space/parking_____

_____time off: weekly_____daily_____

          vacation_____

I, _____, agree to provide the following:
    caregiver

*Yes/No*                          *Specifications*

_____housekeeping_____

_____meal preparation_____

_____transportation_____

_____yardwork or shoveling snow_____

_____laundry_____

_____independent contractor_____

_____personal care_____

          _____

          _____

_____companionship_____

We also agree to the following items:

*Yes/No*                                          *Specifications*

_____ meal planning_____

_____ eating together_____

_____ smoking areas_____

_____ phone sharing_____

_____ visitors: daytime/night-time_____

_____

_____ pets_____

_____ grocery shopping_____

_____ emergency contact list_____

In the event of a health-related emergency we agree to notify the appropriate persons including relatives, doctors, or hospitals and to initiate emergency services to the fullest extent possible.

We also agree that in the event of a hospitalization of the home provider, the caregiver will be able to reside in the home for a period of_____.

We also agree to the following: _____

_____

_____

_____

In the event that an alteration of this agreement is required, or termination of the caregiving match is desired by either party, Project HOME must be notified and a period of_____will be given as notice in advance.

_____     _____
Staff Contact          Phone #        Signature of Home Provider      Date

_____     _____
Signature of Witness        Date      Signature of Caregiver          Date

## AGREEMENT OF NONLIABILITY

The staff of the HOME program or their representatives will act as a referral service to bring together those who have housing and those who are in need of housing or those who are seeking caregivers and those who are seeking caregiving opportunities. The final decision on living or caregiving arrangements will be made by the parties involved. There is no expressed or implied guarantee by Project HOME of the suitability of the match.

It is understood by the undersigned that in no event shall Project HOME or the HOME staff, either individually or as a group, be liable to any party in the Home-sharing or Caregiving arrangement for any liability resulting from Homesharing or Caregiving activities.

It is further understood by the undersigned that Project HOME, its volunteers, and employees shall be held harmless from any and all suits, claims, loss, liability, or damage arising out of or resulting from Project HOME's activities.

_____    _____

Applicant's Signature                                          Date

_____    _____

Witness                                                              Date

*Appendix 2*

# Match Lagtime and Rematches

## HOW LONG DOES IT TAKE TO GET MATCHED?

The simple answer is twenty-eight days, on average. The simple answer, however, is quite inadequate and misleading without further amplification. This section describes how the length of time for getting matched differs for each of the four major groups of applicants, how it has changed over time, and what organizational decisions and applicant characteristics have affected the lag between application and match and why. The applicants to be described include only the 216 who applied during the first through fourth years and who were matched no later than six months after the end of the fourth year.

### The Evidence

Table A2.1, constructed similarly to table 6.1, shows the average time it took to match providers, lodgers, employers, and caregivers during each of the first four years of the program. Some applicants were matched on the day they applied, while others waited literally for years. The median days required to match, at the bottom right of table A2.1, indicates that half of all applicants matched were found a homesharer within 28 days, or 4 weeks, and half after 28 days. The mean lagtime of 97 days, or nearly 14 weeks, and the standard deviation of 163 days reflect the pull of those few applicants who were matched after one or more years' time (about 10 percent of the 216 matched applicants). Although mean scores will be referred to, discussion will focus on the median because of its lower sensitivity to the few extreme scores.

While the numbers of matched applicants in each subgroup is small, especially so in the early years for all groups and in all years for providers, some fairly clear-cut

TABLE A2.1

*Average Time in Days Between Applicant Interview and First Match by Type of Applicant and Year*

| | | | Year | | | |
|---|---|---|---|---|---|---|
| | | 1 | 2 | 3 | 4 | Total |
| **Traditional arrangements** | | | | | | |
| Providers | Md | 202 | 133 | 53 | 93 | 106 |
| | X̄ | 318 | 205 | 151 | 127 | 192 |
| | st.dev. | 323 | 187 | 201 | 160 | 217 |
| | | (6)[a] | (9) | (10) | (7) | (32) |
| Lodgers | Md | 90 | 62 | 30 | 16 | 24 |
| | X̄ | 344 | 90 | 85 | 34 | 91 |
| | st.dev. | 568 | 128 | 138 | 40 | 196 |
| | | (4) | (11) | (15) | (16) | (46) |
| Sharer totals | Md | 178 | 78 | 30 | 31 | 58 |
| | X̄ | 328 | 142 | 111 | 62 | 133 |
| | st.dev. | 407 | 164 | 165 | 100 | 210 |
| | | (10) | (20) | (25) | (23) | (78) |
| **Personal care companion (PCC) arrangements** | | | | | | |
| Employers | Md | 314 | 34 | 37 | 24 | 30 |
| | X̄ | 296 | 97 | 75 | 47 | 81 |
| | st.dev. | 208 | 142 | 112 | 64 | 121 |
| | | (4) | (10) | (19) | (27) | (60) |
| Caregivers | Md | 26 | 22 | 26 | 17 | 20 |
| | X̄ | 30 | 101 | 106 | 54 | 73 |
| | st.dev. | 24 | 171 | 168 | 102 | 132 |
| | | (4) | (10) | (22) | (42) | (78) |
| PCC totals | Md | 68 | 30 | 28 | 19 | 24 |
| | X̄ | 163 | 99 | 92 | 51 | 77 |
| | st.dev. | 197 | 153 | 144 | 89 | 127 |
| | | (8) | (20) | (41) | (69) | (138) |
| Total | Md | 118 | 60 | 29 | 20 | 28 |
| | X̄ | 255 | 120 | 99 | 54 | 97 |
| | st.dev. | 333 | 158 | 151 | 91 | 163 |
| | | (18) | (40) | (66) | (92) | (216) |

[a] Each number in parentheses indicates number of applicants specific to year and applicant group.

patterns emerge. First, and critically important, the lagtime between application and match drops substantially from first to fourth year. The drop in mean lagtime is equally impressive.

The second major pattern observed in table A2.1 is the difference in time required to match among the four groups in general: Clearly the most difficult to match are providers, who, for every time period, take the longest time to match; while caregivers take the least; and lodgers and employers are in the middle but similar to caregivers. The long lagtime in matching providers suggests not only that they are very hard to match but also that Project HOME stays with them as long as it can to find a suitable sharer, resulting in the fairly high match success rate observed in table 6.1.

The final patterns regarding lagtime between application and match are more tentatively offered, because they are based on very small numbers of matched applicants. Nevertheless, it is worth pointing out that, over time, providers and employers show a sharp drop from year one to year two and then a fluctuation (providers) or leveling off (employers); lodgers show a consistent decline from year one to year four; and caregivers are matched quickly no matter when they applied.

The drop in lagtime from first to second years among providers is due probably to the large increase in the numbers of lodger applicants from the second year on. The large drop in lagtime for lodgers implies either that Project HOME is doing a better job of interpreting lodgers' applications—a likely reason for the drop between the first and second years, or that lodgers in later years are better candidates for homesharing than those from the early years—again, a likely explanation for the drop after the first year.

The drop in lagtime for employers, as for providers, is probably explained by an increase in the numbers of potential caregivers. Finally, caregivers have skills in constant demand; although many who profess to caregive appear to be merely lodger applicants who don't want to pay rent or perform services, for those who do in fact have the skills, there is a short waiting period.

Based on the median time it took Project HOME to match the two hundred plus applicants it placed, all matched applicants were divided into those who were matched within four weeks (twenty-eight days) and those whom it took longer to match.[1] The 216 matched applicants were then further divided into providers, lodgers, employers, and caregivers, and for each group all of the predictors from the previous section were cross-tabulated with speed of match. Table A2.2 lists the three most important predictors of getting matched early (within four weeks) separately for each of the four major groups of applicants.

Among the thirty-two *providers*, no characteristic is significantly associated with early matches, in large part because of the group's small size. Nevertheless, three characteristics do have moderate-sized associations and will be mentioned in passing: Providers who don't want to share with children or students, who have had homesharing experience before Project HOME, and who have transportation problems are *most* likely to be matched quickly. Among *lodgers*, good health, a lack of housing problems, and little concern for money matters all help one get matched quickly.

For *employers*, the three most important predictors facilitating early matches appear to have little in common: One facilitator is never having shared before, a second represents a *medium* concern over keeping one's own things, and the third deemphasizes the importance of sharing companionship. The only thread linking them to each other is that they each represent some characteristic or attitude that speaks directly to homesharing. Finally, among *caregivers*, willingness to share with a disabled person, having few friends in the neighborhood, and having little objection to sharer's lifestyle all predict an early match.

While apparently mixed, these findings on applicant characteristics nevertheless provide additional insight into the relative importance of agency effort and individual

TABLE A2.2
*Three Most Important Predictors of Getting Matched Within Four Weeks for Each Applicant Type*

| Providers (N = 32)[a,b] | Lodgers (N = 46)[a] |
|---|---|
| Objects to sharing with students or families with children (d = .29 ns) | Has no physical limitations (d = .53, p < .04) |
| Has transportation problems (d = .29 ns) | Has no housing problems (d = .32, p < .02) |
| Has homeshared prior to Project HOME application (d = .27 ns) | Deemphasizes the importance of money matters (d = .27, p < .05) |

| Employers (N = 60)[a] | Caregivers (N = 78)[a] |
|---|---|
| Has never homeshared prior to Project HOME application (d = .31, p < .02) | Is willing to share with disabled person (d = .40, p < .02) |
| Has medium concern over keeping one's own things (chi$^2$ = 6.7, df = 2, p < .03) | Has few friends in neighborhood (d = .21, p < .01) |
| Deemphasizes the importance of sharing companionship (d = .26, p < .02) | Has little objection to sharer's lifestyle (d = .19, p < .05) |

[a] Number in parentheses refers to total number of applicants from first four years who were matched at least once prior to October 1, 1986 (six months after the end of fourth year).

[b] Primarily because of small sample size, no predictor was statistically significant at .05 level for providers. The three predictors listed showed the strongest associations and were significant near or below the .10 level.

characteristics. In the following discussion, the overall time trend data from table A2.1 and the summary of important applicant characteristics from table A2.2 will be integrated to highlight the keys to getting matched quickly.

## Three Keys to Getting Matched Quickly

Among applicants who get matched, there are certain characteristics increasing the likelihood that they get matched quickly. First, although it is true that lodgers and caregivers are much less likely to get matched than are providers and employers (table 6.1), among all clients who have been matched the movers find partners more quickly than those staying at home (table A2.1). This is not surprising considering that the major objective of Project HOME is to find homesharers or caregivers for elders and disabled individuals who want to stay in their own homes.[2] The large ratio of lodger and caregiver applicants to elderly and disabled applicants, especially after the first year, makes it hard for any one lodger or caregiver to get matched because of the smaller pool of providers and employers; on the other hand, the "ideal" (read: realistic and flexible) lodger and caregiver applicants have a short waiting period because of the pressing needs of Project HOME's main clients.

Related to the relatively quick matches for movers is the second factor distinguishing those who get matched quickly from those who don't: time of application. As shown in table A2.1, applicants from the program's second year on were matched more quickly, on average, than those from the first year. Reasons for increasing efficiency in placing clients would obviously include staff experience and its translation into better client preparation, better insight into what makes "good" homesharing matches, etc. At the same time, the precipitous drop in lagtime between years one and two for providers and employers stems most likely from Project HOME's expanding the pool of lodger and caregiver applicants directly after the program's first year.

The third factor contributing to decreased lagtime between application and match is client flexibility, especially among the lodger and caregiver applicants. From table A2.2 it is clear that lack of physical limitations, lack of perceived problems in housing arrangements at time of application, and not caring about money matters helps lodgers find willing providers quickly. Each of these characteristics suggests a lodger who is unlikely to make serious demands on a home provider and who will be easy to get along with. From the same table, the willingness to share with disabled employers and voicing little objection to potential sharer's lifestyle, characterizing caregivers who are matched quickly, again implies a tolerance commending itself to future employers.

Among providers and employers, some degree of flexibility is also seen in the data from table A2.2. For providers, previous homesharing experience facilitates a quick match, suggesting that the provider who has shared living arrangements before has a more realistic view of what homesharing will involve and therefore will be more flexible in negotiating with a potential sharer. For employers, the deemphasis on sharing companionship helps one get matched quickly, possibly because those employers who are willing to keep some distance between themselves and their caregiver will be seen to be flexible in their willingness to let the caregiver have privacy in the relationship.[3]

# WHO GETS MATCHED MORE THAN ONCE?

Early in Project HOME's existence, it became clear to the director, her staff, the clients, and to the university evaluators that matches were made to be broken. While chapters 7 and 8 will examine the dynamics of matches and rematches involving a variety of clients, it is instructive here to examine which factors, if any, make a person a good candidate for multiple partners. Among the 216 clients who were matched, 51, or 28.2 percent, were matched more than once, including nine who were matched three times, four who were matched four times, five three times, one seven times, and one applicant a total of nine times. Because of the obviously skewed distribution, the following analysis distinguishes those who were matched once only from those who were matched more than once.

## The Evidence

Table A2.3 shows the breakdown by year and applicant type of the percentage of matched applicants who had more than one partner. The data suggest two sets of observations. The first has to do with time trends. While one would expect applicants from the earlier years to have more time to find a second homesharer (and the total percentages by year are consistent with this assumption), a decrease over time in multiple-match applicants occurs clearly only for the providers and lodgers and, to a lesser degree, for the caregivers. Employers, on the other hand, show a contrasting trend: Those who applied in the third and fourth years are, on average, *more* likely to have employed more than one caregiver than those from the first two years of the program. Of course, the small numbers of employer applicants in the first two years makes the figures for those years rather unstable. A second pattern is much more clear cut: Both providers and employers, the two stayer groups, include substantially larger percentages of multiple-partner applicants than do the lodgers and caregivers.

The lack of a decline over time in the percentage of multiple-caregiver employers may be due to a number of factors. After the personal care companion part of Project HOME was begun in earnest during the second and third years, it became apparent that many frail and disabled employers presented serious problems of care for their caregiver companions. As a result, as shown in chapter 8, many personal care companion arrangements became very stressful for even the most experienced and committed caregiver-homesharers. What followed, in many cases, was the caregiver terminating the match and Project HOME rushing to find another caregiver. In other cases, especially since year four, caregiver stress resulted in the call for help in the

TABLE A2.3
*Percent Applicants Matched More Than Once by Type of Applicant and Year*

| | Year | | | | |
| --- | --- | --- | --- | --- | --- |
| | 1 | 2 | 3 | 4 | Total |
| Traditional arrangements | | | | | |
| Providers | 50.0 | 66.7 | 50.0 | 14.3 | 46.9 |
| | (6)[a] | (9) | (10) | (7) | (32) |
| Lodgers | 25.0 | 27.3 | 6.7 | 0.0 | 10.9 |
| | (4) | (11) | (15) | (16) | (46) |
| Sharer totals | 40.0 | 45.0 | 24.0 | 4.3 | 25.6 |
| | (10) | (20) | (25) | (23) | (78) |
| Personal care companion (PCC) arrangements | | | | | |
| Employers | 50.0 | 10.0 | 42.1 | 44.4 | 38.3 |
| | (4) | (10) | (19) | (27) | (60) |
| Caregivers | 25.0 | 40.0 | 27.3 | 16.7 | 23.1 |
| | (4) | (10) | (22) | (42) | (78) |
| PCC totals | 37.5 | 25.0 | 34.1 | 27.5 | 29.7 |
| | (8) | (20) | (41) | (69) | (138) |
| Total | 38.9 | 35.0 | 30.3 | 21.7 | 28.2 |
| | (18) | (40) | (66) | (92) | (216) |

[a] See table A2.1 note.

form of another live-in caregiver during weekends or a caregiver to come in to provide respite care for a few hours a few times a week. When matches were terminated and another caregiver found and when caregivers were provided support services, the employer thus got counted as a client with one or more caregivers.

The generally large percentage of both providers and employers who have had multiple sharers is again probably attributable to Project HOME's stated primary aim to help needy elders and disabled clients remain independent in their own homes. Thus, when a match dissolves, or when respite help is needed, the program staff make their stayer client a top priority. In this case, familiarity breeds, not contempt, but a sense in the program's director and volunteer staff that they are working on behalf of not only a needy client but also someone they have served in the past and don't want to let down. They also are serving a client who is "proven," in the sense that he or she has already been matched once.

In order to look for corroborating evidence to support the above assertions, all possible predictors of whether a client was matched or not were tried as predictors concerning multiple matches. Table A2.4 summarizes the three strongest predictors for each type of client.

Among *providers*, teetotaling, use of senior services, and unwillingness to share

TABLE A2.4
*Three Most Important Predictors of Getting Rematched for
Each Applicant Type*

| Providers (N = 32)[a,b] | Lodgers (N = 46)[a] |
|---|---|
| Does not drink alcohol (d = .54, p < .01) | Believes living situation is too expensive (d = .21, p < .04) |
| Uses senior services (d = .54, p < .02) | Is not seeking a homesharer through other means (d = .20, p < .04) |
| Objects to sharing with disabled person (d = .33, p < .02) | Is willing to share with male or female (d = .17, p < .05) |

| Employers (N = 60)[a] | Caregivers (N = 78)[a] |
|---|---|
| Emphasizes the importance of homesharers helping each other (d = .32, p < .04) | Is willing to cooperate regarding nursing services ($chi^2 = 6.2$, df = 2, p < .05) |
| Cannot drive without help (d = .29, p < .04) | Is not seeking a homesharer through other means (d = .23, p < .04) |
| Is not seeking a homesharer through other means (d = .29, p < .04) | Emphasizes concern over compatibility (d = .14, p < .05) |

[a,b] See table A2.2 notes.

with a disabled lodger were strongly associated with getting matched more than once. Contrary to the table A2.2 results for providers, these predictors are also statistically significant in their effect. Being concerned with expenses, not seeking a sharer through other means, and not being concerned about sharer's gender all increase the likelihood that a *lodger* client will get rematched.

For *employers*, while the specific indicators differ, the general picture is similar to that for providers. Employers who emphasize helping one another, who cannot drive without help, and who are depending on Project HOME alone to find a caregiver are most likely to be rematched. Finally, among *caregivers*, wanting to cooperate on nursing services, depending on Project HOME for finding an employer, and emphasizing concern over compatibility all facilitate finding employers second matches.

## Two Keys to Getting Rematched

In the case of every one of the four types of applicants, two themes stand out as being important in predicting which clients get rematched and which do not. The first is continued need. This is indicated by dependence on Project HOME to find a sharer, which is an important predictor of rematches for all of the applicant groups except providers. Other indicators of need that predict rematches are using senior services (providers), inability to drive without help (employers), and living expense concern (lodgers). Clearly, however measured, those clients who are in need stand a better chance of getting rematched than those who are not.

The second facilitator is attractiveness of the client. This also is measured in a variety of ways, including the absence of a potentially harmful habit like drinking (providers) or flexibility in one's approach to potential sharers: Lodgers who are willing to share with either males or females, employers who emphasize helping one another, and caregivers who are willing to cooperate on nursing services all are implying a flexible approach to homesharing and thus, it would appear, helped in their efforts to get rematched.

Both of these keys are in turn related to the notion of Project HOME's commitment to clients with whom its staff have already worked in various capacities. To the extent that clients previously served by a program manifest serious needs and indicate that the program is their last hope, it is hard to imagine a service program that would not go all out in its efforts to secure relief for those clients. Whether this has any effect on the degree to which other clients are aided by the organization is explored in chapters 9 and 10, which explicitly evaluate all parts of Project HOME.

# Appendix 3

# Follow-Up Interview Schedule for Matched Clients

The following interview schedule is the basis of all the analyses presented in chapters 7 and 8 and some of the analysis in chapter 9. The living situation and HOME services assessments by unmatched and previously matched clients presented in chapter 9 are based on a similar, though less detailed, instrument. To conserve space, the following schedule shows at most two lines for open-ended question responses. In the actual schedule, many more lines were used.

### Project HOME   Follow-up Interview

Original Applicant No. ☐ ☐ ☐ ☐

Name_____

Present Address_____
        Number        Street        (Apt. #)        City        Zip

Telephone_____   _____   _____
        Home                Work        Best time to be reached

### START INTERVIEW HERE

(Introduce yourself if you haven't already done so. Introduce interview you are about to administer by saying:)

I appreciate your letting me ask you some more questions in connection with the

Project HOME program you applied to a while back. The information you gave us at the time of your application was a very important part of efforts to improve the matching process. In a similar way, the information you share with us now is very important. It will be used by the researchers at the University of Vermont to help them and Project HOME understand how to make the matching process work better and to find out how Project HOME has affected its applicants. All of the following information is confidential and will be used for research purposes only. This release form allows the researchers to use the information you give for these purposes only. Your name will not be attached to any of the answers you give me.

(Give applicant release form, let him/her read it over, answer any questions, and make sure it is signed and returned. Thank applicant and begin interview after filling in the following.)

Today's Date _____

               Month           Day           Year

Date of original Project HOME Interview (from office records)

_____

               Month           Day           Year

Sex of respondent     _____ Male    _____ Female

1. Birthdate _____

               Month           Day           Year

2. Birthplace _____

               Town           State

3. Length of time in Vermont _____

    How long have you lived in this home? _____

    Are you a homeowner or seeker? _____

    Are you currently married, widowed, divorced, separated or have you never been married? _____

        How long have you been married, widowed, divorced, etc. _____

## History and Evaluation

(Obtain information on repeat matches also)

4. How long have you been homesharing? _____

_____

5. Discuss the reasons leading up to your decision to homeshare.

_____

_____

6. Did you ever consider or would you have preferred any of the following living arrangements?

Living alone    _____Yes    _____No    comment_____

_____

Moving in with relatives    _____Yes    _____No    comment_____

_____

Relatives moving in with you    _____Yes    _____No    comment_____

_____

Moving to community care home, nursing home, or apartment

_____Yes    _____No    comment_____

_____

Other_____

_____

7. Had you ever homeshared before?    _____Yes    _____No

If yes, discuss the circumstances leading up to the arrangement(s)

_____

_____

8. What part did any of the following play in your decision to homeshare? (discuss previous arrangements as well)

expenses_____

_____

health care_____

_____

tasks of daily living_____

_____

loneliness_____

_____

fear of crime_____

_____

dislike neighborhood_____

_____

inconvenient location_____

_____

home maintenance_____

_____

other_____

_____

9. How did you hear about Project HOME?

_____

_____

10. When you originally contacted Project HOME how likely did you think it was that a homesharer could be found for you? Would you say you thought it was:

    _____very likely?

    _____somewhat likely?

    _____not at all likely?

    Why do you feel that way?_____

    _____

11. After you had been interviewed by Project HOME, how many potential home-sharers did you meet?_____

    How did you feel about the process of introductions?_____

    _____

12. How were you introduced to your present sharer?_____

    _____

13. What made you think this person was right for you?_____

    _____

14. In general, how satisfied are you with your present living arrangements?

    _____very satisfied    _____satisfied    _____not very satisfied

    Discuss_____

    _____

    How is it better or worse than your previous living arrangement?_____

    _____

    _____

15. What do you feel are the major benefits you *receive* from your sharing arrangement?_____

    _____

16. How important are each of the following as benefits you *receive* (R) or resources/ services you *provide* (P)? Check off and discuss all those that apply.

Monthly expenses (be specific as to amounts—include rent, utilities, and taxes): R   P _____

_____

    *Seekers:* How do your present monthly payments for shelter compare with what you paid prior to homesharing? About what proportion of your income before and now goes to shelter? (PROBE) Since you began homesharing how has your economic situation changed, if at all?_____

_____

    *Homeowners:* About what proportion of your income before and now goes to shelter? (PROBE) Since you began homesharing, how has your economic situation changed, if at all?_____

_____

Household tasks (describe)   R   P _____

_____

Health/caregiving tasks (describe)   R   P _____

_____

Home maintenance tasks (described)   R   P _____

_____

Meal preparation (problems sharing kitchen)   R   P _____

_____

Transportation provision (describe how often)   R   P _____

_____

Companionship   R   P _____

_____

Safety/security or emergencies   R   P _____

_____

Other (anything else exchanged?)   R   P _____

_____

17. How satisfied are you with the exchange of services between your housemate and yourself?

        _____very satisfied        _____somewhat dissatisfied

        _____somewhat satisfied      _____very dissatisfied

Why do you feel this way?_____

18. When you first began sharing, what adjustments or compromises, if any, did you have to make when compared with your former lifestyle? _____

    _____

19. Were there any unexpected *benefits or problems* of homesharing that you had not anticipated before you began sharing? (PROBE) have you ever regretted becoming a homesharer? _____

    _____

20. Have you ever felt your privacy or your independence was diminished by the presence of your sharer? Explain. Were there other compensations? _____

    _____

21. Were, or are, any of the following problems in your homesharing situation? If so, please explain.

    difficulty adjusting to other persons routines_____

    _____

    feeling you had to do more than your share_____

    _____

    fear of being stuck for a long time with one person_____

    _____

    problems sharing space or appliances (TV, stove, bath facilities) or furniture

    _____

22. Would you say that your present living arrangement could be described as: businesslike, friendly, familylike, or other_____

    _____

23. Are you presently exploring other housing options or living arrangements?

    _____yes    _____no

    If yes, what are they?_____

    _____

24. How long do you want your present living arrangement to last?

    _____3 months or less    _____2 years or more

    _____about 6 months    _____permanently

    _____about a year

    Why is that?_____

    _____

25. How long do you expect your present living arrangement to last?

    _____ 3 months or less    _____ 2 years or more

    _____ about 6 months    _____ permanently

    _____ about a year

    Why is that? _____

    _____

26. Do you think you might be interested in meeting potential homesharers in the future? (If this one is dissolved)

    _____ yes    _____ no

    Why do you feel that way? _____

    _____

27. Do you feel that the Project HOME program could do any more for you than it has done?

    _____ yes    _____ no

    If yes, what is it they could do? _____

    _____

28. In general, how satisfied are you with the services Project HOME has provided you? Would you say you are

    _____ very satisfied

    _____ somewhat satisfied

    _____ somewhat dissatisfied

    _____ very dissatisfied

    Explain _____

    _____

29. Have you recommended Project HOME to anyone else?

    _____ yes    _____ no

    (If yes, probe for the relationship, i.e., friend, relative, neighbor, etc.)

    _____

    _____

30. If you had *not* been able to find a homesharer, what do you think your living arrangement would be like now? _____

    _____

31. *(For homeowners only)* How important do you feel the homesharing arrangement has been in helping you to continue to live in your own home?

_____

_____

32. Have you ever thought of moving from this house?  _____yes  _____no

    Under what circumstances would you move and where would you move to?_____

_____

33. Are you presently considering alternative living arrangements?

    _____yes  _____no

    If you were to move, what do you think you would miss most about this home and the life you have here?_____

_____

## Meaning of Home

34. The word "home" is one that crops up a lot in our day to day conversation without it ever being questioned very much in sayings such as "home is where the heart is" or "no place like home." Could you tell me what home means to you?

_____

_____

    To what extent is your present residence a "home" for you?_____

_____

    What characteristics does it have or lack that would make it feel like home?

_____

_____

35. Some people say that home can be a reflection or expression of themselves or of their personality. How true do you feel that might be of you?

_____

    What things have you done to make yourself more at home?

_____

_____

*Space*

36. Could you please tell me about the different rooms you've got in this house. What rooms have you and how do you use them?

_____

_____

Which rooms do you like best?

_____

_____

How many bedrooms are there? _____

(Sketch rooms here)




37. (*For homeowners only*) Do you feel that the space in this house is being fully used?
    Explain. _____

    _____

    Are all the bedrooms being used? _____

    _____

    Was the availability of space in this house a major reason for your willingness to homeshare? _____

    _____

38. Which rooms do you almost entirely use for yourself and which rooms do you share with your homesharer (i.e., kitchen, bathroom, bedroom)? _____

    _____

39. Are you satisfied with the way you and your sharer use space in this home?
    Explain. _____

    _____

40. Have you made any changes in living arrangements to accommodate your sharer (i.e., put in a second toilet)? _____

    _____

41. What about the outside. Do you or your sharer use the yard? Please discuss. \_\_\_\_

_____

## Use of Time

42. Think of a typical day—can you tell me what it would be like beginning with when you wake up and going through until you go to bed?

_____

_____

Estimate how many waking hours you spend at home every day.

_____

_____

43. Are there any days of the week that differ from this typical plan? In other words, are there some different activities—either here or outside—that you get involved in? Is your sharer involved? Example: days you shop, weekend activities, etc.

_____

_____

44. About how much of each day do you spend with your homesharer?
    _____ hours

    What do you usually do when you are together with your homesharer?

_____

_____

(PROBE) Watch TV together? Talk together?

_____

_____

How frequently do you talk with your sharer?

_____ every day          _____ one a week or so

_____ several times a week      _____ less than once a week

What kinds of things do you talk about? (PROBE: intimacy of interaction; personal thoughts and feelings; daily events of life; aspects directly related to homesharing arrangement)

_____

_____

Share household chores     _____ Yes    _____ No    comment_____

_____

Eat meals together    _____Yes    _____No    comment_____

Travel outside together    _____Yes    _____No    comment_____

45. Are there any special events throughout the *year* which alter the pattern of day to day/week to week living? (PROBE) Which of these do you particularly look forward to and where/when do they take place? Is your sharer affected by these alterations?

46. *(For homeowners only)* How important is it to you to be the owner of this home? As you have grown older has the home become more or less important to you?

## Social Support

47. In what ways, if any, do neighbors provide support or assistance to you in your present living arrangement? How frequently do you visit with friends? Did you visit this past week? Describe the situation.

48. In what ways, if any, do friends provide support or assistance to you in your present living arrangement. How frequently do you visit with friends? Did you visit this past week? Describe the situation.

49. In what ways, if any, do family members or relatives provide support or assistance to you in your present living arrangement? Did you visit relatives this past week? Describe the situation.

50. What outside community services/groups are most important to you?

51. Do you belong to and regularly attend any community organization? Discuss.

_____

_____

52. Has your reliance on family, friends or neighbors for support or assistance changed since you began homesharing? If so, how has it changed?

_____

_____

53. If you wanted to talk to someone about things that are very personal and private, who would you talk to? (Is it a friend, neighbor, relative, homesharer?)

_____

_____

54. Who are the people you most enjoy getting together with to have fun or relax? (See above)

_____

_____

55. Who are the people that you could call on to give up some of their time and energy to help you take care of something that you needed to do? (PROBE) Things like driving you someplace you needed to go, helping you do some work around the house, going to the store for you, etc.

_____

_____

## Support Networks

56. How many people are presently living here with you? _____

57. If there are people living here with you, please give the following information about each:

| First name or initials | Relationship to you | Age | How long living with him/her |
|---|---|---|---|
| _____ | _____ | _____ | _____ |
| _____ | _____ | _____ | _____ |

58. How many living children do you have? _____

59. How many of your children are living within a day's drive of you? _____
    If you have children within a day's drive of you, please give the following information about each son/daughter:

| First name or initials | Sex | Marital status (single, married widowed, or divorced/ sep.) | How frequently do you see him/her? (daily, weekly, monthly a few times a year, hardly ever) | Does he/she have any children? |
|---|---|---|---|---|
| _____ | _____ | _____ | _____ | _____ |
| _____ | _____ | _____ | _____ | _____ |

60. Do you have any other living relatives (excluding your spouse and children) living within a day's drive of you?_____

    If you have any other relatives living within a day's drive of you please give the following information about each relative:

| First name or initials | Sex | Marital status (single, married widowed, or divorced/ sep.) | How frequently do you see him/her? (daily, weekly, monthly a few times a year, hardly ever) | Relationship to you (e.g., cousin, sister, ect.) |
|---|---|---|---|---|
| _____ | _____ | _____ | _____ | _____ |
| _____ | _____ | _____ | _____ | _____ |
| _____ | _____ | _____ | _____ | _____ |
| _____ | _____ | _____ | _____ | _____ |
| _____ | _____ | _____ | _____ | _____ |

## Services and Health

61. Are you presently participating in any of the following services?

    Visiting Nurses Association (VNA)            Area Agency on Aging (AAA)

    _____yes   _____no                         _____yes   _____no

    Home Delivered Meals                         Retired Senior Vol. Program (RSVP)

    _____yes   _____no                         _____yes   _____no

    Transportation Assistance                    Senior Companion

    _____yes   _____no                         _____yes   _____no

Home nursing            Other

_____yes _____no        _____yes _____no

                                       (please specify)_____

62. Has your use of any of the above services changed (increased, decreased) since you began homesharing?

_____

63. In general, would you say your

| vision is | hearing is | mobility is |
|---|---|---|
| _____excellent? | _____excellent? | _____excellent? |
| _____good? | _____good? | _____good? |
| _____poor? | _____poor? | _____poor? |

64. Here are a list of things that people usually have to do during the day. After each, check the answer which best describes how well you can do the activity. (HAND RESPONDENT CARD #2)

| | Can do Without help | Can do, but need help | Can't do | Who Helps? Equipment Needed? |
|---|---|---|---|---|
| dressing and putting on shoes | _____ | _____ | _____ | _____ |
| bathing | _____ | _____ | _____ | _____ |
| cutting toenails | _____ | _____ | _____ | _____ |
| reading | _____ | _____ | _____ | _____ |
| preparing meals going on walks outside | _____ | _____ | _____ | _____ |
| climbing stairs | _____ | _____ | _____ | _____ |
| cleaning house hearing over the telephone | _____ | _____ | _____ | _____ |
| grocery shopping | _____ | _____ | _____ | _____ |
| riding a bus | _____ | _____ | _____ | _____ |
| driving a car | _____ | _____ | _____ | _____ |

65. Compared with others your age, would you say your health is:

_____better than average?    _____about average?    _____worse than average?

66. How do you feel about your present financial situation?

    _____pretty well satisfied

    _____more or less satisfied

    _____not satisfied at all

67. During the last few weeks, did you ever feel:

    proud because someone complimented you on
    something you had done?                                    _____yes    _____no

    depressed or very unhappy?                                 _____yes    _____no

    bored?                                                     _____yes    _____no

    pleased about having accomplished something?               _____yes    _____no

    on top of the world?                                       _____yes    _____no

    very lonely or remote from other people?                   _____yes    _____no

    so restless that you couldn't sit long in
    a chair?                                                   _____yes    _____no

    that things were going your way?                           _____yes    _____no

    particularly excited or interested in something?           _____yes    _____no

    upset because someone criticized you?                      _____yes    _____no

68. Taking all things together, how would you say things are these days, would you say that you are:

    _____very happy?    _____pretty happy?    _____not too happy?

69. How often do you feel helpless in dealing with the problems of life?

    _____very often    _____often    _____not very often    _____never

70. How many of your friends live in this area or neighborhood?

    _____all    _____most    _____a few    _____none

71. In general, how frequently do you have trouble getting around; that is, how frequently does lack of transportation keep you from doing the things you want to do?

    _____always    _____often    _____sometimes    _____never

72. Highest grade in school for which you got credit?_____

73. What is your employment status?

    _____full-time worker (occupation)_____

    _____part-time worker (occupation)_____

    _____retired

    _____homemaker

_____unemployed, looking for work

_____student

_____other (specify)_____

74. Former occupation_____

75. Spouse's occupation_____

76. Now I'm going to read you a list of sources of income. Tell me if each is a source of income for you or not.

    _____Soc. security     _____Food stamps

    _____S.S.I.           _____Fuel Assistance

    _____Pension        _____Other (Specify_____)

77. (HAND RESPONDENT CARD #1) In which of these groups does your total personal monthly income from all sources fall, before taxes that is? Just tell me the letter.

    1. A    3. C    5. E    7. G

    2. B    4. D    6. F    8. H

78. Have you been hospitalized within the last six months?

    _____yes   _____no

79. Do you have any recurring health problems that affect your activities?

    _____yes   _____no

If yes, what are they?_____

If yes, how do you cope with them?_____

## Interests

80. What activities are important to you? (hobbies, church, and other activities, social engagements, sports, volunteer assignments, etc.)

_____

_____

81. How would you describe your lifestyle? Do you follow a daily routine? Are you neat or sloppy? Easy going? Are you out of your home frequently? Are you a private person? What kind of music do you like? etc.

_____

_____

(Conclude by thanking Respondent for his/her time.)

*Appendix 4*

# Methodological Notes on Follow-Up Samples

## THE CLIENTS WHOSE MATCHES
## WERE EXAMINED

The follow-up interviews of 74 clients, all of whose matches are analyzed in chapter 7 and some of whose are analyzed in chapter 8, were administered during roughly a nine-month period to those clients who were in homesharing matches during the fourth year of the program. The questions were designed to elicit specific information about factors leading to the decision to homeshare and whether alternative arrangements had been considered. Homesharers were also asked how satisfied they were with their present living arrangement, the exchange of services and whether they experienced any problems, compromises or adjustments with their homesharing partner. Considerable additional information was collected on family, friends, neighbors, and community services and Project HOME itself.[1]

Four criteria were used to choose clients to be used in the follow-up sample. Individually, each client had to be in a homesharing arrangement at present and also be receptive to being interviewed in detail. Collectively, the clients had to represent as many different kinds of sharing arrangements as possible and also be as representative as possible of the pool of matched clients from the first four years of the program.

The latter two criteria would appear to be mutually contradictory in the sense that looking for clients in a variety of sharing arrangements might increase the presence of clients with unrepresentative background characteristics. Therefore, the second director was enlisted to help select clients who would meet these criteria. Without her help, it is unlikely that these criteria would have been met.

The director was particularly helpful in suggesting clients who would be willing to submit to much questioning and who represented different kinds of homesharing matches. With respect to the latter, the case studies described in chapter 7 should confirm the success of the director in locating clients whose living arrangements provide important insights into the different kinds of homesharing going on through Project HOME. Finally, while not selected through any random procedure, because of the desire to insure that a wide variety of matches be reflected, the follow-up sample of 74 clients is fairly reflective of the total pool of matched clients from the first four years.

To test for representativeness of this follow-up sample, background characteristics of this group were compared with those of all applicants who had ever been matched during the first four years of the program. First, the sample of 74 was subdivided into providers (n = 14), lodgers (n = 18), employers (n = 22), and caregivers (n = 20), and the 142 (216—74) matched applicants who had not been followed up were likewise divided up into the same groups. Second, the sample and those left out were compared for each of the four groups with respect to the characteristics of gender, age, marital status, education, work status, income, physical limitations, homeownership, and living arrangement prior to match.[2]

The follow-up sample reflects the matched pool of employers, lodgers, and caregivers reasonably well. Minor exceptions are: a lodger sample that is less likely to have been in the work force and is poorer financially than the average lodger who was matched and a caregiver sample that is more likely to be married and have more money than the average caregiver who was matched.

The follow-up sample of providers was less representative in that its members were slightly older, more likely to be widowed, less likely to have been part of the work force, financially better off, more likely to have physical limitations, and more likely to be a homeowner than all other matched providers. Gender, education, and living arrangement prior to match were distributed about the same in both the followed-up and not followed-up provider samples.

Considering that the follow-up sample represents clients who were living in homesharing arrangements during the fourth year of the program only, there is still considerable demographic consistency between this group and all matched clients. Furthermore, the discrepancies in the provider pool will allow some examination of those vulnerable providers who have physical limitations but, while having somewhat higher income than the average matched provider, do not have enough money to pay for caregiver services. This is the group who, it will be remembered from chapter 6, have an extraordinarily difficult time getting matched, so it will be useful to examine the circumstances in the few instances in which matches have been made. Examining homesharing arrangements in which providers with physical limitations have been matched should give important insights concerning the resources these people offer as well as the ones they desire in a sharing arrangement.

# THE CLIENTS WHO PROVIDED EVALUATION INFORMATION

The 148 applicants who provided information for chapter 9 were interviewed at least three months after they initially contacted Project HOME. They are fairly representative of Project HOME's four types of applicants from the first four years, except for time of application and proportion matched. Regarding the former discrepancy, as has already been demonstrated, the program's goals and clientele expanded dramatically during this period, producing the traditional homesharer-personal care companion distinction only after the program's second year. As a result, when follow-up interviews began early in the second year, only mover-stayer and matched-unmatched distinctions were deemed important. Once the two types of sharing arrangements were distinguished in the staff's and our minds, conscious efforts were made to follow up sufficient numbers of personal care companion clients. The result is an overrepresentation of earlier provider and lodger applicants. This is particularly noticeable in the case of never-matched provider applicants, of whom there are many from the first year. Interestingly, employer applicants have been drawn evenly from each of the first four years, although the largest number of them applied during the fourth year. The reason for this apparent anomaly is that resources did not allow any more fourth-year follow-up interviews than those reported here.

What do these above differences translate into with respect to background characteristics? Fortunately, very little. There are *no* statistical differences between those followed up and those not followed up regarding proportion female, educational level, income, or proportion homeowners within any of the four groups. The *only* significant differences are limited to the following: The sample contains a disproportionately greater percentage of older provider applicants, a disproportionately greater percentage of retired and physically disabled lodger applicants, and a disproportionately greater percentage of widowed and married caregiver applicants than in the groups not followed up. Otherwise, the follow-up groups are statistically indistinguishable from those not followed up with respect to background characteristics.

The second "problem," a greater proportion of matched as opposed to unmatched applicants in the follow-up sample, stems from two sources. In the first place, matched clients were intentionally sought out, because a major focus of this research has been to understand what happens in homesharing matches. The results of that effort have been reported in chapters 7 and 8. A second reason was unintended. Never matched applicants, particularly movers, were hard to locate after three months' time. Lodgers, in particular young lodgers, often were no longer living at the address they had given as "current" at time of application; some had found lodging elsewhere in the area without leaving a forwarding address or telephone number, while others had left town.

A separate problem arose with respect to never matched employer and caregiver applicants. First, as shown in table 6.1, there were not nearly as many never matched employer and caregiver applicants as never matched provider and lodger applicants. Second, because the personal care companion applicants who were unmatched tended to cluster in the fourth year, it often was not possible to interview them because insufficient time had elapsed between application and intended follow-up, resource and time exigencies precluding waiting until enough time had passed.

There are also reasons why the numbers of "currently matched" applicants is so high relative to the numbers of those matched but whose matches have dissolved. First, the latter were a small group overall during the first four years because of the small numbers of matches made during the first two years and because many of those matches were still in existence when it was time to interview the clients. Thus, even though the matches may have terminated some time after these clients were interviewed, they are counted as "currently matched," because they *were* matched at the time of interview. Second, after matches dissolved, the mover—as in the case of many never matched movers—often left no forwarding address or telephone number. In a small number of cases, the matches dissolved because of the death of the home provider, preventing us from interviewing the stayer whose match had dissolved. Therefore, the potential numbers of clients whose matches dissolved was very small to begin with and became even smaller because of problems contacting clients involved in such matches.

The result of underrepresentation of never matched applicants and applicants whose matches had dissolved is that the following analysis will be limited to those six groups that are in sufficient numbers to allow some relatively stable comparisons to be made: never matched providers (N = 31), currently matched providers (N = 12), never matched lodgers (N = 18), currently matched lodgers (N = 19), currently matched employers (N = 22), and currently matched caregivers (N = 21). Remaining are six never matched employers, two never matched caregivers and seventeen applicants who had been in matches that were dissolved by the time they were interviewed (five providers, two lodgers, seven employers, and three caregivers). Data from the eight never matched personal care applicants and the seventeen previously matched applicants will be included in all totals reported and in the "never matched," "matched but no longer sharing," and "currently matched" breakdowns, but they will be excluded from further breakdowns into the four types of applicants.

There are two additional caveats regarding the data on the follow-up clients in chapter 9: First, although the applicants in the follow-up sample are drawn relatively evenly from each of the first four years (32, 33, 41, and 42 respectively), the actual number of applications climbed steeply between the second and third years of the program, so that the follow-up sample overrepresents clients from the first two years. When one looks at the proportion of matched applicants by year, it is clear that the first year's contribution to the follow-up sample is largely never matched clients. These individuals are more likely to paint a negative picture of the program for two reasons: For one, of course, they had not found a homesharer by the time they gave the follow-up interview. Logically, one would expect people who ask for a service and don't receive it to be more disappointed than those who do get the service. For another thing, they were applicants at a time during which the director and volunteers were still learning about matching applicants and homesharing in general. Errors of judgment and failure to coordinate follow-up services for applicants by staff are likely to have been much more prevalent during the program's first two years.

A second warning about the data from the evaluation follow-up sample is that many of the questions will contain a large number of missing cases, either because the applicants did not want to answer the questions (a problem encountered in the application interviews as well) or because the reference question for the follow-up question was not asked of the applicants during their particular application interview.

Recall that the application interview underwent several major changes. Therefore, from interview to interview, while new questions were being added, as often old questions were being dropped. In addition, some ten or so of the applicants followed up gave the sketchiest of information, so that for them even basic background data is missing. Fortunately, they are a very small minority.

Despite the problems of too many currently matched applicants overall and too many never matched applicants from the first year in the sample, it is still possible to address important questions about clients' perceptions of Project HOME if clients are separated out by status and whether they had ever been matched when results are reported and if it is remembered that the sample is a fairly accurate portrayal of the first four years' applicants by status.

# Notes

## 1. Homesharing and the Continuum of Care

1. Bed-disability days are defined as days "when a person was kept in bed either all or most of the day because of illness or injury. Includes those work-loss and school-loss days actually spent in bed." U.S Bureau of the Census 1986:101 *fn.* 4

2. Schreter (1986) distinguishes three kinds of shared housing: self-initiated, agency-assisted, and agency-sponsored. The first refers to private arrangements conducted entirely by the sharers, while the third covers group housing that an agency maintains and manages. They will be referred to for comparative purposes, but the main focus of this book is agency-assisted shared housing, which occurs when an agency helps to arrange shared living between two (and sometimes more) individuals in one of the individuals' private residences.

3. This includes Project HOME, the homesharing agency whose organization and clients are analyzed in this book. Project HOME began operation early in 1982.

4. A predecessor to Robins and Howe (1989), Howe et al. (1984) provides some comparative data but focuses primarily on the Madison, Wisconsin program.

## 2. Project HOME

Parts of this chapter have appeared in Danigelis and Fengler (1989).

1. The volunteers, of course, were unpaid, and space was being negotiated with RSVP and the congregate housing corporation in whose building both organizations had offices. Application forms were provided by the university evaluators, and other supplies were relatively inexpensive.

2. For examples of the range of services provided by other homesharing programs,

see Jaffe and Howe (1988) and Shared Housing Resource Center (1988a). Specific programs providing services beyond just matching can be found in Howe and Jaffe (1989), Thuras (1989), and Underwood and Wulf (1989).

3. New issue areas, centering on specific homesharing concerns that either the applicants had been voicing or that the director and her staff had noticed on their own, usually came to the attention of the director and her staff during the interviewing process.

4. In fact, there are two fees. One is an application fee, and the other is a matching fee—the latter to be assessed if the client actually homeshares with another client from the program. Even though the fees are relatively small, the program does waive them if a client asserts that he or she cannot pay.

## 3. Staffing Project HOME

1. The results of the follow-up interviews with unmatched and matched clients alike are analyzed in chapters 7 through 9.

2. In chapter 4, the dynamics surrounding the decision-making process are explored. Of particular importance is how the director's personality and the organization's ethos, which was based on social exchange, together produced the increased involvement of a small core of volunteers in the service delivery of Project HOME.

3. It is not clear why other volunteers did not stay with the program. One possible reason is that they had neither the personal tie to the director nor the desire to make a greater commitment of energy (if not time) to the expanding program. Given the diverse nature of the original volunteers, it is equally likely that they found other volunteer activities to do.

## 4. Organizational Structure, Social Exchange, and Service Delivery

Parts of this chapter have appeared in Danigelis and Fengler (1989).

1. Consequently, Project HOME became well-known among other service providers like the Visiting Nurse Association, area nursing homes, Area Agency on Aging, etc.

2. Certainly there were functional alternatives to what did happen (e.g., RSVP could have taken over the program), so what occurred perhaps was not the *only* solution to Project HOME's early problems. Nevertheless, during this time, no other practical solutions appeared to be available (e.g., RSVP had its hands full trying to maintain its own volunteers on limited resources). See Jaffe's (1989a), Robins and Howe's (1989), and Shared Housing Resource Center's (1988a) descriptions of other models for homesharing program growth.

3. The particular characteristics of stayers and movers and the reasons for their success or lack of success in getting matched are explored in detail in chapters 5 and 6 respectively.

4. Chapter 6 considers the special problems of homeowners in frail health who do not have the material resources to pay for caregiving help in the context of homesharing. These are a particularly disadvantaged group who probably are (to mix

metaphors) "falling through the cracks" of the network of human service programs for elders.

5. In fact, the researchers employed several research assistants during the time of the Andrus grant funding. Those assistants who worked with the director and volunteers will be referred to as "the assistant" because only one served as a contact between the researchers and the program at any time.

6. The city eventually did support the lunches for a period of time. As noted earlier in this chapter, however, the lunch plan was dropped after a while at the request of the volunteers who felt (probably correctly) that an introductory lunch at a neutral site was still stressful for the clients and was only postponing the inevitable.

# 5. Who Wants to Homeshare and Why

1. In each case, factor analysis was used to check the assumptions that each set of questions that logically appeared to measure a single concept should also be included on statistical grounds. All indices, however, were constructed by summing the values of the contributing questions, since the number of value choices was so limited.

2. Given the several changes in the program during the first four years, one would expect that characteristics of stayers and movers change as well. To test this assumption, the characteristics of stayers and movers were considered separately for each year. Of particular interest were any consistent linear trends from first to fourth year. As a rule of thumb, we employ a 10 percent difference: If the percentage of applicants in a particular category for the first year has changed by ten or more percentage points by the fourth year, and if the change represents a consistent increase or consistent decrease, then the first and fourth year percentages are listed. If there is no change as measured by the 10 percent rule, then the table will indicate "no change."

3. See Jaffe (1989b) for an alternative typology emphasizing the transitional nature of homesharing statuses.

4. In fact, comparisons between sharer and PCC applicants among stayers and among movers show a larger number of differences between the two subgroups for each mover and stayer status: In analyses summarized here, it was found that for 41 traits compared there are 25 significant differences among stayers and 16 significant differences among movers. The breakdown by type of characteristic is:

|  | Stayers | Movers |
|---|---|---|
| Background | 4/5 | 3/5 |
| Income and health | 6/9 | 3/9 |
| Living situation | 3/7 | 1/7 |
| Homesharing profile | 3/11 | 4/11 |
| Homesharing expectations | 6/9 | 5/9 |
| Total | 25/41 | 16/41 |

These variations are sufficiently numerous to suggest important differences between types of stayers and between types of movers. Furthermore, the differences also correspond sufficiently well with over-time changes among stayers and among movers to suggest that much of the time change observed is due to the changing relative composition of sharers and PCC applicants among stayers and movers.

## 6. Who Gets Matched and Who Doesn't

1. Secondary issues relate to the duration of the matchmaking process and to its usefulness to clients over a period of time: How long does it take to match applicants, and are there any characteristics affecting the length of time it takes? What is the incidence of rematches, and who is likely to get rematched? These questions are addressed in appendix 2.

2. Maintaining a *balance* of stayer, provider, lodger, employer, and caregiver applicants is a constant problem for Project HOME staff. Overrecruiting of a particular group to redress a current imbalance can easily turn into a future imbalance in the other direction.

3. In fact, the second director has indicated that she believes this was the case on the basis of intake interviews she and her volunteer staff conducted with caregiver applicants.

4. While not statistically significant, the fact that retired caregiver applicants are the best bet to get matched is also consistent with the advantage accruing to being an elderly caregiver applicant.

5. The next chapter will describe the difficulties encountered by provider applicants who, despite wanting more than a business arrangement, did find a homesharer.

6. It is important to remember that expectations of a personal relationship fail to distinguish matched from unmatched caregivers. This is *not* the same as saying that caregivers who expect a personal relationship don't get matched. Both those who want a personal relationship with employer and those who don't want one stand about the same chance of getting matched. For caregivers, expecting to provide services and the importance of money are what distinguish the matched from the unmatched.

## 7. Homesharing Arrangements and the Continuum of Care

A condensed version of this chapter has appeared in Danigelis and Fengler (1990).

1. It should be recalled that all people in the follow-up sample had to have been in a match for at least one month to be included. Thus some of the most unsatisfactory matches, about 20 percent of all matches, have been excluded from evaluation suggesting some bias toward the more satisfactory matches. At the same time, it is important to note that *homesharing matches are made to be broken.* Chapters 9 and 10 will address the question of length of match more systematically. For now, it is important to note that short matches may also be viewed very positively by the participants, even some matches of shorter than a month's duration.

## 8. Frail Elders and Their Caregiving Network

1. The apparent discrepancy in numbers is explained by the fact that some of these matches involve couples as employers and some involve multiple caregivers, as will be seen later in the text.

As was mentioned in the previous chapter, the employers and caregivers interviewed in the follow-up sample are very representative of all employers and caregivers who were matched during the first four years of Project HOME's existence.

2. Quite often, a relative of the elder seeking a caregiver is present during the application process and, in fact, helps the applicant answer the questions asked by the interviewer. While this creates some obvious problems, it is clear that without the relative's help the quality of information would have been quite poor with much vital data omitted. On balance, therefore, we regard the presence of a relative or friend at the application interview to be far more beneficial than harmful.

3. Vermont winters are especially harsh and long, so that spring and fall are often quite fleeting. When frail elders do get out, it is usually during the summer months when weather is cooperative and when neighbors themselves are more likely to be out and around.

## 9. Clients Speak about Project HOME's Service Delivery

1. In fact, cross-tabulation of number of introductions by time of application shows that the proportion of applicants who were introduced to one or more potential sharers increases each year: 54.8 percent in year one, 69.7 percent in year two, 66.7 percent in year three, and 92.5 percent in year four.

## 11. Homesharing: Beyond the 1980s

1. In the latter case, large older homes are converted into six or fewer apartments in which older people can live; these apartments are financed by special state and private sources. What elders like best about these cooperatives are the limited number of apartments in the project, the prospect of a long lease and stable rent, and the high probability of having an important role in decisions affecting their living situation.

## Appendix 2. Match Lagtime and Rematches

1. Other dividing points were tried and found to give results consistent with those reported in the text. Whether one divides length of time getting matched into two categories (results are in table A2.2) or three or four categories, the characteristics predicting quick matches remain pretty much the same.

2. This emphasis on stayers finally received formal recognition during the program's fifth year when the program's mission statement was drawn up. While trying to alleviate the housing "crunch" in the area is mentioned, the number one goal of Project HOME has been and continues to be to help older homeowners remain at home through the provision of acceptable homesharers—be they lodgers or caregivers.

3. Two apparently anomalous findings are worth mentioning here briefly. In chapter 6, it was shown that having serious transportation problems made it impossible for providers to find sharers. At the same time, one of the predictors of early matches for this group appears to be transportation problems. Because no providers

who "always" or "often" have transportation problems were matched, the results in table A2.2, therefore, are based on those provider applicants who had transportation problems "sometimes" or "never," suggesting that the "discrepancy" between tables 6.4 and A2.2 is more apparent than real.

A second problem has to do with previous homesharing experience: Among matched providers, having shared before is an advantage to finding a lodger quickly (a logical occurrence); but, for employers, having shared before is a *hindrance*. In each case, the lack of homesharing experience suggests an especially isolated individual who is quite vulnerable. Vulnerable providers don't get much help from the program, as we have seen earlier, because of the difficulty in attracting lodgers to do more than be a renter. Vulnerable employers, on the other hand, have money to pay caregivers, so their vulnerability works in their favor, because the agency will expend its energy on the employer's behalf with the realistic expectation that an appropriate caregiver will be found.

## Appendix 4. Methodological Notes on Follow-Up Samples

1. Much of this information is important not only for the assessment of the matches discussed in chapters 7 and 8 but also for the evaluation of the program described in chapter 9.

2. The manner in which the follow-up sample was chosen and the relatively small sizes of the groups being compared make statistical tests of significance suspect here. Therefore, chi$^2$ tests of significance and an examination of the magnitude of percentage differences were both used as aids to spotting large discrepancies in background between those included in the follow-up and those not included.

# References

Bengtson, Vern L. and James J. Dowd. 1981. "Sociological Functionalism, Exchange Theory, and Life Cycle Analysis: A Call for More Explicit Theoretical Bridges." *International Journal of Aging and Human Development* 12:55–73.

Blau, Peter. 1964. *Exchange and Power in Social Life.* New York: Wiley.

Blau, Peter. 1977. *Inequality and Heterogeneity: A Primitive Theory of Social Structure.* New York: Free Press.

Brody, Elaine M. 1975. "Intermediate Housing for the Elderly." *The Gerontologist* 15:350–356.

Brody, Elaine M. 1981. "Women in the Middle and Family Help to Older People." *The Gerontologist* 21:471–480.

Butler, N. 1979. "Extended Family Care: An Experimental Alternative to Institutionalization for Elders." Paper presented at the Gerontological Society of America Meeting, Washington, D.C.

Cantor, Marjorie and Virginia Little. 1985. "Aging and Social Care." In Robert H. Binstock and Ethel Shanas, eds., *Handbook of Aging and the Social Sciences.* 2d ed. New York: Van Nostrand Reinhold.

Caraway, Jacqueline and Jan Van Gilder. 1985. "The Role of Lay Volunteers in a Community Hypertension Control Program." *Journal of Voluntary Action Research* 14:133–141.

Carp, Frances M. 1976. "Housing and Living Environments of Older People." In Robert H. Binstock and Ethel Shanas, eds., *Handbook of Aging and the Social Sciences.* New York: Van Nostrand Reinhold.

Chambre, Susan M. 1987. *Good Deeds in Old Age: Volunteering by the New Leisure Class.* Lexington, Mass.: Lexington.

Clipp, Elizabeth C. and Linda K. George. 1990. "Caregiver Needs and Patterns of Social Support." *Journal of Gerontology* 45:S102–S111.

Conrad, William. 1983. *The Effective Voluntary Board of Directors: What It Is and How It Works.* Rev. ed. Athens, Ohio: Swallow Press.

Danigelis, Nicholas L. and Alfred P. Fengler. 1989. "Homesharing Service through Social Exchange: The Case of Project HOME." In Dale J. Jaffe, ed., *Shared Housing for the Elderly.* Westport, Conn.: Greenwood Press.

Danigelis, Nicholas L. and Alfred P. Fengler. 1990. "Homesharing: How Social Exchange Helps Elders Live at Home." *The Gerontologist* 30:162–170.

DePue, Judith D., Barbara L. Wells, Thomas M. Lasater, and Richard A. Carleton. 1987. "Training Volunteers to Conduct Heart Health Programs in Churches." *American Journal of Preventive Medicine* 3:51–57.

Doron, Abraham. 1979. *Social Services for the Aged in Eight Countries.* Jerusalem: Brookdale Institute of Gerontology.

Dorwaldt, Anne L., Laura Solomon, and John K. Worden. 1988. "Why Volunteers Helped to Promote a Community Breast Self-Exam Program." *The Journal of Volunteer Administration* 6:23–30.

Dowd, James J. 1975. "Aging as Exchange: A Preface to Theory." *Journal of Gerontology* 30:584–594.

Dowd, James J. 1980a. "Exchange Rates and Old People." *Journal of Gerontology* 35:596–602.

Dowd, James J. 1980b. *Stratification Among the Aged.* Monterey, Calif.: Wadsworth (Brooks/Cole Series in Social Gerontology).

Edelman, Perry. 1986. "The Impact of Community Care to the Homebound Elderly on Provision of Informal Care." Paper presented at the Gerontological Society of America Meeting, Chicago.

Elder, John P., Carol A. McKenna, Marie Lazieh, Andrea Ferreira, Thomas M. Lasater, and Richard A. Carleton. 1986. "The Use of Volunteers in Mass Screening for High Blood Pressure." *American Journal of Preventive Medicine* 2:268–272.

Fengler, Alfred P. and Nicholas L. Danigelis. 1982. *The Shared Home: Evaluation of a Concept and Its Implementation.* Application to Andrus Foundation.

Fengler, Alfred P., Sheila M. Peace, and Leonie A. Kellaher. 1984. "The Meaning of Home for British Elderly Widowed Homemakers: Consequences for the Decision to Move or to Homeshare." Unpublished paper.

Golant, Stephen M. 1984. *A Place to Grow Old: The Meaning of Environment in Old Age.* New York: Columbia University Press.

Hare, Patrick H. and Margaret Haske. 1984. "Making Housing Work for Home Health Care: Alternative Living Arrangements and Why Hospitals Should Support Them." Unpublished paper.

Harris, Louis (and Associates). 1976. *The Myth and Reality of Aging in America.* Washington, D.C.: National Council on the Aging.

Harris, Louis (and Associates). 1981. *Aging in the '80s: America in Transition.* Washington, D.C.: National Council on the Aging.

Havir, Linda. 1986. "An Evaluation of Older Volunteers as Telephone Interviewers." *Journal of Voluntary Action Research* 15:45–53.

Hickey, J. 1978. "Older Volunteers Use and Learn Special Skills in Seven Model Health Projects." *Hospitals* 52:128–132.

Hobman, David. 1981. *The Impact of Aging: Strategies for Care.* New York: St. Martin's Press.

Holcomb, Briavel and Barbara Parkoff. 1980. "Sex Differences in the Role of Home Place among the Elderly." Paper presented at the Association of American Geographers Meeting, Louisville, Ky.

Holmes, Douglas, Jeanne Teresi, Monica Holmes, Simon Bergman, Yaron Young, and Netta Bentur. 1989. "Informal Versus Formal Supports for Impaired Elderly: Determinants of Choice on Israeli Kibbutzim." *The Gerontologist* 29:195–202.

Homans, George C. 1961. *Social Behavior: Its Elementary Forms.* New York: Harcourt, Brace and World.

Houghland, James G., Jr., Howard B. Turner, and Jon Hendricks. 1988. "Rewards and Impacts of Participation in a Gerontology Extension Program." *Journal of Voluntary Action Research* 17:19–35.

Howe, Elizabeth and Dale J. Jaffe. 1989. "Homesharing for Homecare." In Dale J. Jaffe, ed., *Shared Housing for the Elderly.* Westport, Conn.: Greenwood Press.

Howe, Elizabeth, Barbara Robins, and Dale J. Jaffe. 1984. *Evaluation of Homeshare Program.* Madison, Wis.

Hwalek, Melanie and Elizabeth A. Longley. 1989. "Michigan Match: A Homeshare Experience." In Dale J. Jaffe, ed., *Shared Housing for the Elderly.* Westport, Conn.: Greenwood Press.

International Federation on Ageing. 1979. "Research Studies with Practical Application." *Ageing International* (Winter) 6:23–24.

Jaffe, Dale J. 1989a. "An Introduction to Elderly Shared Housing Research in the United States." In Dale J. Jaffe, ed., *Shared Housing for the Elderly.* Westport, Conn.: Greenwood Press.

Jaffe, Dale J. 1989b. *Caring Strangers: The Sociology of Intergenerational Homesharing.* Greenwich: JAI Press.

Jaffe, Dale J. and Elizabeth Howe. 1988. "Agency-Assisted Shared Housing: The Nature of Programs and Matches." *The Gerontologist* 28:318–324.

Jaffe, Dale J. and Christopher Wellin. 1989. "The Nature of Problematic Homesharing Matches: The Case of Share-A-Home of Milwaukee." In Dale J. Jaffe, ed., *Shared Housing for the Elderly.* Westport, Conn.: Greenwood Press.

Kaminer, Wendy. 1984. *Women Volunteering: The Pleasure, Pain, and Politics of Unpaid Work from 1830 to the Present.* Garden City, N.Y.: Doubleday.

Lawton, M. Powell. 1977. "Environments for Older Persons." *The Humanist* (Sept-Oct), pp. 20–24.

Lawton, M. Powell. 1980. *Environment and Aging.* Monterey, Calif.: Wadsworth (Brooks/Cole Series in Social Gerontology).

Lawton, M. Powell and B. Simon. 1968. "The Ecology of Social Relationships in Housing for the Elderly." *The Gerontologist* 8:108–115.

Leat, Diana. 1983. *A Home from Home: Report of a Study of Short-Term Family Placement Schemes for the Elderly.* Mitcham Surrey, England: Age Concern Research Unit.

Lengermann, Patricia M. and R. A. Wallace. 1985. *Gender in America: Social Control and Social Change*. Englewood Cliffs, N.J.: Prentice-Hall.

Levinson, Marjorie. 1982. "Intergenerational Housemate Matching: An Analysis of the Operation Match Program." Paper presented at the Gerontological Society of America Meeting, Boston.

Liebow, Elliot. 1967. *Tally's Corner: A Study of Negro Streetcorner Men*. Boston: Little, Brown.

Litwak, Eugene. 1985. *Helping the Elderly: The Complementary Roles of Informal Networks and Formal Systems*. New York: Guilford.

Mantell, Joyce, Executive Director, Shared Housing Resource Center. 1988. Personal Communication, November 28.

Mantell, Joyce and Mary Gildea. 1989. "Elderly Shared Housing in the United States." In Dale J. Jaffe, ed., *Shared Housing for the Elderly*. Westport, Conn.: Greenwood Press.

Maatta, Norma, Karen Hornung, Mary Hart, and Karen Primm. 1989. "Homesharing in a Rural Context." In Dale J. Jaffe, ed., *Shared Housing for the Elderly*. Westport, Conn.: Greenwood Press.

McConnell, Stephen R. and Carolyn E. Usher. 1980. *International House-Sharing: A Research Report and Resource Manual*. Los Angeles: University of Southern California Ethel Percy Andrus Gerontology Center.

Miller, Lynn E., Richard M. Weiss, and Bruce V. MacLeod. 1988. "Boards of Directors in Nonprofit Organizations: Composition, Activities, and Organizational Outcomes. *Journal of Voluntary Action Research* 17:81–89.

Mindel, Charles H. 1979. "Multigenerational Family Households: Recent Trends and Implications for the Future." *The Gerontologist* 19:456–463.

Mor, V., C. Gutkin, and M. Seltzer. 1982. "Integration of the Dependent Aged into the Family Life of Personal Care Homes." Unpublished paper. Dept. of Social Gerontological Research, Hebrew Rehabilitation Center for Aged, Boston.

Mukherjee, M. 1982. "House Sharing by Non Relatives in the Private Housing Market." Paper presented at the Gerontological Society of America Meeting, Boston.

Naylor, Harriet H. 1985. "Beyond Managing Volunteers. *Journal of Voluntary Action Research* 14:25–30.

Noelker, Linda and David M. Bass. 1989. "Home Care for Elderly Persons: Linkages Between Formal and Informal Caregivers." *Journal of Gerontology* 44:S63–S70.

O'Bryant, Shirley L. 1983. "The Subjective Value of 'Home' to Older Homeowners." *Journal of Housing for the Elderly* 1:29–43.

O'Bryant, Shirley L. and Susan M. Wolf. 1983. "Explanations of Housing Satisfaction of Older Homeowners and Renters." *Research on Aging* 5:217–233.

Peace, Sheila M. 1981a. " Small Group Living' in Institutional Settings: Alternative Living Arrangements for the Elderly—Part I." *Ageing International* (Spring) 8:13–16.

Peace, Sheila M. 1981b. " 'Small Group Housing' in the Community, Part II: Variations on Sheltered Housing." *Ageing International* (Summer) 8:16–20.

Peace, Sheila (with Charlotte Nusberg). 1984. *Shared Living: A Viable Alternative for the Elderly* Washington, D.C.: International Federation on Ageing.

Peterson, G., D. Abrams, J. Elder, and P. Beaudin. 1985. "Professional Versus Self-Help Weight Loss at the Work Site: The Challenge of Making a Public Health Impact." *Behavior Therapy* 116:213–222.

Pritchard, David C. 1983. "The Art of Matchmaking: A Case Study in Shared Housing." *The Gerontologist* 23:174–179.

Pritchard, David C. and Joelle Perkocha. 1989. "Shared Housing in California: A Regional Perspective." In Dale J. Jaffe, ed., *Shared Housing for the Elderly.* Westport, Conn.: Greenwood Press.

Pynoos, Jon and Arlyne June. 1989. "The Matchmakers of Santa Clara County." In Dale J. Jaffe, ed., *Shared Housing for the Elderly.* Westport, Conn.: Greenwood Press.

Rathbone-McCuan, Eloise E. and Raymond Coward. 1985. "Male Helpers: Unrecognized Informal Supports." Paper presented at the Gerontological Society of America Meeting, New Orleans.

Regnier, Victor. 1981. "Neighborhood Images and Use: A Case Study." In M. Powell Lawton and Sally L. Hoover, eds., *Community Housing Choices for Older Americans.* New York: Springer.

Robins, Barbara and Elizabeth Howe. 1989. "Patterns of Homesharing in the United States." In Dale J. Jaffe, ed., *Shared Housing for the Elderly.* Westport, Conn.: Greenwood Press.

Rosenmayr, L. and E. Kockeis. 1965. *Unwelt und Familie Alter Menshen.* Berlin: Luchterland.

Schreter, Carol A. 1986. "Advantages and Disadvantages of Shared Housing." *Journal of Housing for the Elderly* 3:121–138.

Schreter, Carol and Lloyd Turner. 1986. "Sharing and Subdividing Private Market Housing." *The Gerontologist* 26:181–186.

Seguin, Mary M. 1984. "Social Work Practice with Senior Adult Volunteers in Organizations Run by Paid Personnel." In Florence S. Schwartz, ed., *Voluntarism and Social Work Practice: A Growing Collaboration.* Lanham, Md.: University Press of America.

Shanas, Ethel. 1979. "The Family as a Social Support System in Old Age." *The Gerontologist* 19:169–174.

Shanas, Ethel and George L. Maddox. 1985. "Health, Health Resources and the Utilization of Care." In Robert H. Binstock and Ethel Shanas, eds. *Handbook of Aging and the Social Sciences,* 2d ed. New York: Van Nostrand Reinhold.

Shanas, Ethel, Peter Townsend, Dorothy Wedderburn, Henning Friis, Poul Milhoj, and Jan Stehouwer. 1968. *Old People in Three Industrial Societies.* New York: Atherton Press.

Shared Housing Resource Center. 1988a. *Survey of Shared Housing Programs in the States: A Summary of Findings.* Philadelphia: Shared Housing Resource Center.

Shared Housing Resource Center. 1988b. "Volunteers Help Shared Housing Grow." *Shared Housing Quarterly* (Fall) 5:1–3.

Sherwood, Sylvia, Vincent Mor, and Claire Gutkin. 1980. "The Family and Placement of Eligible Applicants into Doms (Board and Care Homes)." Paper presented at the Gerontological Society of America Meeting, San Diego.

Smith, David Horton. 1985. "Volunteerism: Attracting Volunteers and Staffing

Shrinking Programs." In Gary A. Tobin, ed., *Social Planning and Human Service Delivery in the Voluntary Sector.* Westport, Conn.: Greenwood Press.

Spence, David H. 1989. "Ontario's Homesharing Program." In Dale J. Jaffe, ed., *Shared Housing for the Elderly.* Westport, Conn.: Greenwood Press.

Streib, Gordon F. 1978. "An Alternative Family Form for Older Persons: Need and Social Context." *Family Coordinator* 27:413–420.

Streib, Gordon F., W. Edward Folts, and Mary Anne Hilker. 1984. *Old Homes— New Families: Shared Living for the Elderly.* New York: Columbia University Press.

Struyk, Raymond J. and Beth Soldo. 1980. *Improving the Elderly's Housing.* Cambridge, Mass.: Ballinger.

Sussman, Marvin B. 1985. "The Family Life of Old People." In Robert H. Binstock and Ethel Shanas, eds. *Handbook of Aging and the Social Sciences.* 2d ed. New York: Van Nostrand Reinhold.

Thornton, Patricia and Jeanette Moore. 1980. *The Placement of Elderly People in Private Households: An Analysis of Current Provision.* Leeds, England: University of Leeds Department of Social Policy and Administration Research.

Thuras, Paul D. 1989. "Habits of Living and Match Success: Shared Housing in Southern California." In Dale J. Jaffe, ed., *Shared Housing for the Elderly.* Westport, Conn.: Greenwood Press.

Treas, Judith. 1977. "Family Support Systems for the Aged." *The Gerontologist* 17:486–491.

Underwood, Janet B. and Connie Wulf. 1989. "Share-A-Home of Wichita." In Dale J. Jaffe, ed., *Shared Housing for the Elderly.* Westport, Conn.: Greenwood Press.

U.S. Bureau of the Census. 1986. *Statistical Abstract of the United States, 1987.* 107th ed. Washington, D.C.: U.S. Department of Commerce.

U.S. General Accounting Office. 1977. *Home Health: The Need for a National Policy to Provide for the Elderly.* Washington, D.C.: Report # HRD78–19.

U.S. Senate Special Committee on Aging. 1985. *America in Transition: An Aging Society.* 1984–85 edition. Washington, D.C.: GPO.

Vander Zanden, James W. 1984. *Social Psychology.* 3d ed. New York: Random House.

Vermont Office on Aging. 1988. *Characteristics and Needs of Older Vermonters.* Waterbury, Vt.: State of Vermont.

Watts, Ann DeWitt and Patricia Klobus Edwards. 1983. "Recruiting and Retaining Human Service Volunteers: An Empirical Analysis." *Journal of Voluntary Action Research* 12:9–21.

Weil, Marie. 1984. "Involvement of Senior Citizens in Needs Assessment and Service. Planning." In Florence S. Schwartz, ed., *Voluntarism and Social Work Practice: A Growing Collaboration.* Lanham, Md.: University Press of America.

Weber, Max. 1947. *The Theory of Social and Economic Organization.* Trans. by A. M. Henderson and Talcott Parsons. New York: Free Press.

Welfield, I. and Raymond Struyk. 1979. *Occasional Papers in Housing and Community Affairs. Vol. 3: Housing Options for the Elderly.* Washington, D.C.: GPO.

Wheeler, Rose. 1982. "Staying Put: A New Development in Policy?" *Ageing and Society* 2:299–329.

# Index